Abdominal Gray Scale Ultrasonography

Wiley Series in Diagnostic and Therapeutic Radiology

Luther W. Brady, M.D., Editor
Professor and Chairman, Department of Therapeutic Radiology and Nuclear Medicine, Hahnemann Medical College and Hospital, Philadelphia, Pennsylvania

TUMORS OF THE NERVOUS SYSTEM
Edited by H. Gunter Seydel, M.D., M.S.

CANCER OF THE LUNG
By H. Gunter Seydel, M.D., M.S.
Arnold Chait, M.D.
John T. Gmelich, M.D.

CLINICAL APPLICATIONS OF THE ELECTRON BEAM
Edited by Norah duV. Tapley, M.D.

NUCLEAR OPHTHALMOLOGY
Edited by Millard Croll, M.D.
Luther W. Brady, M.D.
Paul Carmichael, M.D.
Robert J. Wallner, D.O.

HIGH-ENERGY PHOTONS AND ELECTRONS:
Clinical Applications in Cancer Management
Edited by Simon Kramer, M.D.
Nagalingam Suntharalingam, Ph.D.
George F. Zinninger, M.D.

TRENDS IN CHILDHOOD CANCER
Edited by Milton H. Donaldson, M.D.
H. Gunter Seydel, M.D., M.S.

ORBIT ROENTGENOLOGY
Edited by Peter H. Arger, M.D.

ABDOMINAL GRAY SCALE ULTRASONOGRAPHY
Edited by Barry B. Goldberg, M.D.

Abdominal Gray Scale Ultrasonography

Edited by

Barry B. Goldberg, M.D.

Professor of Radiology
Director, Division of Diagnostic Ultrasound
Thomas Jefferson University Hospital
Philadelphia, Pennsylvania

A WILEY MEDICAL PUBLICATION
JOHN WILEY & SONS
New York / London / Sydney / Toronto

Copyright © 1977, by John Wiley & Sons, Inc.

All rights reserved. Published simultaneously in Canada.

No part of this book may be reproduced by any means, nor
transmitted, nor translated into a machine language without the written permission of the publisher.

Library of Congress Cataloging in Publication Data:

Main entry under title:

Abdominal gray scale ultrasonography.

  (Wiley series in diagnostic and therapeutic radiology)
(A Wiley medical publication)
  Includes bibliographical references and index.
  1. Diagnosis, Ultrasonic.   2. Abdomen—Radiography.
I. Goldberg, Barry B.   [DNLM: 1. Ultrasonics—
Diagnostic use.   2. Abdomen.   WI900 Al33]

RC944.A18   617′.55′0754   77-5889
ISBN 0-471-01510-5

Printed in the United States of America

10 9 8 7 6 5 4 3 2 1

Contributors

Kenneth W. Albertson, M.D., Assistant Professor of Radiology, University of California at San Diego

Ernest N. Carlsen, M.D., Ph.D., Associate Professor of Radiology, Loma Linda University; Director of Diagnostic Ultrasound, Loma Linda Medical Center, Loma Linda, California

Bruce D. Doust, M. B., Associate Professor of Radiology, Medical College of Wisconsin; Director of Ultrasound, Milwaukee County Medical Complex, Milwaukee, Wisconsin

Roy A. Filly, M.D., Assistant Professor of Radiology, University of California at San Francisco; Picker Scholar, James Picker Foundation; Chief, Section of Ultrasound Diagnosis, University of California Medical Center, San Francisco, California

Barry B. Goldberg, M.D., Professor of Radiology; Director, Division of Diagnostic Ultrasound, Thomas Jefferson University Hospital, Philadelphia, Pennsylvania

R. E. Grahame, M.D., M.Sc., Associate Professor and Acting Head, Department of Anatomy, Faculties of Medicine and Dentistry, University of Manitoba, Winnipeg, Manitoba

George R. Leopold, M.D., Professor of Radiology; Head, Division of Ultrasound, University of California at San Diego

E. A. Lyons, M.D., F.R.C.P.C., Director, Section of Ultrasound, Health Sciences Center, Winnipeg, Manitoba

Gordon S. Perlmutter, M.D., Clinical Associate Professor of Radiology, Temple University Health Sciences Center, Philadelphia, Pennsylvania; Director, Ultrasound Section, The Reading Hospital, West Reading, Pennsylvania

Howard M. Pollack, M.D., Professor of Radiology, University of Pennsylvania Hospital and School of Medicine, Philadelphia, Pennsylvania

Kenneth J. W. Taylor, M.D., Ph.D., Associate Professor of Diagnostic Radiology; Head, Ultrasound, Yale University School of Medicine, New Haven, Connecticut

*to my parents,
wife, and children*

Preface

Diagnostic ultrasound has advanced rapidly in the past several years due to the introduction of more sophisticated equipment. Progress in this young field is demonstrated most dramatically by the rapid acceptance and utilization of gray scale two-dimensional ultrasonography. The advantage of this mode of display over previous ones lies in its superior ability to depict information making it easier to interpret the images obtained. Of course, other advances have occurred including improved transducers and the introduction of real-time ultrasound. In this rapidly changing and advancing field of medicine, the literature soon becomes outdated, while general principles remain unchanged. In this book, we have attempted to cover, as thoroughly as possible, the utilization of gray scale two-dimensional ultrasonography of the abdomen. Ample use is made of illustrations to support the text. Throughout, the images displayed are in gray scale with either a black or a white background.

In keeping with recent efforts toward general standardization of the methods of display of ultrasonograms, all longitudinal images are displayed as if one were looking at the patient from the right. Thus, caudad is always on one's right-hand side as one faces the image, and cephalad is to one's left. (H) is used to indicate the direction of the head. Transverse ultrasonograms always are displayed as if one is looking up from the patient's feet toward his head. As a result, all ultrasonograms obtained in the supine position are displayed with the right side of the patient on one's left as the illustration is viewed. (R) is used to designate the right side of the body and (L) the left side. For ultrasonic images obtained in the prone position, usually for evaluation of the retroperitoneal and kidney areas, the left side of the patient is on one's left as the illustration is viewed. Other views in the erect or decubitus position also will be displayed and appropriately labeled or described in the legend for that illustration. Labeling of organs usually is described in the legend or, if repeated within the chapter, will be noted in the first set of figures.

This book is intended as a reference for those who are presently working with ultrasound as well as for those who are interested in entering the field of ultrasound. It should be of interest to both physicians and sonographers (technologists). Physicians in other specialities, interns, residents, and student technologists also may find this book of interest as a guide to which ultrasonic studies can be performed successfully and as a basis for a more thorough understanding of the capabilities and imaging characteristics of this new and rapidly developing field of medical diagnosis.

BARRY B. GOLDBERG

Philadelphia, Pennsylvania

Acknowledgments

The authors wish to thank the following individuals whose help has made this book possible: Ruth Shapiro, Dot Reilly, Victoria Babcock, and Diana Lawrence for assistance in the typing and preparation of the manuscript; Sandra Hagen-Ansert, Jerome Tymkiw, Randy Kemberling, Linda McKay and Cheryl Wilson for their invaluable assistance in performing many of the ultrasonic studies; and Robert Waxham, Jagdish Patel, M.D., Carl Rubin, D. O. and Jack Breckenridge, M.D. for reviewing portions of the manuscripts. I particularly wish to thank William Burke, medical illustrator, for his invaluable assistance in arranging and photographing the ultrasonograms reproduced in this book. While credit for illustrations used will be given in each section, I specifically want to thank the following for the use of their illustrations: William F. Sample, M.D., from the University of California, Los Angeles; Ernest Carlsen, M.D. from Loma Linda University Medical Center, Loma Linda, California; Robert Bard, M.D. from Alta Bates Hospital, Oakland, California; Martin I. Resnick, M.D., William H. Boyce, M.D. and James W. Willard from Bowman Gray School of Medicine, Winston-Salem, North Carolina; Jerry Rosenbaum, M.D. from the Wilmington Medical Center, Wilmington, Delaware; and Michael Geller, M.D., from Allentown–Sacred Heart Hospital, Allentown, Pennsylvania.

I would also like to thank E. I. du Pont de Nemours & Company, Incorporated, for their support in the publication of the color plates in Sectional Abdominal Anatomy.

BARRY B. GOLDBERG

Contents

1
Physics of Gray Scale

Gordon S. Perlmutter, M.D.
Clinical Associate Professor of Radiology
Temple University Health Sciences Center
Philadelphia, Pennsylvania

Director, Ultrasound Section
The Reading Hospital
West Reading, Pennsylvania

Ernest N. Carlsen, Ph.D., M.D.
Associate Professor of Radiology
Loma Linda University

Director of Diagnostic Ultrasound
Loma Linda Medical Center
Loma Linda, California

This chapter will deal primarily with the physical aspects of gray scale imaging. The discussion assumes that the reader is conversant with the basic principles of ultrasound. These fundamentals have been covered in several excellent articles (1–5) to which the reader is referred.

To deal with gray scale ultrasound, it is first necessary to understand the intensity spectrum of a standard ultrasound signal. The intensity of a sound signal is measured in decibels. A decibel is defined as 10 times the $\log_{10}$ of the difference in the intensity of two signals. Thus, the intensity difference in decibels between two signals one of which is twice as intense as the other would be 3 decibels.

Assume

$$I_2 = 2 \times I_1$$

and

$$db = 10 \times \log_{10} \frac{I_2}{I_1}$$

then

$$db = 10 \times \log_{10} \frac{2}{1}$$

$$db = 3$$

A 10-decibel difference in signal strength is equivalent to a tenfold difference in intensity. The intensity of an ultrasound signal is given as approximately 100 decibels with the strongest signal being approximately 10 billion times more intense than the weakest signal (Figure 1). From a practical standpoint, it is impossible to obtain an ultrasound imaging system having the capability of displaying more than 50–60 decibels in signal intensity. The ability of a piece of equipment to display signals of varying amplitude is classified as the dynamic range of the equipment. The dynamic range of the standard methods used to display and record ultrasound signals is as follows:

Gray scale scan converter	30 decibels
Cathode ray tube (CRT)	20 decibels
Television monitor	20 decibels
Photographic film	10–20 decibels
Bistable storage scope	0–5 decibels

It can be seen from these dynamic ranges that one limiting factor in reproducing the ultrasound intensity spectrum with conventional non-gray scale equipment is the restricted dynamic range of the bistable scope. In fact, any one information point on the surface of this type of scope is either illuminated at full brightness or is unilluminated; hence, the term *bi*stable. Any ultrasound signal above a threshold intensity causes a given point on the bistable scope to be fully illuminated, whereas any signal below this threshold renders the point unilluminated. The relative intensity difference of echoes cannot be displayed on the bistable scope whether they are above or below the threshold. Another limitation of the bistable scope is the low resolution afforded by the approximately 0.5–1 mm spot size of the picture elements on the surface of the bistable tube (Figure 2).

Because of these severe limitations in bistable imaging, alternative approaches that would afford both higher resolution and greater dynamic range were sought. Two dif-

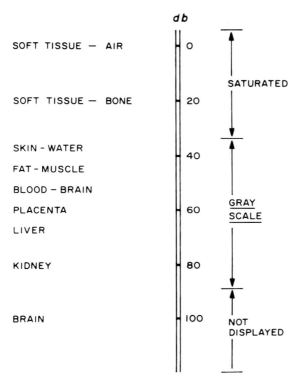

Figure 1.   Ranges of amplitudes of echoes from interfaces encountered in the body.

ferent approaches to solving this problem have been taken—nonstorage gray scale imaging and storage gray scale imaging.

NONSTORAGE GRAY SCALE IMAGING

Nonstorage gray scale imaging exploits the much broader dynamic range of a cathode ray tube (CRT) as compared to a bistable storage tube. As noted previously, the CRT has an estimated dynamic range of approximately 20 decibels. Stated differently, any one point on the surface of the cathode ray tube can be illuminated to any of approximately 10 varying degrees of brightness, or shades of gray, recognizable and distinguishable by the human eye. Although the dynamic range of the CRT display represents an approximately fivefold increase over the bistable scope, it is still unable to display the full intensity range of echoes contained in a 60-decibel ultrasound signal. It becomes necessary, therefore, to somehow compress or funnel the 60-decibel intensity spectrum of the ultrasound signal into a more restricted 20-decibel format. A simple method would be to divide the 60-decibel signal into three 20-decibel segments, displaying one-third of the signal at any given time. This, of course, requires the simultaneous rejection of two-thirds of the information content of the signal, which is considered unacceptable. Another approach is to electronically compress the 60-decibel signal spectrum into a 20-decibel format. In practice, sometimes this is accomplished by passing the ultrasound signal through a device such as a logarithmic amplifier, or its equivalent, which amplifies the sound signals as a function of their intensity; the weaker signals

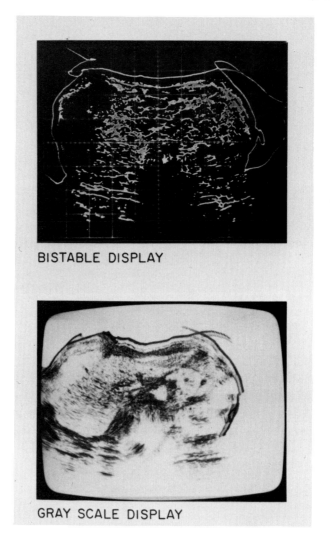

BISTABLE DISPLAY

GRAY SCALE DISPLAY

Figure 2.   Examples of bistable and gray scale images demonstrating the relatively restricted dynamic range and resolution of the bistable scans.

being more highly amplified than the stronger ones. This is done in such a way that the weakest signals are brought within a 20-decibel range of the strongest signals, thereby matching the ultrasound signals with the dynamic range of the cathode ray tube on which they are to be displayed. This type of logarithmic amplification is used not only in nonstorage gray scale displays but also as a means of compressing the sound signal for matching with the storage gray scale units to be discussed in the next section.

The compressed sound signal is then fed into the cathode ray tube which displays the sound signal in approximately 10 shades of gray. The CRT display is a real-time, non-storage display such that, at any moment in time, a line of dots of varying brightness is displayed in the same spacial orientation as the transducer. There is no means of storing these signals, however, once the transducer is moved to a different orientation.

Therefore, it is necessary to devise a means of storing and integrating all these instantaneous one-line displays in order to form a two-dimensional cross-sectional scan as a permanent record. The means most commonly used is a time-exposure photograph with the photographic film functioning as the storage device, often called the open-shutter technique. Since the brightness of any line or point on the photographic film is a function not only of the brightness of the dots on the oscilloscope but also of the amount of time these points are illuminated, it becomes necessary to devise a complex scanning method that essentially illuminates all points on the CRT for approximately the same period of time. This can be accomplished with contact scanners by sweeping the scanning transducer in a sectoring motion across the patient in such a way that each sector begins with the scanning transducer out of contact with the patient and terminates with the transducer out of contact with the patient (Figure 3). By scanning the patient with a fixed velocity of sectoring motion and a fixed sectoring interval, it is possible to produce excellent gray scale nonstorage scans. Fulfilling these scan requirements, however, is extremely difficult with a manually operated scanning arm. To some extent, this problem has been solved by the use of some type of automated scanning device that carefully

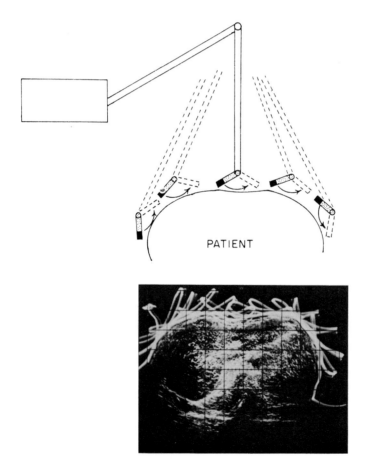

Figure 3. This is a schematic of the sector scanning method with the open-shutter technique. An example of a typical scan also is shown.

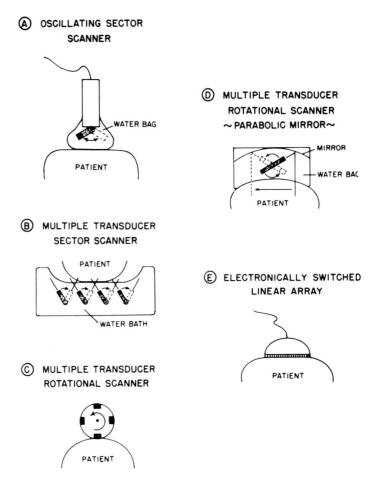

Figure 4.   Examples of various automatic scanning devices.

controls the scanning motion of the transducer in order to illuminate all points on the CRT for a given and fixed interval of time. This prevents overwriting which results when points on the CRT are illuminated for unequal time durations.

Several experimental units using automated scanning arms have been devised dating back to the units developed by Howry, Holmes, and Kossoff in the 1960s (6). Commercially available units taking advantage of nonstorage gray scale imaging coupled with mechanisms for automated scanning come in several forms. These include oscillating sector scanners, multiple transducer sector scanners, multiple transducer rotational scanners, and parabolic-mirror-equipped multiple transducer rotational scanners (Figure 4). It should be noted that whenever there is a large mechanical scanning motion of the transducer, it is necessary to couple this moving transducer to the patient by means of a water bath. Electronically timed switching of a linear array of transducers, either in a phased or nonphased mode is yet another method of controlling the scanning motion (Figure 4). Linear or phased-array transducers can be used in direct contact with the patient, eliminating the need for an intervening water bath. The reader is referred to Chapter 2 for a more detailed description of these types of instrumentation.

One last point to be made about using a nonstorage CRT display is the fact that the spot size of picture elements on the surface of a CRT is 0.25 to 0.5 mm with a marked improvement in image resolution possible compared to the bistable scope.

STORAGE GRAY SCALE IMAGING

At the heart of storage gray scale imaging is the scan converter unit. Similar to the photographic film used in nonstorage gray scale imaging, the scan converter tube acts as the storage device for building up a two-dimensional cross-sectional scan. Unlike methods based on photographic film, however, it is possible to observe the scan being built up in real time rather than having to wait for termination of the time exposure and development of the film, as is true of the open-shutter technique.

To understand how this works, it is necessary to have a basic understanding of the operation of a scan converter tube. The scan image is impressed onto the imaging surface of the scan converter tube by a stream of electrons accelerated across the tube from an electron gun at the back of the tube. The imaging surface of the scan converter tube is composed of a 1000×1000 matrix of elements, often silicone dioxide, rather than image phosphors as on the surface of the CRT. These silicone dioxide elements are able to store electrical charges that vary in degree from element to element. It is possible to operate a scan converter tube in such a way that any particular storage element does not accumulate electron charges additively during the writing process but rather accepts only the most intense signal presented to it. In this mode of operation, referred to as peak detection mode, it is possible to overwrite areas of the scan without creating serious image degradation (Figure 5).

So far we have discussed only the "write" mode of the scan converter tube. Since the surface of the tube is not composed of phosphors, it is not possible to view the surface of the scan converter tube directly and see an illuminated image on it. To display the image, it is necessary to operate the tube in the "read" mode in which a stream of electrons is directed against the charged silicone dioxide image surface but at a different voltage than in the "write" mode. The beam of electrons is either attracted or repelled by the imaging surface depending on the charge accumulated by the silicone dioxide elements. These repelled electrons are then collected on a grid. The sweep of the electron

SCAN CONVERTER TUBE

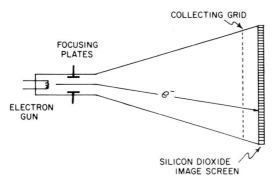

Figure 5.   Diagrammatic representation of a scan converter tube.

gun in the "read" mode of the scan converter tube is synchronized with the raster of a standard 525-line commercial television monitor. It is possible therefore to transfer the data stored on the scan converter tube to an electron gun in the television monitor. In other words, the latent image on the scan converter is reconstructed as a visible image on the surface of the television tube. In practice, the "write" and "read" modes of the scan converter tube can be operated simultaneously, permitting on-line viewing of the scan.

Similar to the nonstorage display scope (CRT), the scan converter-television monitor system is able to display approximately 10 detectable shades of gray. The resolution of the system is limited by the spot size of the electron beam (approximately 0.125 mm in diameter) which results in a matrix of approximately 1000 × 1000 elements. The small spot size permits a several-fold improvement in resolution over the bistable unit and, for practical purposes, the resolution is probably as good as that of nonstorage CRT images.

The dynamic range of the scan converter-television chain is a function of its weakest link, which is the 20-decibel dynamic range of the television monitor. Therefore it is necessary to match the much larger dynamic range of the scan converter tube, usually advertised at approximately 30 decibels, with the more restricted 20-decibel range of the television monitor. Several different image processing methods are being employed by varying manufacturers for this purpose. One manufacturer matches the dynamic range of the ultrasound signal to the 30-decibel range of the scan converter tube and then uses an "image processor" to variably compress and select that portion of the scan converter image to be displayed on the television monitor. Another manufacturer divides or quan-

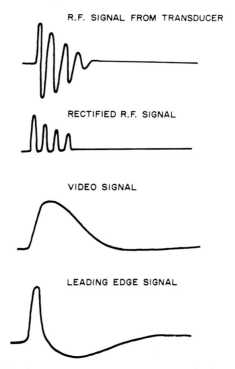

Figure 6.   Wave diagrams demonstrating various methods of signal processing.

tifies the 60-decibel sound signal into eight or nine discrete steps and assigns each step an appropriate shade of gray (7). Yet another manufacturer mixes a video signal display with the leading edge type of signal employed with bistable scopes and produces a composite signal that is impressed on the scan converter-television system (Figure 6). There are good and bad features associated with each type of signal processing that go beyond the scope of this chapter. Suffice it to say that the type of imaging format that is considered most acceptable is usually a matter of personal preference.

The possibility of digitizing the ultrasound signal and then using a digital microprocessor or computer in place of the scan converter is being explored actively. Machines using this type of image storage format are to be anticipated in the near future (8–10).

Once the ultrasound signal has been converted to a television format, it is possible to use many of the peripheral units developed for commercial television for storing, processing, and displaying the ultrasound image. These include videotape and videodisc storage, TV-compatible character generators for adding alpha numeric data to the scans, and television image processing units for varying the polarity, contrast, brightness, and other parameters of the scan. In most laboratories, the permanent storage of the ultrasonic scans is achieved by taking a photographic picture of the surface of the television monitor.

GRAY SCALE IMAGE RECORDING

The most extensively used method of recording the gray scale image, whether it be on a CRT or on a television monitor, is the use of photographic film. The type of photographic film most commonly used is self-developing film. Self-developing film provides almost immediate picture images but has the disadvantage of high contrast and narrowed latitude. Single emulsion photographic film has superior dynamic range as compared to self-developing film; specifically, it has less contrast and wider latitude. Similarly, photographic film has better resolution characteristics than self-developing film. The difficulty with photographic film, whether it is roll film or cut film, is that dark room facilities and automatic processing are required. From the standpoint of cost, it is possible to reproduce ultrasound images on photographic film at approximately one-quarter to one-eighth the cost of using self-developing film. Nevertheless, self-developing film remains the most prevalent form of ultrasound recording, primarily because of the convenience afforded by its simple and rapid self-developing process.

As mentioned earlier, it is possible with the television format in storage gray scale imaging to employ television-compatible peripheral units such as videotape and videodisc recorders for storage of ultrasonic scans. Because of the cost of videodiscs and the inconvenience of retrieving images from videotape, these methods of storage usually are employed only for short-term purposes. Image decay from videotape and videodisc storage, although present, is minimal for all practical purposes.

REFERENCES

1. Ziskin MC: Basic physics, in Goldberg BB, et al: *Diagnostic Uses of Ultrasound.* New York, Grune & Stratton, 1975, pp 1–30.
2. Ziskin MC: Instrumentation, in Goldberg BB, et al: *Diagnostic Uses of Ultrasound.* New York, Grune & Stratton, 1975, pp 31–70.

3. Carlson EN: Ultrasonic physics for the physician—a brief review. *J Clin Ultrasound* **3:**69, 1975.

4. Baker DW: Physical and technical principles, in King DL (ed): *Diagnostic Ultrasound.* St. Louis, C. V. Mosby, 1974, pp 16–51.

5. Wells PNT: *Physical Principles of Ultrasound Diagnosis.* New York, Academic Press, 1969.

6. Holmes JH: Historical prospectives, in King DL (ed): *Diagnostic Ultrasound.* St. Louis, C.V. Mosby, 1974, pp 1–15.

7. Busey HW, Rosenblum LH: Physical aspects of gray scale ultrasound, in White D (ed): *Ultrasound in Medicine,* vol. 1. New York, Plenum Press, 1975, pp 559–566.

8. Carlsen EN, Slater, JM, Nielsen IR, et al: An ultrasound/computer/video display and storage system. *J Clin Ultrasound* **1:**236, 1973.

9. Schorum SW, Fidel H: The Phosonic SM: a computer-controlled ultrasound image forming system. Presented at the World Federation for Ultrasound in Medicine and Biology (WFUMB), San Francisco, 1976.

10. Ophir, J, Goldstein A: The principles of digital scan conversion and their application to diagnostic ultrasound. WFUMB, San Francisco, 1976.

2
Gray Scale Instrumentation

Ernest N. Carlsen, Ph.D., M.D.
Associate Professor of Radiology
Loma Linda University

Director of Diagnostic Ultrasound
Loma Linda Medical Center
Loma Linda, California

Gordon S. Perlmutter, M.D.
Clinical Associate Professor of Radiology
Temple University Health Sciences Center
Philadelphia, Pennsylvania

Director, Ultrasound Section
The Reading Hospital
West Reading, Pennsylvania

Several types of gray scale ultrasound machines are now either on the market or under development for marketing in the near future. The various approaches that different manufacturers have employed in developing gray scale imaging will be described, but no attempt will be made to judge the various claims and counterclaims made by the manufacturers regarding the performance characteristics of their machines. Parameters for evaluating machines including dynamic range, gray scale, and resolution have been mentioned in the previous chapter. It behooves anyone intending to purchase an ultrasound machine to require the manufacturers to provide specifications on each parameter before purchasing a unit.

NONSTORAGE GRAY SCALE INSTRUMENTS

The principles of operation of nonstorage gray scale equipment have been outlined in the previous chapter. Two major groupings of machines in this category are those employing mechanical scanning techniques and those employing electronic scanning techniques.

Mechanical nonstorage gray scale ultrasound units use several methods for moving the transducer over the area of interest. One unit developed by George Kossoff and associates at the Ultrasonics Institute (formerly Commonwealth Acoustic Laboratories) in Australia, mechanically and synchronously sweeps eight transducers in a sector motion across the area of interest (1). The use of eight transducers allows for rapid scanning with approximately 1 second required for a full scanning pass. The images are integrated and stored on photographic film from a CRT by an open-shutter photographic technique. Images are in gray scale. The mechanically controlled motion of the transducers prevents image overwriting. The overlapping sectoring motion of the transducers permits detection of specular reflectors within the body that are not in the plane of the transducer array (Figure 1).

Another approach to mechanical scanning has been developed by Dr. Holm and his group at the Gentofte Hospital in Copenhagen, Denmark (2). This unit employs four transducers embedded within the circumference of a small wheel with the transducers oriented at 90-degree angles to each other (Figure 2). As the wheel turns, each transducer in turn is activated as it comes in contact with the patient's skin. A repetitive simple sector scan is thus achieved. By rotating the wheel in excess of four cycles/second, it is possible to develop a frame repetition rate of 16 frames/second or greater

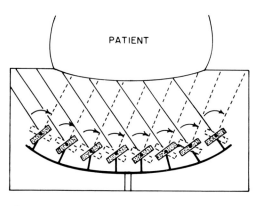

Figure 1. Multiple transducer sector scanner.

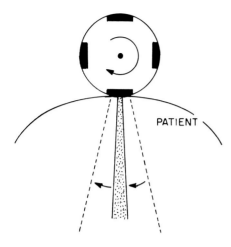

Figure 2.   Multiple transducer rotational scanner.

which allows for visual fusion of the images and real-time viewing. Unlike the unit previously described which uses a water bath to accomplish acoustic coupling between the active surface of the transducers and the patient, this transducer assembly operates in direct contact with the patient.

A somewhat less complicated means of moving a transducer in a sector sweeping motion has been developed by Bronson and Turner (3). In this unit a single transducer oscillates in a reciprocating motion with sufficient rapidity to allow for real-time imaging of the patient. A water bath coupling system within a hand-held housing is utilized to separate the gross mechanical oscillations of the transducer from the patient. A closely related type of imaging unit in which the oscillating transducer is applied directly to the patient is currently being marketed by several manufacturers particularly for cardiac imaging. Oscillating units of the water bath type are used primarily in ophthalmology and the evaluation of superficial masses (Figure 3).

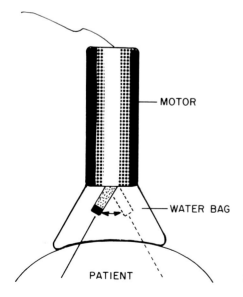

Figure 3.   Oscillating sector scanner.

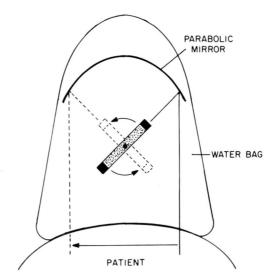

Figure 4.   Multiple transducer rotational scanner with parabolic mirror.

Another approach to a mechanical real-time gray scale unit employs a principle in which rotating transducers are contained within a water-filled housing (Figure 4). In this unit there are two transducers opposed to each other by 180 degrees. A parabolic mirror focusing system converts the rotatory motion of the transducer to a linear sweep motion across the patient. The rotation rate is approximately seven cycles/second allowing for approximately 14 repetitive images/second which is close to the visual fusion rate. The rotating transducers are coupled to the patient by an intervening water bath that is contained in a housing along with the transducers and the parabolic mirror.

Another approach developed to produce real-time gray scale scans uses a linear array of transducers that are electronically sequentially pulsed, in essence duplicating the effect of mechanically moving a single transducer across an area of interest. One of the first units of this type was developed by Dr. Bom of Holland for use in cardiac evaluation (4). This unit consists of a linear array of 20 transducers that are consecutively pulsed to produce a frame repetition rate of 150 frames/second (Figure 5). A similar

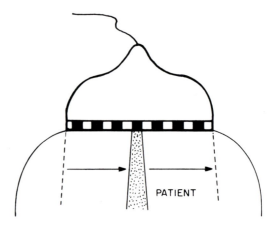

Figure 5.   Electronically switched linear array.

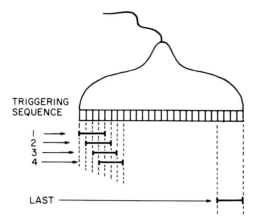

Figure 6.   An example of a multiplexed triggering sequence for a linear transducer array.

approach has been taken by others in developing a real-time unit with a linear array of 64 transducers that are multiplexed, or pulsed in groups, at a frame repetition rate of 40 frames/second, again producing a real-time gray scale image (Figure 6). With this type of unit, the length of the linear array determines the length of the field of view. In order to image a cross-sectional width of 10 cm, for instance, it is necessary to have a linear array of transducers 10 cm long.

It is possible, however, to have a linear array of transducers that can be triggered at

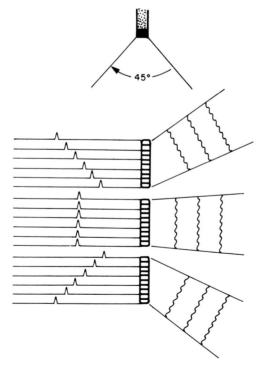

Figure 7.   An example of a phased linear array demonstrating varying beam direction as a result of phase changes in the triggering sequence

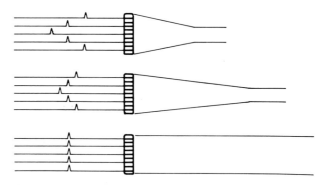

Figure 8.   Dynamic focusing resulting from phase changes in the triggering sequence.

varying phases to each other in such a way that the sound beam sweeps through an arc of 45 to 90 degrees from the surface of the transducer array (Figure 7). This allows for sector viewing over a distance greater than the length of the transducer array. A phased-array unit has been developed by Dr. Thurstone at Duke University (5). This type of unit is particularly useful in cardiac scanning since it is possible to take advantage of the acoustic window created by a rib interspace by placing in it a compact linear array of transducers that are phased in such a way as to provide a 45- to 90-degree angle of view from the skin surface. Several units employing the phased-array principle have been developed. One of the difficulties inherent in linear array transducer systems is poor lateral resolution of the sound beam. By using the phase firing principle, it is also possible to focus the sound beam at varying depths producing what has been termed "dynamic focusing" (Figure 8).

STORAGE GRAY SCALE INSTRUMENTS

As mentioned in the previous chapter, at the heart of all storage gray scale units is the scan converter. The principle of operation of all scan converter units is identical. To date no ultrasonic manufacturer makes his own scan converter, but instead purchases it from one of two major manufacturers. By using a scan converter and interfacing electronics for signal processing and compression it is possible to upgrade a conventional bistable B-scan ultrasound unit to gray scale capability. The operation of the scanning arm is the same as with conventional bistable scanning; however, the scanning technique tends to vary in that less sectoring and overwriting is required with gray scale scanning (Figure 9) (6). While the scan converter units are nearly identical in all gray scale storage equipment, the methods of image processing employed in conjunction with the scan converter are different. The methods of image processing used by the various manufacturers are considered proprietary information and details are often sketchy. Examples of the different types of signal processing employed by the various manufacturers have been given in the previous chapter and include image quantification, variable gray scale window and width control, signal mixing, and digital format. Other types and combinations of image processing methods probably are used as well. In spite of all the ballyhoo about the various image processing methods, the critical factor is the production of an ultrasonic image that has good diagnostic quality and is easy to

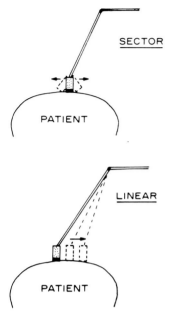

Figure 9. Upper diagram demonstrates typical sector scanning technique and lower diagram, linear technique which is used more commonly with a gray scale storage instrument.

interpret. Ultimately, the choice of imaging format becomes a matter of personal preference.

CONCLUSION

Different approaches used by several manufacturers have been outlined in this chapter for producing gray scale ultrasound images of diagnostic quality. Great strides have been made in the past few years in improving the diagnostic quality of the ultrasonic image, and even greater improvements are to be anticipated in the foreseeable future. As important as it is to obtain a good quality ultrasonic image, it is equally or even more important to be able to interpret the information that is available on the gray scale scan. To be sure, "You can't hit what you can't see," but on the other hand, "You can't hit what you do see if you don't understand what it is you are looking at."

REFERENCES

1. Kossoff G, Carpenter DA, Robinson DE et al: Octoson—a new rapid general purpose echoscope, in White D, Barnes R (eds): *Ultrasound in Medicine,* vol. 2. New York, Plenum Press, 1976, pp. 330–340.

2. Holm HH, Kristensen JK, Pedersen JF, et al: A new mechanical real-time contact scanner. *Ultrasound Med Biol* **2**:19, 1975.

3. Bronson NR: An ophthalmological ultrasonoscope. *Trans Amer Acad Ophthal Otolaryngol* **71**:360, 1967.

4. Bom N, Lancee CT, Honkoop J: Ultrasonic viewer for cross-sectional analysis of moving cardiac structures. *Biomed Eng* **6**:500, 1971.

5. von Ramm OT, Thurstone FL: Thaumascan: design considerations and performance characteristics. *J Clin Ultrasound* **2**:251, 1974.

6. Carlsen EN: Gray scale ultrasound. *J Clin Ultrasound* **1**:190, 1973.

3
Normal Vessels

Roy A. Filly, M.D.
Assistant Professor of Radiology
University of California at San Francisco

Picker Scholar, James Picker Foundation

Chief, Section of Ultrasound Diagnosis
University of California Medical Center
San Francisco, California

Barry B. Goldberg, M.D.
Professor of Radiology
Director, Division of Diagnostic Ultrasound
Thomas Jefferson University Hospital
Philadelphia, Pennsylvania

Recent improvements in ultrasound equipment, particularly gray scale image processing, have made it possible to identify a large number of vascular structures within the abdomen. The aorta and inferior vena cava can be seen with considerable clarity in all patients in whom interposed bowel gas does not prevent their visualization. The major systemic veins draining into the inferior vena cava and arteries arising from the aorta are often identified on good quality static gray scale images. The extrahepatic tributaries of the portal venous system can be traced through the abdomen. Intraparenchymal vessels, particularly in the liver, also are identifiable (1, 2).

A thorough knowledge of these vascular channels is necessary in order to avoid confusion with pathologic structures and to diagnose abnormalities of the vascular system itself. Major vessels serve as useful anatomic landmarks.

The relationships of vessels to one another can be demonstrated noninvasively. Using rapid B-scan (real-time) instrumentation, it is possible to demonstrate motion patterns (3, 4). Ultrasonic imaging of abdominal vascular channels will become increasingly important in the future since experimental Doppler equipment shows promise for measuring specific vessel blood flow (5).

The technique for obtaining satisfactory images, the usefulness of the procedure, and reasons for considering ultrasonography as a primary study in evaluating the major abdominal vessels will be discussed in this chapter and in the next one.

TECHNIQUE

The patient is placed in the supine position with adequately supported arms and legs to provide as much relaxation of the abdominal wall musculature as possible. Since interposed bowel gas is the primary cause for failure in evaluation of intraabdominal vessels, it is generally advisable for the patient to fast prior to the examination. Swallowed air tends to increase the amount of gas within the stomach and bowel. A similar precaution is to avoid performing the examination after a barium study. Barium, a colloid suspension, prevents penetration of the ultrasonic beam by producing multiple reflections that interfere with the evaluation of structures that are located beneath the barium (6).

Scans in the parasagittal planes are made using a single sweep of the transducer beginning in a subcostal position and arching the transducer from an anterior and cranial direction to a posterior and caudal direction (Figure 1). Whenever possible, scans should be performed in suspended maximum inspiration. In addition to the obvious benefit of decreasing image degradation from respiratory motion, maximum inspiration causes upper abdominal viscera to descend from beneath the rib cage. The writing speed of most modern gray scale equipment will permit completion of the scan during the breath-holding time of all but the most dyspneic patients.

Single pass or sector scans are of considerable importance in depicting small vascular structures. Compound movements of the transducer or repetition of sector passes tend to degrade the sonographic image because of the inherent motion of vascular structures even when respiration is suspended. Scan intervals are usually 1 to 2 cm depending on the size of the patient. However, in obtaining detailed sonograms of small vascular structures even slight changes in the position of the scanning arm may improve visualization. Compound scan techniques should not be abandoned; however, they are usually unnecessary. Those situations in which compound motions of the transducer will be helpful generally are not difficult to assess in the individual scanning situation.

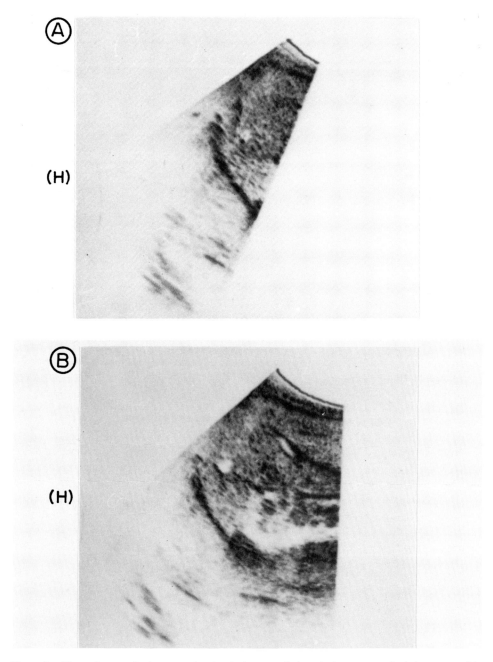

Figure 1. Three photographs demonstrating the single pass technique during a parasagittal ultrasonographic section of the right hepatic lobe (V = vein). (*Continued on next page.*)

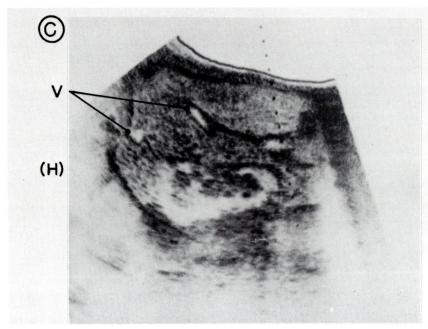

Figure 1. (Continued)

Hard and fast rules for adjustment of time gain compensation are impractical because of the great variation in optimum machine settings from patient to patient. When scanning parenchymal organs one generally adjusts time gain compensation factors to record a uniform distribution of low amplitude parenchymal echoes from the abdominal solid viscera.

A note of caution is advised when one is employing the gray scale B-scan mode of display for visualization of small vascular structures. Weak echoes (the lightest shades of gray) will tend to appear within what one would normally expect to be an echo-free lumen. These echoes should not be misinterpreted as arising from clots, which tend to produce echoes of slightly greater intensity. In most instances, these artifactual intralumenal echoes are due to reverberations. A major cause of these spurious, apparently intralumenal, echoes is the fact that gray scale sonograms invariably are performed at rather high receiver amplification and transducer output in order to record low amplitude parenchymal echoes. These "high gain" settings yield electronic noise and an increased propensity to record reverberations. Decreasing the overall system gain while increasing time compensated gain may alleviate this difficulty.

Another important reason for the appearance of these spurious echoes is the poor lateral resolution of the ultrasonic beam. This results in echoes being recorded at the same level as the vessel from soft tissues that actually surround the vessel lumen. Thus, there is a tendency for the normally echo-free lumen to appear partially or completely filled with low amplitude reflections, particularly if the vessels are smaller than the width of the ultrasonic beam. The effective beam width is widened by high gain machine settings typical of gray scale scans. The closer the ultrasonic transducer is to the area of interest, the less the divergence of the ultrasonic beam and the greater its ability to delineate structures. As a result, the thinner the patient, the easier it is to obtain images of smaller vascular structures and, similarly, images that are free of spurious echoes.

Usually it is not possible to complete a cross-sectional scan of the upper abdomen with a single sector pass of the transducer. Rather, a single arc of the transducer is made between the costal edges in the desired transverse plane. The scan is completed subsequently by compound scan technique between the ribs (Figure 2). It is important to not redirect the transducer beam toward the midabdominal vessels already depicted by the single sector pass when using the compound scan technique to image between the ribs since the image quality may be reduced significantly.

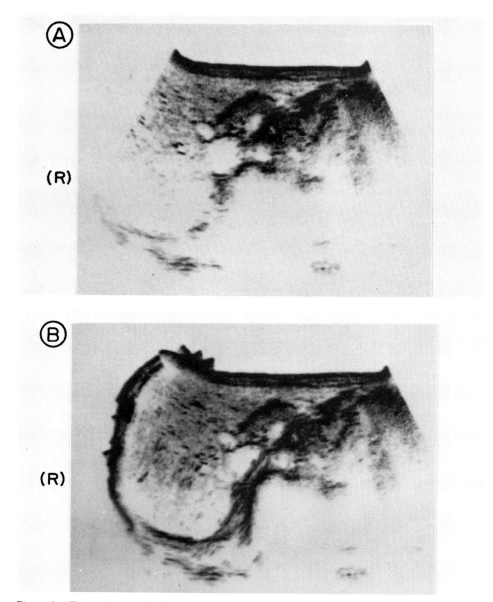

Figure 2. Three photographs demonstrating the technique for cross-sectional sonograms of the upper abdomen. *A*. A single sector sweep is made between the costal margins. The scan is completed by compound scan technique through the intercostal spaces (B and C). (*Continued on next page.*)

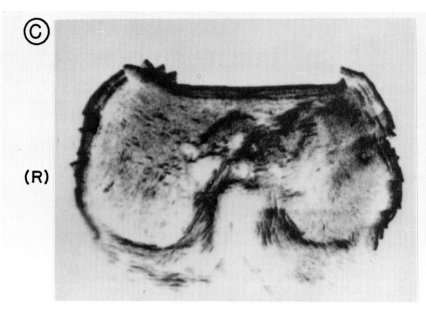

Figure 2.   (Continued)

A useful method for depicting a vascular structure of specific interest is to abandon the concept of obtaining a complete transverse or parasagittal section scan in every instance. A limited sector scan (Figure 3) performed immediately over the vessel of interest is the most successful technique for imaging vessels of small caliber. The transducer is moved in a short arc directing the ultrasonic beam toward the structure to be visualized. This technique reduces scanning time and enables the examiner to select the optimum vantage point for transducer placement. Bone and gas artifacts are frequently avoided. One can "work around" interfering gas containing bowel loops with this simple and effective technique.

The rate of transducer motion across the skin is important but somewhat less critical than optimizing the gain function curve or employing a sector scan technique. Only by experience can one determine the optimal speed of transducer motion since it is a highly visual phenomenon and varies with the gain function curve, transducer frequency, and patient body habitus. The inherent "writing speed" of the equipment in use is often a limiting factor.

Proper selection of transducers will improve significantly detailed visualization of small vascular structures. A general rule in transducer selection is to use the highest frequency transducer that will fulfill the requirement to penetrate the organ or anatomic region under study. When difficulty is encountered in recording low amplitude parenchymal echoes in the far field, the temptation is to change immediately to a transducer of lower frequency. Often, the more satisfactory solution is to select a transducer with a wider crystal diameter rather than a transducer of the same crystal diameter but lower frequency. Focused transducers generally produce higher quality images of vascular structures if the vessel falls within the zone of optimal beam focusing. Thus, it is advisable to have a variety of transducers available that have zones of focus at varying distances from the piezoelectric crystal.

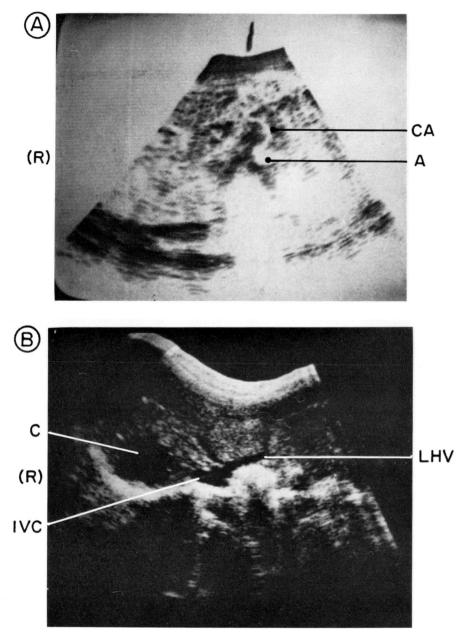

Figure 3.   Limited sector scans performed to visualize optimally: *A.* the celiac axis bifurcation (CA) and *B.* the entrance of the left hepatic vein (LHV) into the inferior vena cava (IVC) (R = right; A = aorta; C = incidental hepatic cyst).

Real-time ultrasonographic units are very helpful in the evaluation of abdominal vessels (3, 4, 7). Phased array, dynamically focused real-time ultrasonographic systems provide very high resolution images of abdominal vessels. However, the less expensive linear array real-time imaging transducer systems are also valuable for rapid identification of vessels and the recording of their wall motion. A significant advantage of real-time sonographic systems is the rapidity with which vessels can be identified. Similarly, the course of a vessel can be traced quickly and the transducer subsequently reoriented along the longest axis of the vessel. The vessel axis then can be marked on the skin. If desired, static gray scale images of the vessel then can be obtained by orienting the transducer movement along this predetermined scanning plane. When marking the skin, a wax pencil is useful since acoustic coupling agents tend to prevent other types of skin markers from visibly adhering to the skin surface.

In normal individuals, both systemic and portal venous structures dilate with respiratory maneuvers which increase intrathoracic pressure. These respiratory variations in venous caliber are valuable in differentiating arteries from veins.

Doppler ultrasonography is useful in demonstrating the presence and direction of flow in a vessel (5). In the future, the use of combined B-scan and Doppler instrumentation (duplex systems) should result in dramatically improved assessment of flow dynamics within blood vessels. When narrowing or occlusion is suspected, pulsed Doppler, which can be gated to measure a specific vessel depicted on the B-scan image, may be employed to display flow patterns and velocity in the diseased vessel.

NORMAL VENOUS ANATOMY

Inferior Vena Cava and Iliac Veins

The inferior vena cava (IVC) forms at the confluence of the right and left common iliac veins. It courses cranially anterior to the right side of the vertebral column. In the upper abdomen the IVC is not situated immediately anterior to the surface of the spine but courses anteriorly in intimate contact with the hepatic parenchyma until it passes through the caval hiatus of the diaphragm to enter the right atrium (Figure 4). In the midportions of the abdomen the inferior vena cava displays a horizontal course, while in the upper abdomen it turns anteriorly to join the right atrium. The caliber of the inferior vena cava increases as the blood from the renal veins admixes with that of the lower extremity venous return.

If there is no interposed bowel gas, the vena cava can be recorded consistently from the diaphragm to its bifurcation. The initial ultrasonograms usually are obtained in longitudinal planes of section starting to the right of the midline. The vena cava is most readily demonstrated when the patient is asked to suspend respiration after deep inspiration. The Valsalva maneuver frequently helps but may sometimes hinder the demonstration of the IVC if the abdomen is expanded during the procedure. The transducer movement for a longitudinal scan usually is begun at the xyphoid sweeping in a caudal direction to the level of the umbilicus. Transverse scans of the inferior vena cava are obtained at 1 to 2 cm scanning intervals from the xyphoid to its bifurcation (Figure 5).

Normal respiratory variation in the caliber of the IVC is visualized most readily on real-time sonography. Conventional M-mode scans are satisfactory for recording

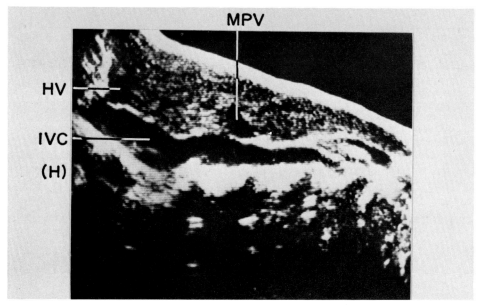

Figure 4. Parasagittal ultrasonogram of the inferior vena cava (IVC) demonstrating that the IVC turns anteriorly in the upper abdomen to join the right atrium. (HV = hepatic vein; MPV = main portal vein; H = head). (Reproduced from *Journal of Clinical Ultrasound* with permission.)

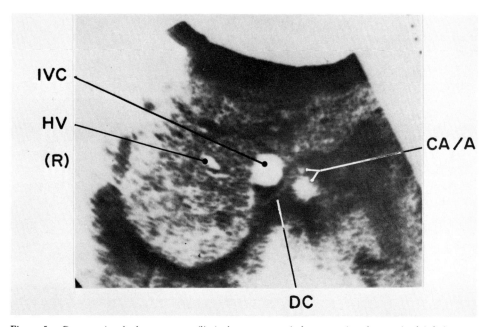

Figure 5. Cross-sectional ultrasonogram (limited sector sweep) demonstrating the proximal inferior vena cava (IVC) in intimate contact with the hepatic parenchyma (HV = hepatic vein; R = right; CA/A = origin of celiac axis from the aorta immediately caudal to the termination of the diaphragmatic crus (DC)).

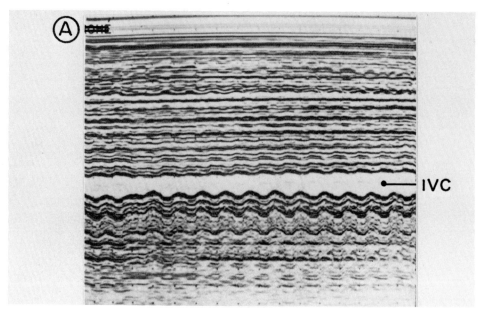

Figure 6. *A.* M-mode recording of the inferior vena cava (IVC) with the patient in expiration. The caliber of the IVC is narrow and transmitted cardiac pulsations are moderately prominent. *B.* During a Valsalva maneuver the IVC distends and pulsations are dampened. *C.* By angling the transducer cranially the ultrasonic beam intersects the right atrium (RA).

respiratory motions or transmitted cardiac pulsations to the IVC (Figure 6). The characteristic patterns of movement of the IVC near the right heart can be quickly learned and employed both in the anatomic identification of the IVC and in the detection of pathologically altered venous pressures and flow volumes.

The caliber of the IVC, as visualized on sonograms, varies dramatically in normal individuals. Undoubtedly, the degree of Valsalva effort varies and accounts for many of the changes noted. Nonetheless, petite females may show a very prominent IVC while this vessel may be difficult to demonstrate in robust males.

Interestingly the larger common iliac vessels are demonstrated less frequently than the smaller external iliac veins. The external iliac veins are not infrequently identified when scanning low in the pelvis through the distended urinary bladder (Figure 7). Conversely, the larger common iliacs often are obscured by bowel gas.

Renal Veins

The entrances of the renal veins into the inferior vena cava are recognized frequently on static gray scale B-scans. The left renal vein exits the left renal sinus and takes a generally transverse course toward the abdominal midline. The vein crosses anterior to the aorta in the crook formed by the superior mesenteric artery to enter the anterior and medial aspect of the inferior vena cava (Figure 8). The right renal vein, of course, has a much shorter anatomic course. The right renal vein exits the right renal sinus and courses anteriorly and slightly medially to enter the posterior and lateral aspect of the inferior vena cava.

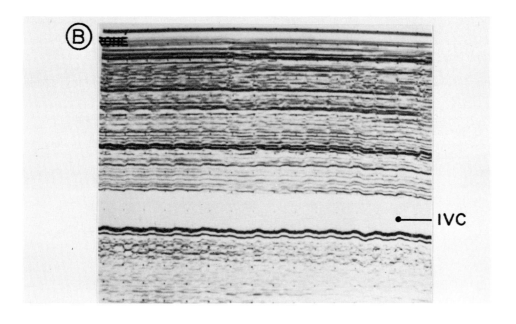

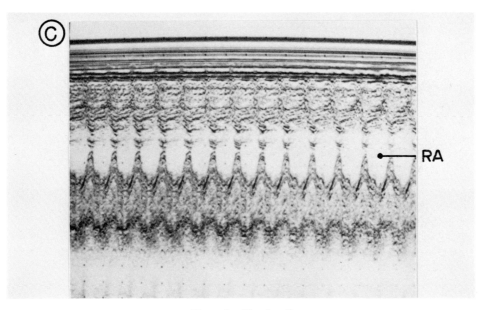

Figure 6. (Continued)

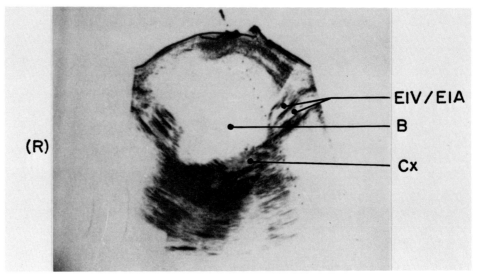

(R)

EIV/EIA

B

Cx

Figure 7. A transverse ultrasonogram in the low pelvis demonstrates the external iliac vein and artery (EIV/EIA) by angling the ultrasonic beam through the urine distended bladder (B) (R = right; Cx = cervix).

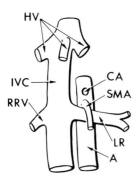

Figure 8. Diagram illustrating the course of the left renal vein (LR) and its relationship to the anterior surface of the aorta (A) and the origin of the superior mesenteric artery (SMA). (HV = hepatic veins; IVC = inferior vena cava; RRV = right renal vein; Ca = celiac axis). Reproduced from *Journal of Clinical Ultrasound* with permission.

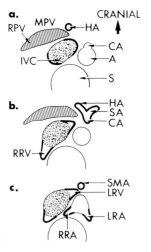

Figure 9. Diagram of cross-sectional vessel anatomy in an idealized patient. *A.* Cranial to the entrance of the renal veins the inferior vena cava (IVC) is large and displays smooth contours. The margins of the IVC that are altered by the entrance of the renal veins are highlighted (RPV = right portal vein; MPV = main portal vein; HA = hepatic artery; CA = celiac axis; A = aorta; S = spine). *B.* The posterolateral margin of the IVC "dips" posteriorly at the entrance of the right renal vein (RRV) (SA = splenic artery). *C.* The anteromedial margin of the IVC extends to the left at the entrance of the left renal vein (LRV) just caudal to the origin of the superior mesenteric artery (SMA) (LRA and RRA = left and right renal arteries, respectively). *D.* Inferior to the entrance of the renal veins the IVC again displays smooth contours but is smaller in caliber. Reproduced from *Journal of Clinical Ultrasound* with permission.

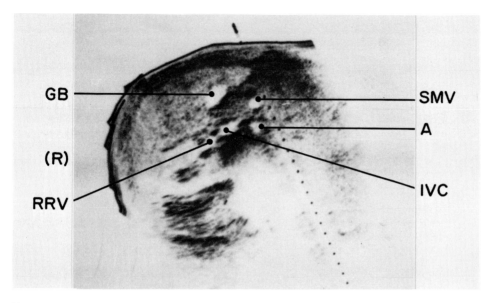

Figure 10. *A.* Cross-sectional ultrasonogram of the right (R) upper abdomen demonstrating the right renal vein (RRV) entering the posterolateral aspect of the inferior vena cava (IVC) (A = aorta; SMV = superior mesenteric vein; GB = gallbladder). The head of the pancreas (unlabeled) is contained in the triangle of gallbladder, IVC, and SMV.

The locations of these large systemic veins are identified by the distinctive alteration in the contour of the inferior vena cava noted on cross-sectional echograms traversing the entrances of these vessels. Figure 9 illustrates the alteration in the contour of the IVC as seen in transverse sections in an idealized paient. Cranial to the entrance of the renal veins the inferior vena cava is large in caliber and displays smooth contours. Figure 9*B* illustrates that the posterior-lateral margin of the inferior vena cava "dips" posteriorly at the entrance of the right renal vein. The cross-sectional echogram in Figure 10 demonstrates the right renal vein causing this typical alteration in the contour of the inferior vena cava. Figure 9*C* diagramatically illustrates that the anterior-medial border of the inferior vena cava appears to extend to the left denoting the entrance of the left renal vein. At times, a considerable length of the left renal vein can be seen crossing the aorta. Figures 11*A* and *B* depict representative sonograms of the proximal left renal vein.

The IVC increases in caliber superior to the entrance of the renal veins. The large volume of blood returning from the kidneys to the inferior vena cava accounts for this difference. Longitudinal scans of the inferior vena cava frequently demonstrate this caliber change to best advantage (Figure 12).

Extrahepatic Portal Venous System

While there are a variety of contributing vessels to the portal venous system, the main portal vein is formed at the confluence of the splenic (SV) and superior mesenteric veins (SMV) (Figure 13). The splenic vein exits the splenic hilus and follows a transverse

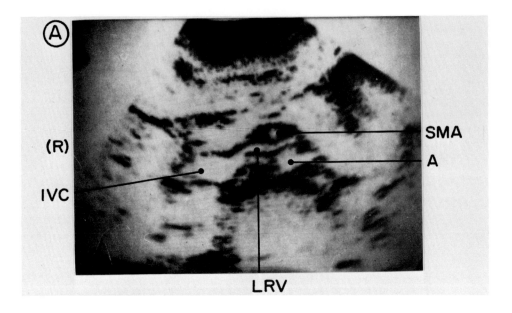

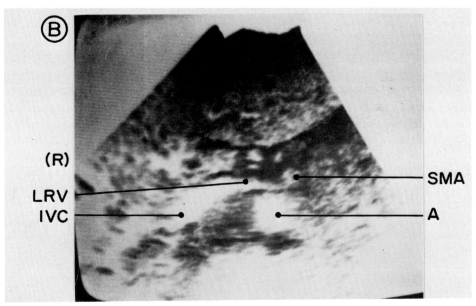

Figure 11. *A.* Cross-sectional limited sector sweep demonstrating a "thin" left renal vein (LRV) entering the anteromedial aspect of the inferior vena cava (IVC) after coursing between the aorta (A) and superior mesenteric artery (SMA). The splenic-portal confluence and the origin of the left renal artery are displayed but not labeled (R = right). *B.* Larger left renal vein (LRV) demonstrated on a limited sector sweep. The LRV responds to a Valsalva maneuver as do other abdominal veins (R = right; SMA = superior mesenteric artery; A = aorta). The superior mesenteric vein is depicted but not labeled.

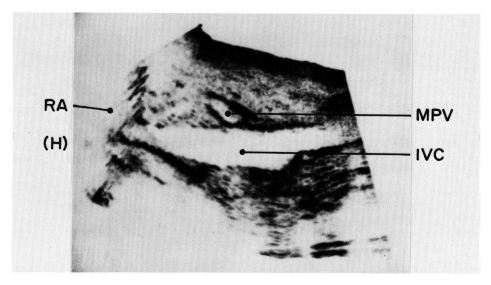

Figure 12. Parasagittal scan through the inferior vena cava (IVC) demonstrating the increase in caliber of the proximal IVC after the entry of the renal veins (H = head; RA = right atrium; MPV = main portal vein).

course through the left upper quandrant to join the SMV near the midline. Throughout its course, the splenic vein relates to the posterior and superior aspect of the pancreatic body and tail. Conversely, the superior mesenteric vein travels a longitudinal course through the abdomen. It frequently is found directly in the midline in a position anterior to the inferior vena cava and the aorta. From the confluence of the splenic vein with the superior mesenteric vein the main portal vein then courses in a cranial and slightly rightward direction. Upon entering the porta hepatis, it divides into the more cranial and smaller left portal vein and the larger and more caudal right portal vein. During its course, the main portal vein is closely related to the anterior surface of the inferior vena cava. Indeed, the relationship is so intimate that the portal vein and inferior vena cava frequently appear to share a common wall as visualized on ultrasonograms. The pancreatic head lies caudal to the main portal vein and lateral to the SMV.

The splenic vein is best demonstrated on transverse ultrasonograms (Figure 14A). It can be identified most commonly as it passes anterior to the abdominal aorta before it joins the main portal vein. The superior mesenteric artery and the celiac axis, which

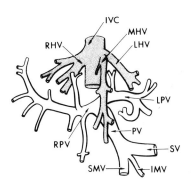

Figure 13. Diagram illustrating the arrangement of the hepatic veins and intra- and extrahepatic portal veins in an idealized subject. The vessels are not necessarily drawn in their true proportional anatomic size (IVC = inferior vena cava; RHV, MHV, LHV = right, "middle," and left hepatic veins, respectively; PV, LPV, RPV = main, left, and right portal veins, respectively; SMV = superior mesenteric vein; IMV = inferior mesenteric vein; SV = splenic vein). (Reproduced from *Journal of Clinical Ultrasound* with permission.)

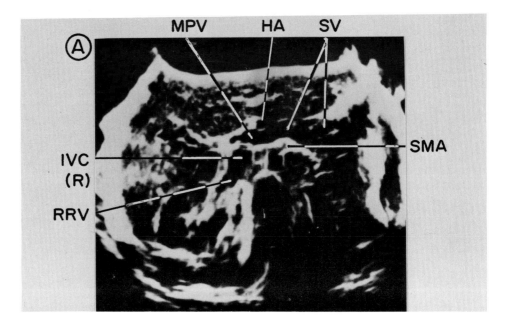

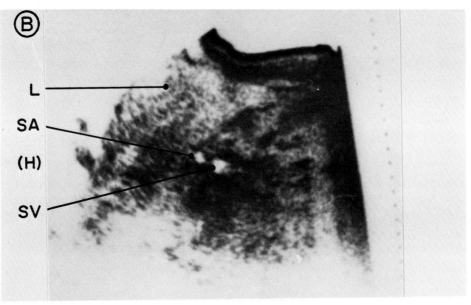

Figure 14.   *A*. Cross-sectional scan at the level of the splenic-portal confluence. This confluence is frequently identified anterior to the origin of the superior mesenteric artery (SMA) (IVC = inferior vena cava; RRV = right renal vein; MPV = main portal vein; SV = splenic vein; HA = hepatic artery). *B*. Parasagittal scan immediately to the left of the spine demonstrating the larger and more caudal splenic vein (SV) and the smaller and more cranial splenic artery in a patient with splenomegaly (H = head; L = liver). (Reproduced from *Journal of Clinical Ultrasound* with permission.)

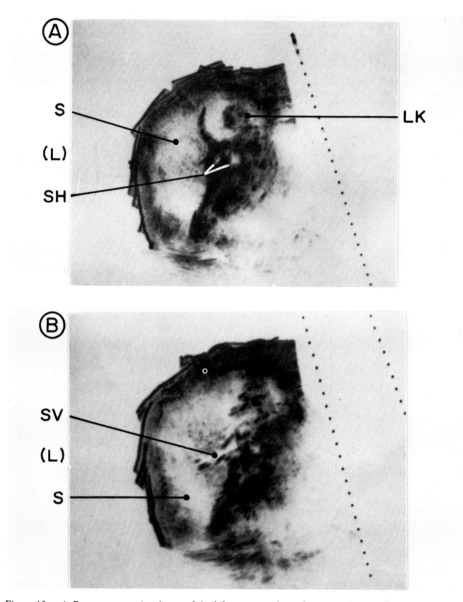

Figure 15. *A.* Prone cross-sectional scan of the left upper quadrant demonstrating vessels in the splenic hilus (SH). The spleen is enlarged (S) (L = left; LK = left kidney). *B.* Scan obtained 1 cm cranial to that in Figure 15*A* demonstrates the splenic vein (SV) exiting the enlarged spleen (S).

will be discussed in detail later, are useful landmarks in the identification of the position of the confluence of the splenic vein with the portal vein. The craniocaudal location of this confluence varies from its most typical position just cephalad to the take off of the superior mesenteric artery to a position just caudal to the bifurcation of the celiac axis. The course of the splenic vein, as with any other vessel, varies so that small degrees of obliquity may be helpful in demonstrating the splenic vein if the initial transverse scan is inadequate. It also may be helpful to position the ultrasonic beam perpendicular to the aortic walls rather than the abdominal wall, which in this anatomic location may be somewhat scaphoid, angling downward from the xyphoid. The splenic vein is usually smaller than the superior mesenteric vein and, of course, the main portal vein. The larger diameter of the portal vein is the result of the additional influx of blood from the superior mesenteric vein. Thus, at the junction of the splenic vein and the portal vein, an obvious widening is demonstrated. The splenic vein often is identified on parasagittal sonograms near its confluence with the portal vein usually in a position anterior to the aorta. Occasionally, the SV can be traced to the left of the spine particularly when the spleen is enlarged pathologically (Figure 14*B*).

It is sometimes possible to detect the origin of the splenic vein at the splenic hilus. Again, this is most frequently seen when the spleen is enlarged pathologically (Figure 15). Since bowel gas frequently overlies the left side of the abdomen, supine scans routinely fail to demonstrate the origin of the splenic vein. Increasing success can be obtained by scanning the patient in the prone position through the left flank and directing the transducer toward the splenic hilus.

The superior mesenteric vein lies to the right of the superior mesenteric artery (Figure 16). Near the origin of the superior mesenteric artery the superior mesenteric vein is also more anteriorly located. More distally in the abdomen, the superior mesenteric artery and vein have a parallel and side-by-side course. Differentiation of the superior mesenteric artery and vein will be discussed later.

The best ultrasonic approach for visualization of the superior mesenteric vein is on parasagittal sections (Figure 17). Parasagittal scans at short intervals are obtained from the midpoint of the inferior vena cava to the lateral aspect of the aorta. If there is no

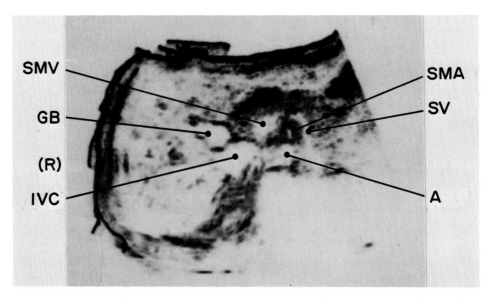

Figure 16. Partial cross-sectional scan near the origin of the superior mesenteric artery (SMA). Fewer echoes are seen in the hepatic parenchyma than is optimal since the "gain" was decreased to eradicate spurious echoes in the lumens of the smaller vessels. The superior mesenteric vein (SMV) is larger than the SMA and at this level is also slightly anterior. Echogenic pancreatic tissue between the vessels and left hepatic lobe is unlabeled (R = right; GB = gallbladder; A = aorta; IVC = inferior vena cava; SV = splenic vein).

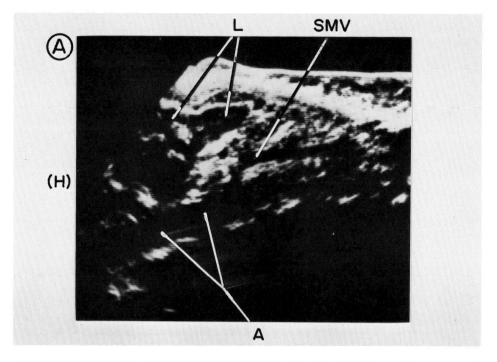

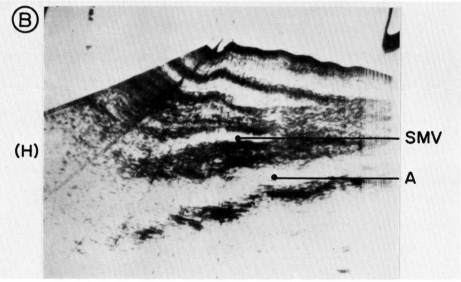

Figure 17. *A*. Parasagittal scan near the abdominal midline. The scan is oblique to the course of the aorta (A); thus only the proximal aorta is visualized. The scan was obtained through the long axis of the superior mesenteric vein (SMV). The splenic vein (unlabeled) is "cut" through its short axis (L = liver). *B*.In this individual the superior mesenteric vein (SMV) courses more directly anterior to the aorta (A). (Figure 17*A* reproduced from *Journal of Clinical Ultrasound* with permission.)

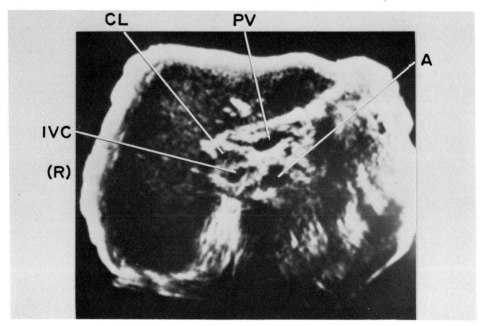

Figure 18.   Cross-sectional scan near the confluence of the splenic vein and portal vein (PV). It is unusual for the caudate lobe (CL) to be interposed between the inferior vena cava (IVC) and portal vessels this far caudal in the abdomen (A = aorta). (Reproduced from *Journal of Clinical Ultrasound* with permission.)

interfering bowel gas the superior mesenteric vein will be identified within this anatomic region.

The caudate lobe of the liver, situated just cranial to the bifurcation of the main portal vein, may separate the vena cava from the portal vein. However, it is unusual for the portal vein to be separated from the IVC throughout its entire course by the caudate lobe (Figure 18). The relationship of the caudate lobe of the liver to the portal vein usually is demonstrated best in a longitudinal plane through the inferior vena cava. As previously discussed, the portal venous system in normal individuals also responds to respiratory variation in intrathoracic pressure.

Intraparenchymal Hepatic and Portal Veins

Four tubular fluid-filled structures enter or leave the liver. These are the hepatic and portal veins, the hepatic artery, and the bile ducts. The intraparenchymal hepatic arteries and bile ducts are not visible on sonograms of normal individuals although the extrahepatic components of these structures occasionally are demonstrated. Conversely, the major branches of the portal and hepatic veins are visible within the liver parenchyma of the vast majority of patients scanned with gray scale ultrasonography.

Variation of the hepatic venous anatomy is the rule rather than the exception. A typical arrangement of the major radicles is depicted in Figure 13. These consist of a right, middle, and left hepatic vein. The major components of the right hepatic vein are visible on virtually all sonograms of the liver. The middle hepatic vein is seen in most patients. The smaller left hepatic vein is usually not visualized during routine scanning

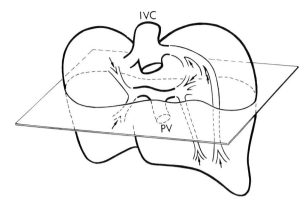

Figure 19.   Diagram illustrating that the angle formed by the branching of portal and hepatic veins cranial to a plane of section through the bifurcation of the main portal vein is a clue to which venous system the smaller vessel belongs.

procedures. It is not unusual to see second order and sometimes third order branching of the larger right hepatic veins.

The hepatic veins are recognized most readily on longitudinal sections of the liver. Major components of the hepatic venous system also can be identified on transverse scans obtained at the level of the xyphoid particularly when the transducer is angulated in a cranial direction.

The sine qua non for recognition of hepatic venous channels is to trace the vessel to its entry point in the inferior vena cava or, in the case of smaller branches, to trace them to known major hepatic venous trunks. This task is tedious and generally unnecessary when certain basic patterns and principles have been recognized.

The hepatic veins drain cephalad toward the diaphragm and then dorsomedially toward the inferior vena cava. Four anatomic features distinguish the hepatic veins. These features enable one to recognize hepatic venous radicles on individual transverse or longitudinal section sonograms. All large venous trunks situated close to the diaphragm may be considered to represent hepatic veins. Hepatic veins increase in caliber as the vessel approaches the diaphragm or the right atrial-inferior vena caval (RA-IVC) junction. Hepatic veins are not surrounded by bright acoustical reflections although a slight amount of acoustical enhancement may be noted along the posterior aspect of the vessel. The fourth differentiating feature will be discussed separately.

Conversely, portal veins become smaller in caliber as they progress centrifugally from the porta hepatis. Thus, in contrast to hepatic veins, large venous radicles situated near the porta hepatis or venous radicles that increase in caliber as they approach the porta hepatis represent portal veins. Characteristically, portal veins are ringed by high amplitude acoustical reflections presumably arising from the fibrous tissues that surround the portal triad as it courses through the liver substance.

If a plane is cut transversely through the liver at the bifurcation of the portal vein (Figure 19) it can be seen that the angle formed by the branching of portal veins cranial to this plane will point inferiorly or inferomedially. Conversely, the angle formed by the branching of hepatic venous radicles will point superiorly or superomedially. Caudal to this plane, the angles formed by the branching of both the hepatic and portal veins point in similar directions. Representative sonograms of hepatic veins are seen in Figure 20.

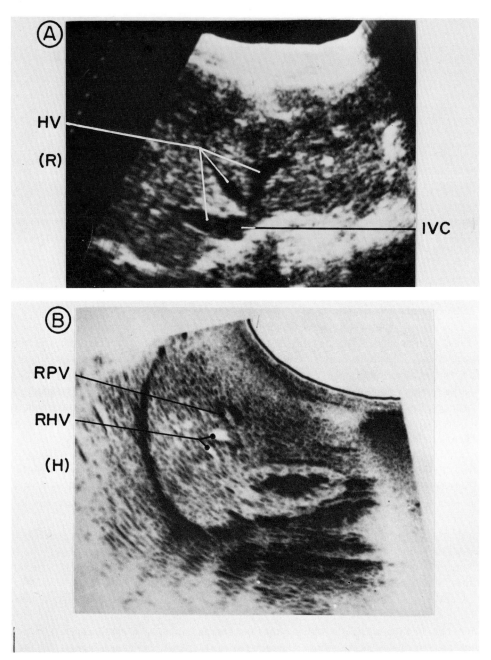

Figure 20. *A.* Limited cross-sectional single sector sweep angled cranially from the xyphoid demonstrating three large hepatic veins (HV) joining the inferior vena cava (IVC). *B.* Parasagittal scan of the right hepatic lobe demonstrating second order branches of the right hepatic vein (RHV). Note that the right portal vein (RPV) is ringed by bright reflections while the hepatic veins are not. *C.* Parasagittal sonogram medial to that of Figure 20*B*. Two large branches of the right hepatic vein (RHV) are seen adjacent to the diaphragm. Note that even though these hepatic venous branches are larger than the right portal vein (RPV) the latter vessel is much more conspicuous since it is ringed by bright echoes. An intrahepatic venous radicle (HV) is recognized

40

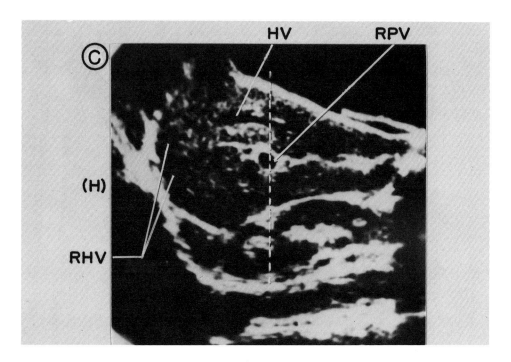

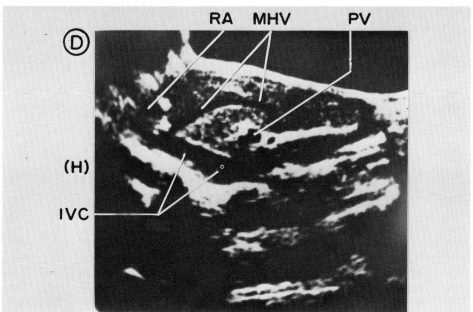

easily as an hepatic vein since its caliber increases as it approaches the diaphragm and the angle formed at its branch point aims toward the diaphragm. The dashed line represents the plane of section in Figure 19. *D.* Parasagittal scan through the IVC at the junction with the right atrium (RA). The "middle" hepatic vein (MHV) enters the anterior surface of the IVC (PV = portal vein). (Figures 20*C* and *D* reproduced from *Journal of Clinical Ultrasound* with permission.)

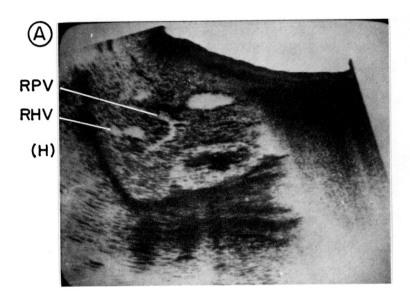

RPV
RHV
(H)

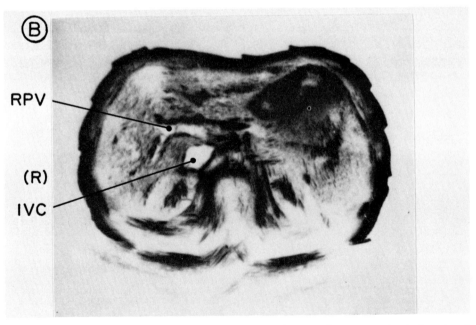

RPV
(R)
IVC

Figure 21. *A.* Parasagittal scan through the right hepatic lobe demonstrating two second order branches of the right portal vein (RPV) (H = head; RHV = right hepatic veins). *B.* Cross-sectional sonogram through the long axis of the right portal vein (RPV) also demonstrating some second order branches. Note that the angle formed by the branch point aims toward the porta hepatis and that the portal vessels are surrounded by bright echoes (IVC = inferior vena cava). *C.* Parasagittal scan through the IVC. The left portal vein (LPV), "cut" through its short axis, is small and more anterior and cranial than the main portal vein (MPV) (H = head; MHV = "middle" hepatic vein). *D.* Cross-sectional scan demonstrating the left portal vein (LPV). Note that the proximal LPV demonstrates an echo-free lumen while the course of the distal LPV is recognized only by bright periportal echoes (R = right; A = aorta).

42

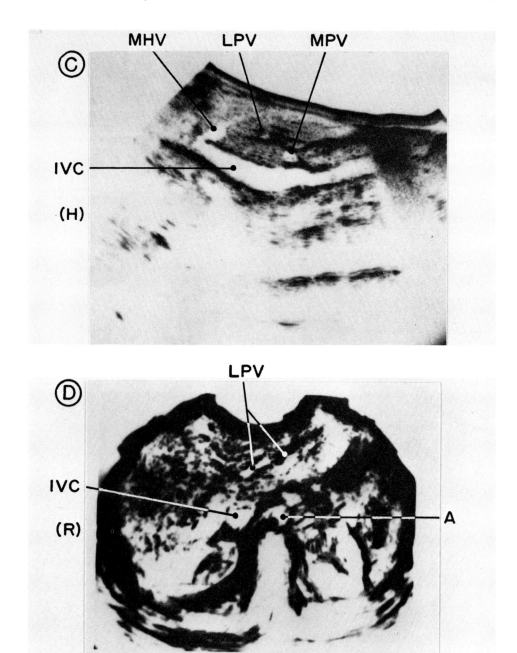

Figure 21.   (Continued)

The major portal venous structures, the right and left portal veins, course through the liver transversely. Thus, in parasagittal scans the major portal radicles are depicted in planes traversing their shortest axis (Figure 21*A* and *C*). Greater lengths of the portal veins are depicted on transverse planes of sections (Figure 21*B* and *D*).

Although similar criteria are employed in the recognition of the portal veins as with the hepatic veins, the reference point for the portal system is the porta hepatis while that for the hepatic veins is the diaphragm or the RA-IVC junction.

The right portal vein is the more easily recognizable of the two major intrahepatic portal trunks. Of all branch vessels in the abdomen, the right portal vein probably is demonstrated the most consistently. While there is considerable minor variation in the course of the right portal vein its recognition usually does not constitute a significant problem. The right portal vein extends into the hepatic parenchyma from the right lateral aspect of the main portal vein. Anatomically, any intraparenchymal segment of the portal venous system lying to the right of the lateral aspect of the inferior vena cava is a branch of the right portal system.

The left portal vein is seen as a narrow caliber trunk coursing transversely through the left hepatic lobe on cross-sectional scans. Usually its course, when viewed from the porta hepatis into the parenchyma of the left hepatic lobe, is from a posterior to a more anterior position. Because the vessel is small in caliber, the lumen is frequently obliterated with false internal echoes. However, the bright echoes that surround the portal veins serve as a landmark to demonstrate the position and course of the left portal vein. In the region of the porta hepatis, the left portal sometimes combines with two or three smaller portal radicles to form a confluence (Figure 22).

The confluence of the left and right portal veins in the porta hepatis at the bifurcation of the main portal vein similarly shows moderate variation from patient to patient. Nonetheless, the main portal vein is recognized easily by its relationship to the anterior surface of the inferior vena cava (Figure 23). While some portion of the caudate lobe may interpose between the portal system and the inferior vena cava, this generally does not constitute a problem in recognition of the portal vein. Since this confluence is seen consistently in nearly all patients, it requires only a short period of observation to

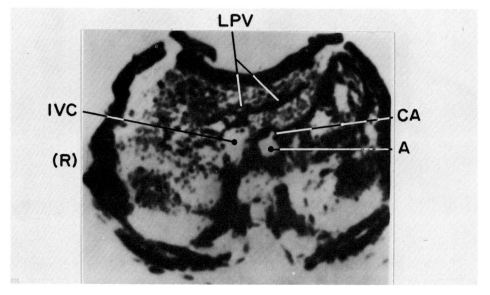

Figure 22.   Cross-sectional sonogram demonstrating a confluence of small portal vessels near the origin of the left portal vein (LPV) (R = right; IVC = inferior vena cava; A = aorta; CA = origin of the celiac axis). (Reproduced from *Journal of Clinical Ultrasound* with permission.)

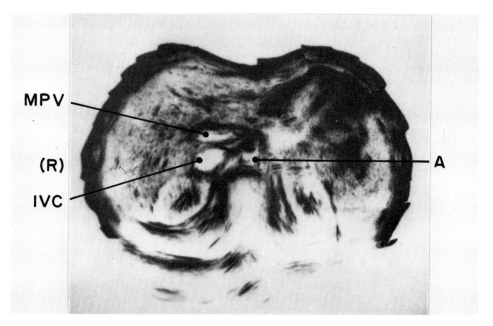

Figure 23. The main portal vein (MPV) that courses from right to left is "cut" obliquely in this transverse scan. Note the intimate contact of the MPV and inferior vena cava (IVC). The unlabeled left portal vein is recognizable by the bright echoes surrounding it (R = right; A = aorta).

become familiar with the minor degrees of variation noted at the junction of the two major intrahepatic portal radicles. Familiarity with these minor pattern variations is becoming increasingly important as ultrasonography is employed more and more in differentiating obstructive from nonobstructive jaundice. Dilated biliary radicles also become confluent in the porta hepatis, usually in a position anterior to the portal vessels (Figure 24). The ability to recognize an alteration in the known patterns of confluence of the portal vessels will enable ready recognition of the abnormally dilated biliary trunks at the porta hepatis.

ABDOMINAL ARTERIES

The Aorta and Iliac Arteries

The aorta enters the abdominal cavity through the aortic hiatus and proceeds caudally in a position anterior to the vertebral column and to the left of the midline. It bifurcates into the common iliac arteries at a level slightly cranial to the umbilicus. In the normal patient the aorta is related intimately to the anterior surface of the vertebral column throughout its course. Only an abnormal situation will alter this relationship. The proximal aorta is more posterior than the distal aorta. If the lumbar lordosis is prominent this appearance will be striking in longitudinal ultrasonograms of the aorta. Since all normal individuals have some degree of lumbar lordosis the proximal abdominal aorta is invariably more posterior in position than the distal abdominal aorta. This anatomic appearance helps to distinguish the abdominal aorta from the infe-

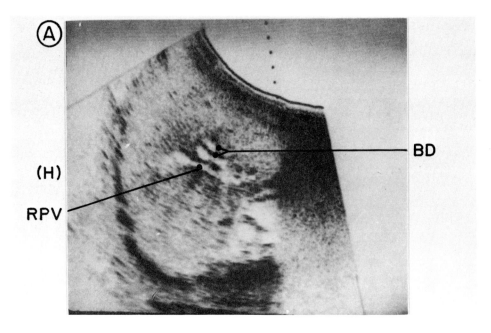

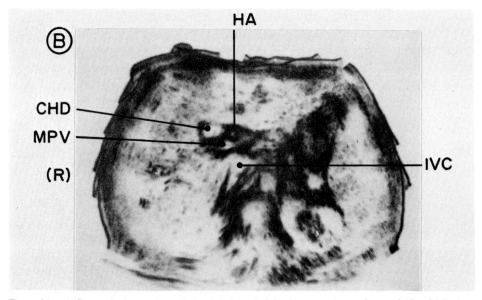

Figure 24. *A*. Parasagittal scan through the right hepatic lobe demonstrating a cluster of dilated bile ducts (BD) surrounding the right portal vein (RPV). Incidental hydronephrosis (H = head). *B*. Transverse scan demonstrating the anatomic arrangement of the vessels in the hepatoduodenal ligament in a patient with extrahepatic biliary obstruction. The portal vein (MPV) is posterior; the common hepatic duct (CHD) is anterior and lateral; the hepatic artery (HA) is anterior and medial (R = right; IVC = inferior vena cava).

rior vena cava which, as discussed previously, courses more horizontally through the abdomen and then turns anteriorly to join the right atrium. These major abdominal vessels also differ in the character of their pulsations. The abdominal aorta is pulsatile throughout its entire length while the inferior vena cava tends to show transmitted pulsations from the right atrium only in its more proximal abdominal segment. The relationship of the portal vein to the inferior vena cava also serves to distinguish the vena cava from the aorta.

Normal values have been established for the lumen size at various points along the aorta from the xyphoid to its bifurcation (8). In the normal individual the aorta shows a gradually tapering lumenal dimension as it proceeds distally in the abdomen. Normal lumen diameters as established by ultrasonographic measurements at the xyphoid, at the umbilicus, and at two points between (usually above and below the levels of the renal arteries) are listed in Figure 25 (8). The ultrasonic results were compared with contrast aortographic measurements. The ultrasonic and roentgenographic measurements of aortic diameter demonstrated no significant differences when x-ray magnification factors were taken into account. Thus, ultrasound can be employed as a noninvasive tool to determine the lumenal dimensions of the normal abdominal aorta.

If interposed bowel gas does not present a problem, the abdominal aorta invariably can be recorded throughout its entire length in the abdomen. Unfortunately, it is usually impossible to visualize the aorta from the axillary (side) view or from a prone position since bowel gas and interposed ribs in the former and the spine in the latter prevent transmission of the sound beam.

The iliac arteries arise from the aortic bifurcation angling away from the abdominal midline (Figure 26). Usually, it is difficult to visualize any significant portion of these vessels. The iliac vessels descend into the pelvis where branches are given off to pelvic organs, after which they terminate at the inguinal ligament becoming the common femoral arteries. Overlying bowel is abundant in this region of the abdomen and usually precludes accurate recording of the common iliac arteries. Employing gray scale ultrasound, there is a greater chance of recording at least the proximal portions of the

	--------- Diameter (mm) ---------			
	At 11th Rib	Above Renal Arteries	Below Renal Arteries	At Bifurcation of Aorta
Aortography Results Steinberg et al. (transverse lumen diameter in mm corrected for magnification)	24	21	19	17
Aortography Results Goldberg et al. : Ten cases (AP lumen diameter corrected for magnification)	25	22	19	15
Ultrasonic Results Goldberg et al. : Ten cases (AP lumen diameter)	23	20	18	15

Figure 25. Comparison of measurement of the lumen of normal aortas by ultrasound and arteriographic techniques.

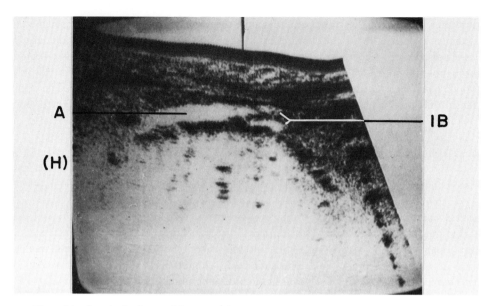

Figure 26.   Longitudinal scan of the aorta (A) demonstrating the iliac bifurcation (IB) (H = head).

iliac vessels. In pregnant patients, the iliac vessels are seen frequently since the gravid uterus displaces interfering bowel loops. In a similar fashion to the external iliac veins described above, the external iliac arteries are not infrequently seen when scanning the pelvis through the filled urinary bladder (Figure 7). It is difficult to record long lengths of either iliac artery because of interposed bowel gas and the difficulties encountered when attempting to align the transducer to the long axis of the vessel.

The Major Visceral Arteries

One or more and occasionally all the major visceral arteries can be recognized on high quality gray scale sonograms. Arteries that can be visualized include the celiac axis (CA), the superior mesenteric artery (SMA), and the right and left renal arteries (RRA and LRA). The hepatic artery, splenic artery, gastroduodenal artery, and inferior mesenteric artery are seen with considerably less frequency. The celiac and superior mesenteric arteries usually can be demonstrated on both cross-sectional and longitudinal sectional scans when bowel gas does not preclude their recognition. The renal, hepatic and splenic arteries are recognized on cross-sectional scans and only uncommonly are depicted on longitudinal sectional scans. The inferior mesenteric artery has been noted only on longitudinal scans.

These arteries can be grouped conveniently into those arising from the anterior surface of the abdominal aorta—the celiac, superior mesenteric, and inferior mesenteric arteries—and those arising from the lateral and posterolateral aspect of the abdominal aorta—the left and right renal arteries. Lumbar arteries which also arise from the lateral and posterolateral aspects of the abdominal aorta are difficult or impossible to recognize with confidence.

The most easily located and recorded branch of the aorta is the superior mesenteric artery. Anatomically, it arises just distal to the origin of the celiac trunk. The artery

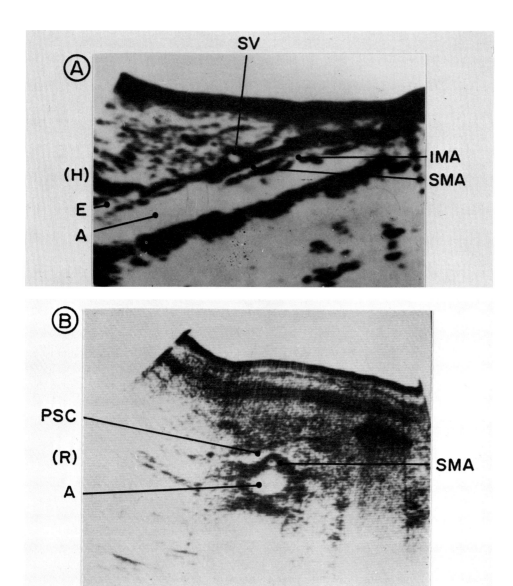

Figure 27. *A*. Longitudinal scan of the abdominal aorta (A) demonstrating the superior (SMA) and inferior (IMA) mesenteric arteries. The relationship of the splenic vein (SV) to the origin of the SMA can be seen (H = head; E = esophagus—abdominal segment). *B*. Limited sector sweep near the origin of the SMA causing a "bubblelike" distortion of the anterior aortic wall (A) (PSC = portal-splenic confluence; R = right). *C*. Slightly caudal, the SMA appears as an echo-free "ring" anterior to the aorta (A) (R = right; GB = gallbladder; RRV = right renal vein; IVC = inferior vena cava). The portal-splenic confluence and left renal arteries are not as clearly visible but present on this scan (unlabeled). (Figure 27*A* reproduced from *Radiologic Clinic of North America* with permission.) (*Continued on next page.*)

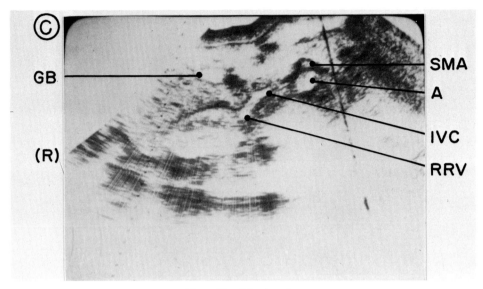

Figure 27.   (Continued)

travels in a generally caudal direction where it gives off branches to pancreas and to the
bowel. The superior mesenteric artery usually is located immediately anterior to the
aorta (Figure 27A). However, there is a moderate anatomic variation in its course. Not
infrequently, the SMA courses obliquely either to the right or left of the aorta. Thus, a
longitudinal ultrasonogram through the abdominal aorta may record only a portion of
the SMA.

Once longitudinal scans have been obtained, transverse scans can be recorded. One
normally begins just above the origin of the superior mesenteric artery and proceeds
caudally at 1-cm intervals. The origin of the superior mesenteric artery lies posterior to
the body of the pancreas. As it courses caudally the SMA exits from its position posterior to the pancreatic body to lie medial to the head of the pancreas. Distal to the
pancreatic head the SMA rarely if ever is recorded on transverse ultrasonograms.

The relationship of the superior mesenteric artery to the aorta can be demonstrated
and alterations in this normal relationship caused by pathologic processes can be
determined. Limited single sweep linear scanning is particularly helpful in demonstrating the superior mesenteric artery on cross-sectional images. Excess motion of the
transducer often will obliterate the relatively small echo free lumen of the SMA.

The relationship of the left renal vein to the origin of the superior mesenteric artery is
a helpful landmark for determining the point of origin of the SMA. Similarly, the
confluence of the splenic and portal veins provides a useful anatomic landmark in many
individuals. Cross-sectional scans through the origin of the superior mesenteric artery
may produce a "bubblelike" distortion of the anterior surface of the aorta (Figure 27B).
However, the SMA more often is recognized in cross-sectional scans as a small, echo
free "ring" anterior to the aorta (Figure 27C).

Because of the intimate relationship of the superior mesenteric vein and superior
mesenteric artery confusion in distinguishing these two vascular structures sometimes
arises. Several points are helpful in making this distinction: (a) the superior mesenteric
vein is considerably larger in caliber than the SMA; (b) respiratory variation in lumen
diameter of the SMV can be identified, as is true of any venous structure; (c) the SMA,

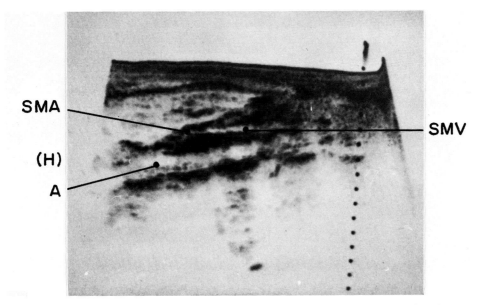

Figure 28. In this longitudinal scan the superior mesenteric artery (SMA) appears to abruptly widen as it courses distally. The plane of section has crossed slightly from left to right so that cranially the SMA is depicted, but as the transducer moved caudally the superior mesenteric vein (SMV) was depicted (H = head; A = aorta).

as seen on longitudinal scans, tends to angle away from the abdominal aorta, while the SMV tends to parallel the course of the aorta or even course anteriorly away from the aortic lumen near the confluence of the SMV with the portal vein; (d) identification of the confluence of the SMV and portal vein or the origin of the SMA from the aorta provides unequivocal identification of these structures. Occasionally, parasagittal planes of section may cross from the SMA to the SMV creating a particularly confusing image (Figure 28).

Celiac Axis

It is possible to record the celiac axis and some of its major branches in a moderately high percentage of patients in whom bowel gas has not interfered with penetration of the ultrasonic beam. The superior mesenteric artery is usually located first due to the relative ease with which it can be recorded. The celiac axis can then be sought just cephalad to the origin of the SMA.

The main trunk of the celiac axis takes a generally vertical course from the anterior surface of the aorta and then divides in a "winglike" pattern into the hepatic and splenic arteries proceeding to the right and left, respectively (Figure 29). The hepatic component courses anterior to the main portal vein while the splenic component curves posteriorly and leftward in its course toward the splenic hilus. These arterial structures are dipicted on cross-sectional scans obtained just cranial to the confluence of the splenic and portal veins. The main hepatic artery lies ventral to the portal vein in 91 percent of individuals (9). Its continuation toward the liver sometimes is recognized in cross-sectional scans as a discretely rounded, echo-free structure touching the anterior surface of the main portal vein (Figure 14). Celiac-mesenteric trunks have been demonstrated sonographically (Figure 29).

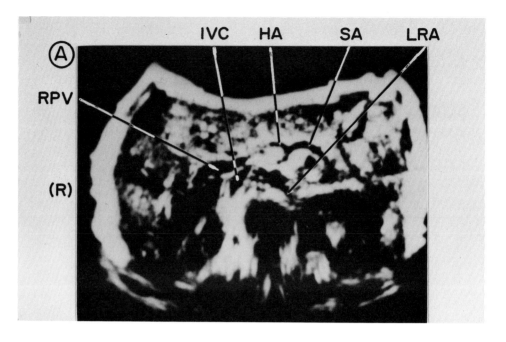

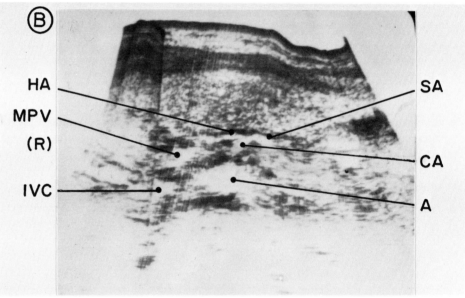

Figure 29. *A.* Cross-sectional scan demonstrating the "winglike" bifurcation of the celiac axis into the right hepatic component (HA) and the left splenic component (SA) (R and L = right and left, respectively; RPV = right portal vein; IVC = inferior vena cava; LRA = left renal artery). *B.* Similar scan to Figure 29*A* in a different patient demonstrating a more flattened celiac axis (CA) bifurcation. Note that the hepatic component (HA) courses to a position anterior to the main portal vein (MPV) (R = right; IVC = inferior vena cava; SA = splenic artery). *C.* Longitudinal scan demonstrating the origin of the celiac axis (CA) from the anterior surface of the aorta (A) (H = head; LPV = left portal vein). *D.* Longitudinal scan demonstrating a celiacomesenteric trunk (CMT). Several branches of the celiac component are depicted (CB). The relationship of the splenic vein (unlabeled) is seen (A = aorta; SMA = superior mesenteric artery). (Figures 29*A* and *D* were reproduced from *Journal of Clinical Ultrasound* with permission.)

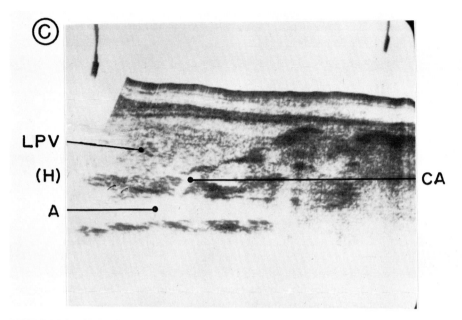

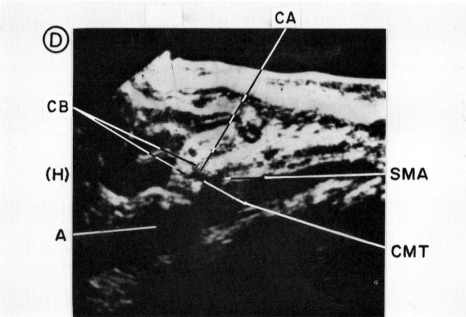

Figure 29.   (Continued)

The lumen of the celiac axis appears to be only slightly larger than that of the superior mesenteric artery, but enough ultrasonic data have not as yet been gathered to compare it with known anatomic and arteriographic measurements.

The gastroduodenal artery has been recorded on transverse and longitudinal scans of the pancreatic parenchyma (10). Identification of this small vessel provides precise anatomic localization of the pancreatic head. Unfortunately, it is exceedingly difficult to record this small arterial branch.

Inferior Mesenteric Artery

The inferior mesenteric artery (IMA) is much more difficult to visualize ultrasonically than the superior mesenteric artery or the celiac axis. Only rarely is the inferior mesenteric artery recorded. When seen, it is recognized on longitudinal scans (Figure 27). Its origin from the anterior surface of the aorta is seen at a variable distance caudal to the origin of the superior mesenteric artery. The inferior mesenteric artery tends to lie close to the anterior wall of the abdominal aorta. This vessel has a variable course and it is difficult to demonstrate any significant length of IMA unless it happens to lie in a longitudinal plane directly anterior to the aorta. In this situation it is seen as a small elongated tubular structure caudad to the SMA.

Renal Arteries

The renal arteries arise from the lateral or posterolateral walls of the abdominal aorta. They usually originate just caudal to the origin of the superior mesenteric artery. The right renal artery courses posterior to the inferior vena cava and anterior to the vertebral column in a posterior and slightly caudal direction (Figure 30). The left renal artery, arises from the left lateral or posterolateral aortic wall and courses anterior to the psoas muscle to enter the left renal sinus (Figure 31). Accessory renal arteries, which have variable points of origin, have never been successfully demonstrated ultrasonographically.

The renal arteries are best seen on transverse ultrasonograms, although occasionally a segment of the right renal artery coursing posterior to the inferior vena cava is demonstrated on a longitudinal ultrasonogram. Again, the origin of the superior

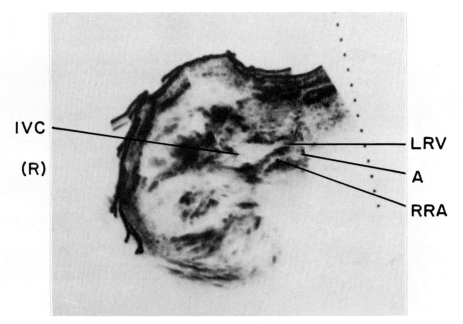

Figure 30.   Cross-sectional scan of the right side of the abdomen (R) demonstrating the right renal artery (RRA) coursing between the inferior vena cava (IVC) and the spine (A = aorta; LRV = left renal vein).

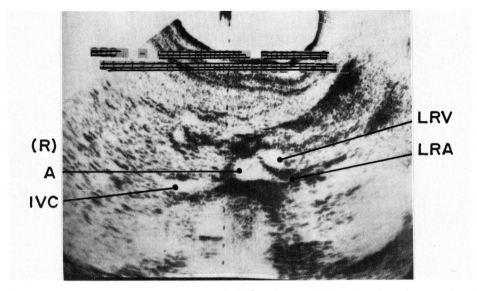

Figure 31.   Cross-sectional scan demonstrating the left renal artery (LRA) arising from the posterolateral aspect of the aorta (A) (R = right; LRV = left renal vein, IVC = inferior vena cava).

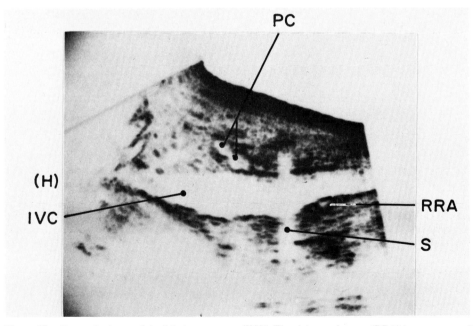

Figure 32.   Parasagittal scan of the inferior vena cava (IVC). The right renal artery (RRA) is seen as a small "ring" posterior to the IVC. Gas in the gastric antrum casts a small acoustic shadow (S) (H = head; PC = portal confluence in the porta hepatis).

55

mesenteric artery is employed as an anatomic landmark. Transverse scans are begun at this level and subsequent ultrasonograms are recorded at small increments in a caudad direction. The left renal artery has a much shorter course than the right and is generally more difficult to demonstrate. Slight obliquity of the transducer plane is often helpful in demonstrating a greater length of these vessels.

A segment of the right renal artery occasionally is demonstrated on longitudinal scans of the inferior vena cava. It can be recognized as a small ringlike structure just behind the posterior margin of the inferior vena cava (Figure 32). If identified on the longitudinal scan, the skin can be marked with a wax pencil to serve as a reference point for a transverse scan.

Occasionally, tubular branching structures are noted within the renal sinuses. Three tubular fluid-filled structures traverse the renal sinus; the renal veins, renal arteries, and calyceal infundibuli. It is usually impossible to distinguish which structure has been recorded on a given ultrasonographic scan.

SUMMARY

Gray scale ultrasonography has proved to be an important tool in the demonstration of various intraabdominal vessels, both venous and arterial. The relationship of vessels to one another can be demonstrated noninvasively. Using real-time gray scale instrumentation, it is possible to display patterns of vessel motion. M-mode ultrasonic display enables one to record motion patterns for analysis. Experimental pulsed Doppler equipment, in combination with gray scale B-scanning, also shows promise in being able to measure vessel flow. Further refinements in equipment design, possibly coupled to computers, should further decrease the need to invasively image abdominal vascular structures.

REFERENCES

1. Carlsen EN, Filly RA: Newer ultrasonographic anatomy in the upper abdomen: I. The portal and hepatic venous anatomy. *J Clin Ultrasound* **4**:85–90, 1976.

2. Filly RA, Carlsen EN: Newer ultrasonographic anatomy in the upper abdomen: II. The major systemic veins and arteries with a special note on localization of the pancreas. *J Clin Ultrasound* **4**:91–96, 1976.

3. Winsberg F, Cole CM: Continuous ultrasound visualization of the pulsating abdominal aorta. *Radiology* **103**:455–457, May 1972.

4. Weill F, Eisenscher A, Aucant D, Bourgoin A, Gallinet D: Ultrasonic study of venous patterns in the right hypochondrium: An anatomical approach to differential diagnosis of obstructive jaundice. *J Clin Ultrasound* **3**:23, 1975.

5. Mozersky DJ, Hokanson DE, Baker DW, Sumner DS, Strandness DE: Ultrasonic arteriography. *Arch Surg* **103**:663–667, December 1971.

6. Leopold GR, Asher WM: Deleterious effects of gastrointestinal contrast material on abdominal echography. *Radiology* **98**:637–640 March 1971.

7. Weill F, Maurat P: The sign of the vena cava: echotomographic illustration of right cardiac insufficiency. *J Clin Ultrasound* **2**:27–32, 1974.

8. Goldberg BB, Ostrum BJ, Isard HJ: Ultrasonic aortography. *JAMA* **198**:4 353–358, October 1966.

9. Grant JCB: *An Atlas of Anatomy*. The Williams and Wilkins Co., Baltimore, 1962, figure 144 (n.p.).

10. Sample FW: Technique for the improved delineation of normal anatomy of the upper abdomen and high retroperitoneum with grey scale ultrasound. Presented at the 62nd Scientific Assembly of the RSNA. November, 1976.

Sectional Abdominal Anatomy

E. A. Lyons, M.D., F.R.C.P.C.
Director, Section of Ultrasound
Health Sciences Center
Winnipeg, Manitoba

R. E. Grahame, M.D., M.Sc.
Associate Professor and Acting Head
Department of Anatomy
Faculties of Medicine and Dentistry
University of Manitoba
Winnipeg, Manitoba

This section of the book is a small tribute to that which is consistent and perfect—the human body. The entire book is a large collection of the best gray scale images that can be produced by today's level of ultrasonic instrumentation. As has been witnessed in the past 10 years, the prize pictures of the present rapidly become hopelessly unacceptable studies in the future.

The following pages display selected anatomical sections and labelled line diagrams. No representative ultrasound scans were used due to a space restriction as well as a strong feeling that even the best examples would only be a compromise on what we eventually will be capable of producing given the proposed, rapid advances in instrumentation. Anything short of an exact duplication of the anatomical specimen would be a compromise. Post mortem scans were attempted and were found to be unsatisfactory, due to an abundance of very strong interfaces, probably associated with changes in the fat planes. We were fortunate in that each post mortem specimen was received in the anatomy department within 24 hours of his or her demise. The criteria for our selection included the restrictions that no prior surgery had been performed and that the individuals should have expired from causes which would not irrevocably distort their abdominal anatomy. Each one does, however, exhibit some deviations from the norm and these are indicated on the line diagrams by an asterisk (*). To prepare the body, a special declotting solution was used to flush out the system and pulmonic vessels, followed by the introduction of red or blue latex solutions into the arteries or veins respectively.

In diagnostic ultrasound and, to a lesser extent, in computerized tomography, recognition of the position of upper abdominal vessels is a great aid in delineating pathology.

A major advantage of this over other texts is that the user has greater ability to recognize readily arteries and veins by their artificial coloring and all other organs by their natural coloring.

The large number of structures labelled required the use of abbreviations. Because no standard nomenclature of anatomical abbreviations exists, one was created.

All of the individuals used in the following pages donated their bodies to the Anatomy Department at the Health Sciences Center in Winnipeg. This program was successfully initiated and promoted by Professor I. M. Thompson, Professor Emeritus and head of the Department of Anatomy, University of Manitoba, Winnipeg. We are indebted to him for his efforts and to the many individuals who have recognized the value of this program and have contributed to its success.

Finally, we would like to express our deepest appreciation to the Medical Photography Department for its superb work, to Mr. Syd Bradbury for preparing the specimens, and to the Department of Anatomy for their continuing support and cooperation.

Color photographs have been reproduced with the permission of C. V. Mosby Co. From Lyons, EA: *Color Atlas of Sectional Anatomy,* 1977. In press.

ABBREVIATIONS

ACCESS. SPL.	ACCESSORY SPLEEN
ACET.	ACETABULUM
ADD. BREV. M.	ADDUCTOR BREVIS MUSCLE
ADD. GP. M.	ADDUCTOR GROUP MUSCLES
ADD. MAG. M.	ADDUCTOR MAGNUS MUSCLE
ANT. EXT. VEN. PLEXUS	ANTERIOR EXTERNAL VENOUS PLEXUS
ANT.-LAT. ABD. M.	ANTEROLATERAL ABDOMINAL MUSCLES
ANT. LONG. LIG.	ANTERIOR LONGITUDINAL LIGAMENT
ANT. RECT. SH.	ANTERIOR RECTUS SHEATH
AO.	AORTA
AO. ANEUR./THROMB.	AORTIC ANEURYSM (MURAL THROMBUS)
APON. EXT. OBL.	APONEUROSIS OF EXTERNAL OBLIQUE MUSCLE
APOPH. JT.	APOPHYSEAL JOINT
ASC. COLON	ASCENDING COLON
AZ. V.	AZYGOS VEIN
B. DUCT	BILE DUCT
CATH.	CATHETER
CATH. BULB	CATHETER BULB
CAUD. EQ.	CAUDA EQUINA
C. B. D.	COMMON BILE DUCT
CEC.	CECUM
CEL. A.	CELIAC ARTERY
C. I. A. & V.	COMMON ILIAC ARTERY AND VEIN
C. MED.	CONUS MEDULLARIS
CORP. CAV. (CLIT.)	CORPUS CAVERNOSUM (CLITORIS)
CORP. CAV. PEN.	CORPUS CAVERNOSUM PENIS
CORP. CAV. (URET.)	CORPUS CAVERNOSUM (URETHRAL PORTION)
COST. CART.	COSTAL CARTILAGE
COSTO-DIAPH. REC.	COSTO-DIAPHRAGMATIC RECESS
CRUS. DIAPH.	CRUS OF DIAPHRAGM
C. V. JT.	COSTOVERTEBRAL JOINT
D. D. P. V.	DEEP DORSAL PENILE VEIN
DESC. COLON	DESCENDING COLON
DIAPH.	DIAPHRAGM
D. R. GANG.	DORSAL ROOT GANGLION
DUOD.	DUODENUM
DUOD. BULB.	DUODENAL BULB
E. I. A.	EXTERNAL ILIAC ARTERY
E. I. V.	EXTERNAL ILIAC VEIN
EMPH. BULLA	EMPHYSEMATOUS BULLA
EPICARD. FAT	EPICARDIAL FAT
ERECT. SP. M.	ERECTOR SPINAE MUSCLES
ES. A.	ESOPHAGEAL ARTERY

ESOPH.	ESOPHAGUS
EXT. OBL. M.	EXTERNAL OBLIQUE MUSCLE
FALC. LIG.	FALCIFORM LIGAMENT
FISS. LIG. TERES.	FISSURE FOR LIGAMENTUM TERES
F. P. A.	FIRST PERFORATING ARTERY
F. TERM.	FILUM TERMINALE
F. V.	FEMORAL VEIN
GASTROLIEN. LIG.	GASTROLIENAL LIGAMENT
G. BLAD.	GALL BLADDER
G. D. A.	GASTRODUODENAL ARTERY
GEM. M.	GEMELLI MUSCLES
G. E. VESSELS	GASTROEPIPLOIC VESSELS
GL. MAX. M.	GLUTEUS MAXIMUS MUSCLE
GL. MED. M.	GLUTEUS MEDIUS MUSCLE
GL. MIN. M.	GLUTEUS MINIMUS MUSCLE
GR. OMENT.	GREATER OMENTUM
H. A.	HEPATIC ARTERY
H. A. (BR.)	BRANCH OF HEPATIC ARTERY
H. DUCT	HEPATIC DUCT
HEMIAZ. V.	HEMIAZYGOS VEIN
H. FLEX. (ASC. COLON)	HEPATIC FLEXURE (ASCENDING COLON)
H. V.	HEPATIC VEIN
I. I. V. (BR.)	BRANCH OF INTERNAL ILIAC VEIN
I. L. A. & V.	ILIOLUMBAR ARTERY & VEIN
ILIAC. M.	ILIACUS MUSCLE
ILIUM	ILIUM
I. M. A.	INFERIOR MESENTERIC ARTERY
I. M. V.	INFERIOR MESENTERIC VEIN
INF. ART. PROC.	INFERIOR ARTICULAR PROCESS
INF. PUB. RAM.	INFERIOR PUBIC RAMUS
INTERCOST. A. & V.	INTERCOSTAL ARTERY & VEIN
INTERCOST. M.	INTERCOSTAL MUSCLES
INTERV. DISC.	INTERVERTEBRAL DISC
INTERV. FOR.	INTERVERTEBRAL FORAMEN
INT. OBL. M.	INTERNAL OBLIQUE MUSCLE
I. V. C.	INFERIOR VENA CAVA
JEJ.	JEJUNUM
L1	LUMBAR VERTEBRA (1st)
LAB. MAJ.	LABIUM MAJORUM
LAM.	LAMINA
LAT. DORSI. M.	LATISSIMUS DORSI MUSCLE
L. C. I. A.	LEFT COMMON ILIAC ARTERY
L. C. I. V.	LEFT COMMON ILIAC VEIN
LEV. ANI. M.	LEVATOR ANI MUSCLE
L. G. A. (BR.)	BRANCH OF LEFT GASTRIC ARTERY
LIN. ALBA	LINEA ALBA
L. OMENT.	LESSER OMENTUM

L. O. V.	LEFT OVARIAN VEIN
L. R. A.	LEFT RENAL ARTERY
L. R. V.	LEFT RENAL VEIN
LT. SUPRAR. GL.	LEFT SUPRARENAL GLAND
LT. SUPRAR. V.	LEFT SUPRARENAL VEIN
LUMBAR N.	LUMBAR NERVE
LUM. PL.	NERVE OF LUMBAR PLEXUS
LYM. N.	LYMPH NODE
NUC. PULP.	NUCLEUS PULPOSUS
OBT. EXT. M.	OBTURATOR EXTERNUS MUSCLE
OBT. FOR.	OBTURATOR FORAMEN
OBT. INT. M.	OBTURATOR INTERNUS MUSCLE
OMENT. BUR.	OMENTAL BURSA
PAMP. PLEX.	PAMPINIFORM PLEXUS
PANC.	PANCREAS
PANC. (BODY)	PANCREAS (BODY)
PANC. (HEAD)	PANCREAS (HEAD)
PAR. PERIT.	PARIETAL PERITONEUM
PAR. PL.	PARIETAL PLEURA
PECT. M.	PECTINEUS MUSCLE
PERICARD. EFF.	PERICARDIAL EFFUSION
PERICARD. FAT.	PERICARDIAL FAT
PERIREN. FAT.	PERIRENAL FAT
PERIT. CAV.	PERITONEAL CAVITY
PHRENIC V.	PHRENIC VEIN
PIR. M.	PIRIFORMIS MUSCLE
PL. CAV.	PLEURAL CAVITY
PL. REC.	PLEURAL RECESS
PROST.	PROSTATE
PS. MAJ. M.	PSOAS MAJOR MUSCLE
PUBIS	PUBIS
P. V.	PORTAL VEIN
PYL.	PYLORUS
QUAD. LUMB. M.	QUADRATUS LUMBORUM MUSCLE
R. A.	RENAL ARTERY
R. C. I. A.	RIGHT COMMON ILIAC ARTERY
R. C. I. V.	RIGHT COMMON ILIAC VEIN
RECT. ABD. M.	RECTUS ABDOMINUS MUSCLE
RECT. SH.	RECTUS SHEATH
REN. PYR.	RENAL PYRAMID
RETROP. FAT	RETROPUBIC FAT
R. O. A. & V.	RIGHT OVARIAN ARTERY & VEIN
R. R. A.	RIGHT RENAL ARTERY
R. R. V.	RIGHT RENAL VEIN
RT. COR. LIG.	RIGHT CORONARY LIGAMENT
RT. GAST. A. & V.	RIGHT GASTRIC ARTERY & VEIN
RT. SUPRAR. GL.	RIGHT SUPRARENAL GLAND
RT. TRIANG. LIG.	RIGHT TRIANGULAR LIGAMENT

R. V. SEPT.	RECTOVAGINAL SEPTUM
SAC. CANAL	SACRAL CANAL
SEM. VES.	SEMINAL VESICLES
SER. ANT. M.	SERRATUS ANTERIOR MUSCLE
SER. POST. INF. M.	SERRATUS POSTERIOR INFERIOR MUSCLE
S. G. A. & V.	SUPERIOR GLUTEAL ARTERY & VEIN
SIG. COLON	SIGMOID COLON (FECES)
S. M. A.	SUPERIOR MESENTERIC ARTERY
S. M. V.	SUPERIOR MESENTERIC VEIN
SP. CORD	SPINAL CORD
SPERM. CORD	SPERMATIC CORD
SPH. ANI EXT.	SPHINCTER ANI EXTERNUS
SPH. ANI INT.	SPHINCTER ANI INTERNUS
SPL. A.	SPLENIC ARTERY
SPL. A. (BR.)	BRANCH OF SPLENIC ARTERY
SPL. FLEX. (DESC. COLON)	SPLENIC FLEXURE (DESCENDING COLON)
SPL. V.	SPLENIC VEIN
SP. PROC.	SPINOUS PROCESS
ST. GAST. A. & V.	SHORT GASTRIC ARTERY & VEIN
SUP. ART. PROC.	SUPERIOR ARTICULAR PROCESS
SUP. EPIG. A. & V.	SUPERIOR EPIGASTRIC ARTERY & VEIN
SUP. PUB. RAM.	SUPERIOR PUBIC RAMUS
SYMPH.	SYMPHYSIS
SYMP. TR.	SYMPATHETIC TRUNK
T12	THORACIC VERTEBRA (12th)
TEST.	TESTES
THOR. DUCT	THORACIC DUCT
T. ILEUM	TERMINAL ILEUM
TRANS. ABD. M.	TRANSVERSUS ABDOMINUS MUSCLE
TRANS. COLON	TRANSVERSE COLON
TRAP. M.	TRAPEZIUS MUSCLE
URIN. BLAD.	URINARY BLADDER
U. R. POUCH	UTERORECTAL POUCH
UT. CX.	UTERINE CERVIX
UT. FUND.	UTERINE FUNDUS
U. V.	UTEROVESICAL POUCH
VAG.	VAGINA
VAG. N.	VAGUS NERVE
VERT. CAN.	VERTEBRAL CANAL
VISC. PERIT.	VISCERAL PERITONEUM
VISC. PL.	VISCERAL PLEURA
XIPHOID PROC.	XIPHOID PROCESS

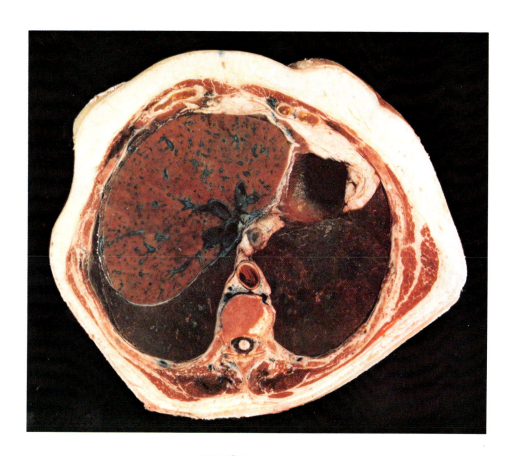

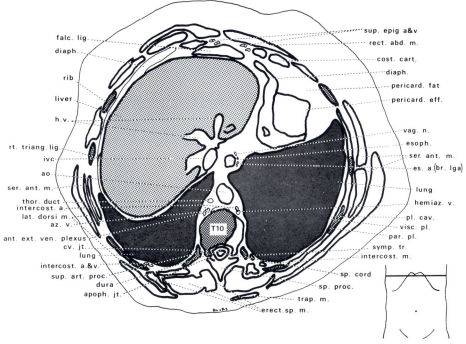

falc. lig.
diaph.
rib
liver
h.v.
rt. triang. lig.
ivc
ao
ser. ant. m.
thor. duct
intercost. a.
lat. dorsi m.
az. v.
ant. ext. ven. plexus
cv. jt.
lung
intercost. a.&v.
sup. art. proc.
dura
apoph. jt.

sup. epig a&v
rect. abd. m.
cost. cart.
diaph.
pericard. fat
pericard. eff.
vag. n.
esoph.
ser. ant. m.
es. a.(br. lga)
lung
hemiaz. v.
pl. cav.
visc. pl.
par. pl.
symp. tr.
intercost. m.
sp. cord
sp. proc.
trap. m.
erect.sp. m.

T10

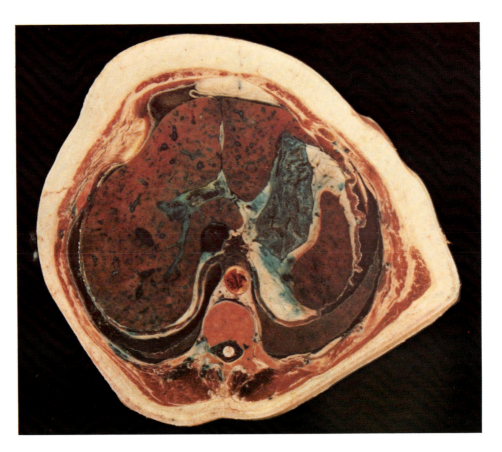

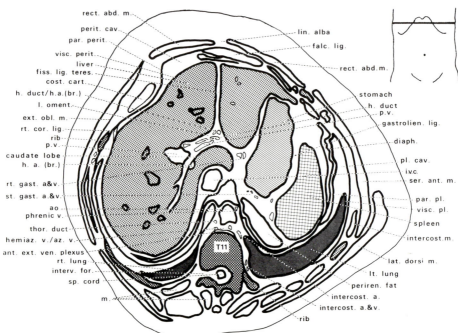

rect. abd. m.
perit. cav.
par. perit.
visc. perit.
liver
fiss. lig. teres.
cost. cart.
h. duct/h.a.(br.)
l. oment.
ext. obl. m.
rt. cor. lig.
rib
p.v.
caudate lobe
h. a. (br.)
rt. gast. a.&v.
st. gast. a.&v.
ao
phrenic v.
thor. duct
hemiaz. v./az. v.
ant. ext. ven. plexus
rt. lung
interv. for.
sp. cord
m.

lin. alba
falc. lig.
rect. abd.m.
stomach
h. duct
p.v.
gastrolien. lig.
diaph.
pl. cav.
i.v.c.
ser. ant. m.
par. pl.
visc. pl.
spleen
intercost.m.
lat. dorsi m.
lt. lung
periren. fat
intercost. a.
intercost. a.&v.
rib

T11

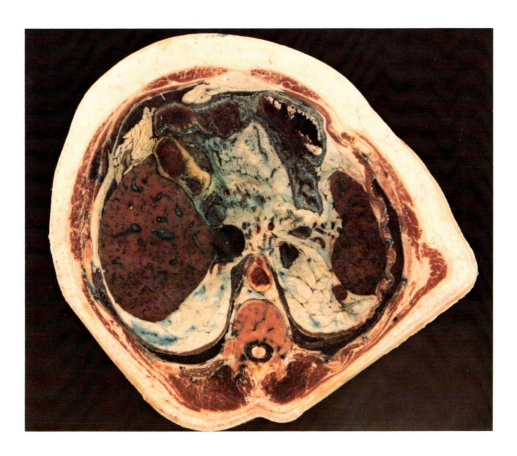

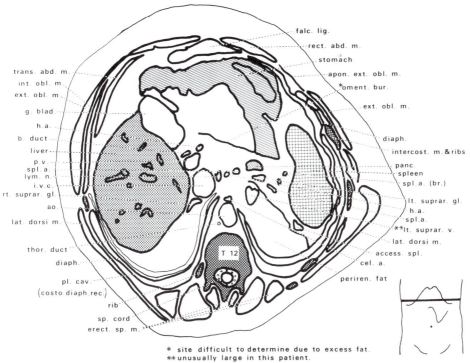

	falc. lig.
	rect. abd. m.
	stomach
trans. abd. m.	apon. ext. obl. m.
int. obl. m.	*oment. bur.
ext. obl. m.	ext. obl. m.
g. blad.	
h.a.	diaph.
b. duct	intercost. m. & ribs
liver	panc.
p.v.	spleen
spl. a.	spl.a. (br.)
lym. n.	
i.v.c.	lt. suprar. gl.
rt. suprar. gl.	h.a.
ao.	spl.a.
lat. dorsi m.	**lt. suprar. v.
	lat. dorsi m.
thor. duct	access. spl.
diaph.	cel. a.
pl. cav.	periren. fat
(costo.diaph.rec.)	
rib	
sp. cord	
erect. sp. m.	

T 12

* site difficult to determine due to excess fat.
**unusually large in this patient.

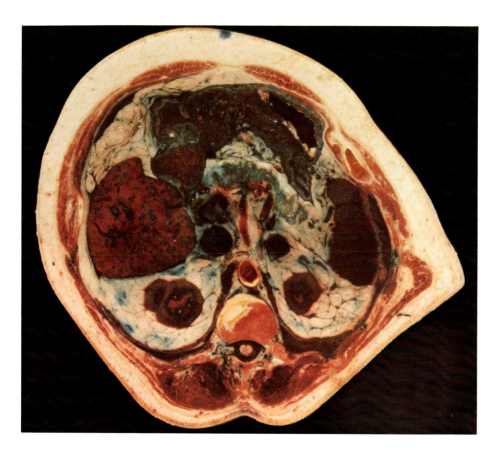

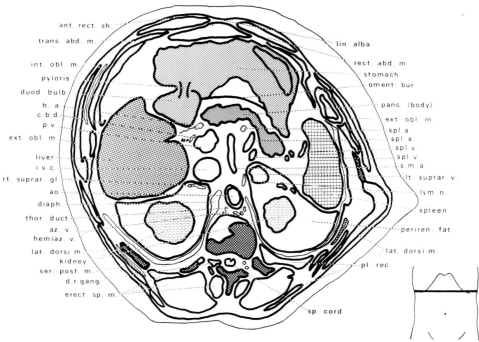

ant. rect. sh.
trans. abd. m.
int. obl. m.
pyloris
duod. bulb
h. a.
c.b.d.
p.v.
ext. obl. m.
liver
i.v.c.
rt. suprar. gl.
ao
diaph
thor. duct
az. v.
hemiaz. v.
lat. dorsi m.
kidney
ser. post. m.
d.r.gang.
erect. sp. m.

lin. alba
rect. abd. m.
stomach
oment. bur.
panc. (body)
ext. obl. m.
spl. m.
spl. a.
spl. v.
s.m.a.
lt. suprar. v.
lym. n.
spleen
periren. fat
lat. dorsi m.
pl. rec.

sp. cord

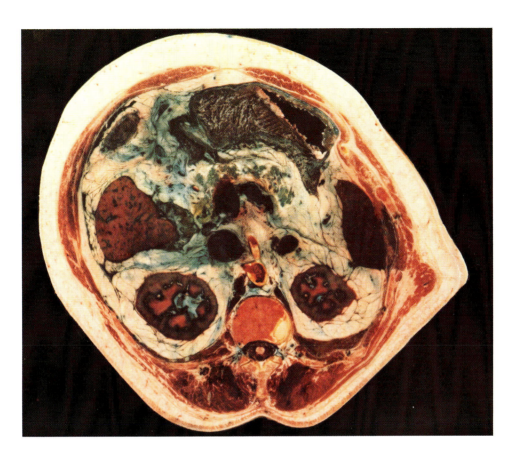

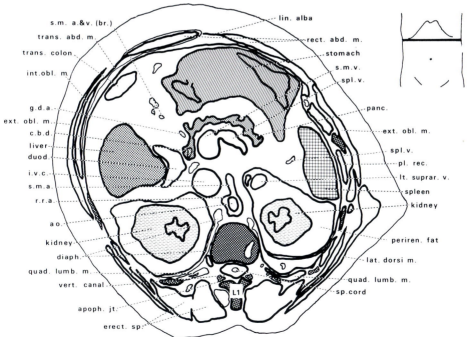

s.m. a.&v. (br.)

trans. abd. m.

trans. colon

int.obl. m.

g.d.a.

ext. obl. m.

c.b.d.

liver

duod.

i.v.c.

s.m.a.

r.r.a.

ao.

kidney

diaph.

quad. lumb. m.

vert. canal

apoph. jt.

erect. sp.

lin. alba

rect. abd. m.

stomach

s.m.v.

spl. v.

panc.

ext. obl. m.

spl. v.

pl. rec.

lt. suprar. v.

spleen

kidney

periren. fat

lat. dorsi m.

quad. lumb. m.

sp.cord

L1

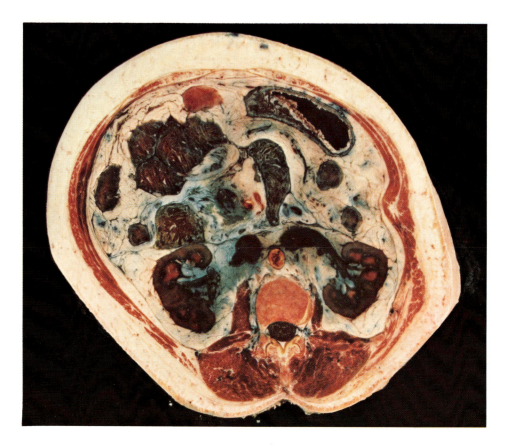

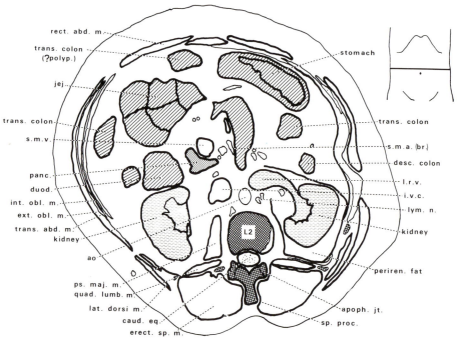

rect. abd. m

trans. colon
(?polyp.)

jej

trans. colon

s.m.v.

panc.

duod.

int. obl. m.

ext. obl. m.

trans. abd. m.

kidney

ao

ps. maj. m.

quad. lumb. m.

lat. dorsi m.

caud. eq.

erect. sp. m.

stomach

trans. colon

s.m.a. (br.)

desc. colon

l.r.v.

i.v.c.

lym. n.

kidney

periren. fat

apoph. jt.

sp. proc.

L2

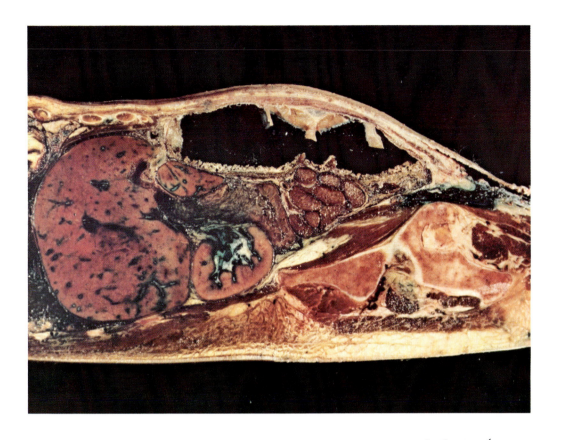

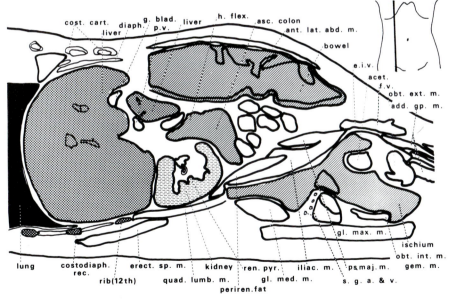

cost. cart.   diaph. g. blad. liver h. flex. asc. colon

liver   p.v.   ant. lat. abd. m.

bowel

e.i.v.

acet.

f.v.

obt. ext. m.

add. gp. m.

gl. max. m.

ischium

obt. int. m.

lung   costodiaph.   erect. sp. m.   kidney   ren. pyr.   iliac. m.   ps.maj.m.   gem. m.

rec.   s. g. a. & v.

rib(12th)   quad. lumb. m.   gl. med. m.

periren.fat

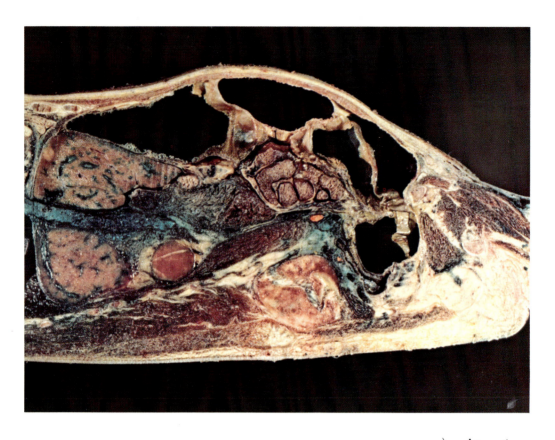

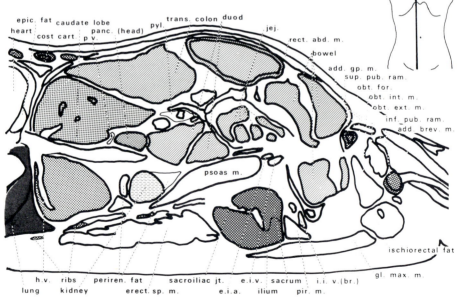

epic. fat caudate lobe trans. colon duod
heart cost cart panc. (head) pyl. jej. rect. abd. m.
p v. bowel
add. gp. m.
sup. pub. ram.
obt. for.
obt. int. m.
obt. ext. m.
inf. pub. ram.
add. brev. m.

psoas m.

ischiorectal fat

gl. max. m.

h.v. ribs periren. fat sacroiliac jt. e.i.v. sacrum i.i. v.(br.)
lung kidney erect. sp. m. e.i.a. ilium pir. m.

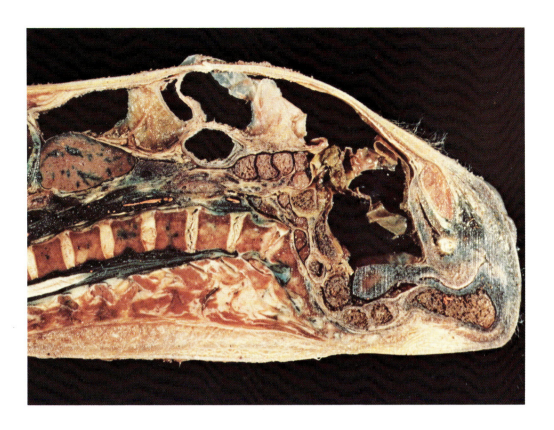

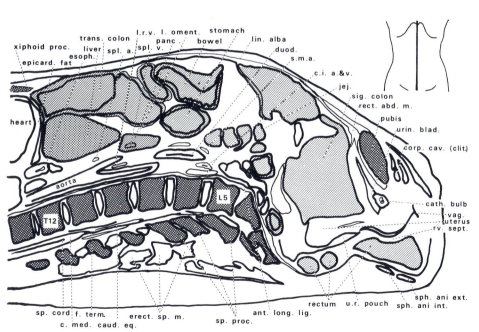

xiphoid proc.

epicard. fat

trans. colon

liver

esoph.

spl. a.

l.r.v. l. oment.

panc

spl. v.

stomach

bowel

lin. alba

duod.

s.m.a.

c.i. a.&v.

jej.

sig. colon

rect. abd. m.

pubis

urin. blad.

corp. cav. (clit.)

heart

aorta

L5

T12

cath. bulb

vag.

uterus

rv. sept.

rectum

u.r. pouch

sph. ani ext.

sph. ani int.

sp. cord

f. term.

c. med. caud. eq.

erect. sp. m.

sp. proc.

ant. long. lig.

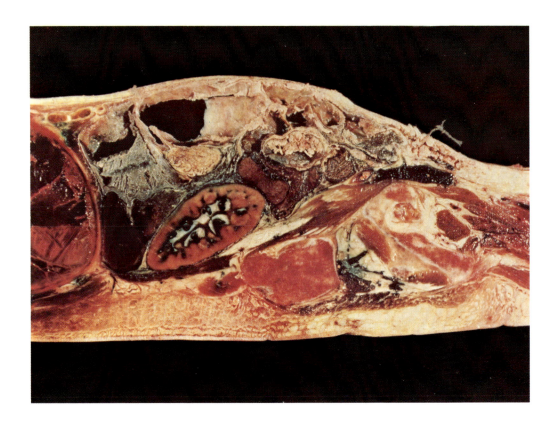

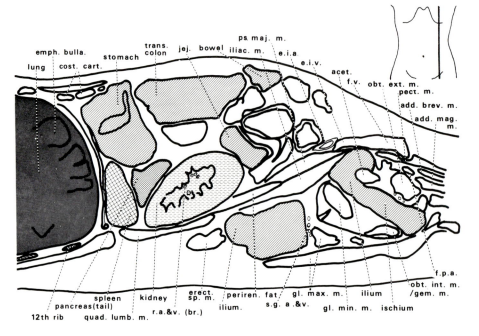

4
Abnormal Vessels

Roy A. Filly, M.D.
Assistant Professor of Radiology
University of California at San Francisco
Picker Scholar, James Picker Foundation
Chief, Section of Ultrasound Diagnosis
University of California Medical Center
San Francisco, California

Barry B. Goldberg, M.D.
Professor of Radiology
Director, Division of Diagnostic Ultrasound
Thomas Jefferson University Hospital
Philadelphia, Pennsylvania

Ultrasonic aortography is a valuable diagnostic procedure in the evaluation of the abdominal aorta (1–11). In many institutions it has become the procedure of choice whenever an abdominal aortic aneurysm is suspected. Prior to the advent of ultrasound, the only noninvasive means of confirming the presence of a clinically suspected noncalcified aortic aneurysm was the use of nuclear scans. Contrast aortography was employed for definitive evaluation. As a result, many patients in whom an aneurysm was suspected clinically were found to have a normal or relatively normal aorta after arteriography. Aortosonography has decreased dramatically the use of other diagnostic methods in the initial evaluation of the abdominal aorta (12, 13).

It is fair to state that the diagnosis of abdominal aortic aneurysm is not particularly difficult. The clinical assessment of the abdominal aorta in experienced hands is highly accurate. A significant percentage of abdominal aortic aneurysms contain sufficient calcification to enable a diagnosis to be made from supine and lateral radiographs of the abdomen. Isotope angiography, an essentially noninvasive technique, has been used successfully for the detection of abdominal aortic aneurysm. Arteriography, in addition to its high diagnostic accuracy in the detection of abdominal aortic aneurysm, also provides useful information concerning the branches of the abdominal aorta. Although aortosonography was a late comer in the diagnostic armamentarium for assessment of aneurysms, its broad clinical acceptance is a testament to the specificity and sensitivity of this modality in the detection and diagnosis of aortic aneurysms.

The accuracy of ultrasound in the evaluation of the aorta for significant dilatation has been reported to be as high as 98.6 percent, which is equal to and, in fact, exceeds the reported accuracy rates for other diagnostic procedures including the invasive variety (14). With aortosonography, the overall dimensions of an aneurysm can be displayed easily. Additionally, information about internal structure, such as a clot or dissection, often can be determined (15, 16). Evaluation of the abdominal aorta is obtained quickly and noninvasively. Serial evaluation of patients treated nonoperatively is readily obtainable.

TECHNIQUE

The technique for visualization of the aorta, vena cava, and smaller vascular structures within the abdomen has been discussed in the previous chapter. Techniques that are of use when a pathologic condition is suspected or detected are considered in this section.

The search for abnormalities of the abdominal aorta usually is begun with longitudinal scans. Optimally, one should begin the examination with real-time sonography which enables the examiner to determine quickly the course of the abdominal aorta (particularly if it is tortuous). Real-time sonography also provides a rapid appraisal of the motion dynamics of the abdominal aorta (17).

In addition to B-scan techniques, it is useful to obtain A-mode point readings. A-mode can be particularly helpful for estimating lumenal and overall diameters. The point of maximum aortic diameter is first determined by B-scan technique. An A-mode reading then is obtained from the designated area at a relatively low receiver sensitivity so only the strongest echos are recorded (Figure 1). The aortic walls produce high amplitude reflections that are not suppressed by a decrease in gain. This allows precise measurement of the aortic diameter. TM-mode (time-motion; M-mode) technique can be used to demonstrate the expansile motion of the vessel at any particular point (Figure 2). In general, the younger the patient, the easier it is to record arterial expansile

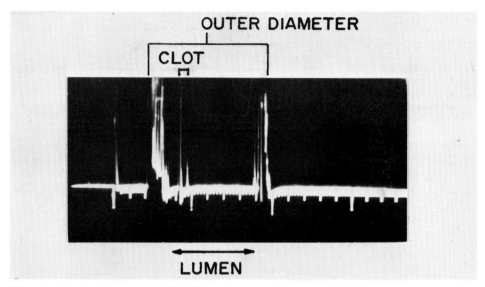

Figure 1. A-mode ultrasonogram defines the maximum aortic outer diameter as well as the lumen. Note the weaker echoes anteriorly from the clot.

motion during systole. An aorta with advanced atherosclerotic changes or aneurysmal dilatation tends to show little or no expansile motion. Care should be taken when obtaining an M-mode tracing not to press too firmly on the anterior abdominal wall, otherwise, the transducer will move with each expansile motion of the anterior aortic wall. If the movement of the transducer is similar to the excursion of the anterior wall of the aorta, the M-mode recording will appear to show dampened anterior wall motion,

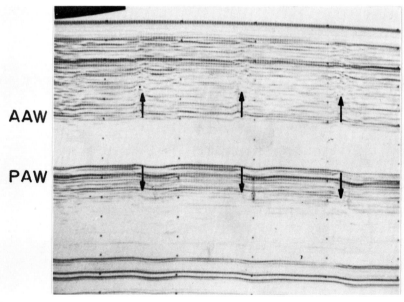

Figure 2. TM-mode ultrasonogram demonstrates the expansile wall motion (arrows) of a minimally dilated abdominal aorta (AAW = anterior aortic wall; PAW = posterior aortic wall).

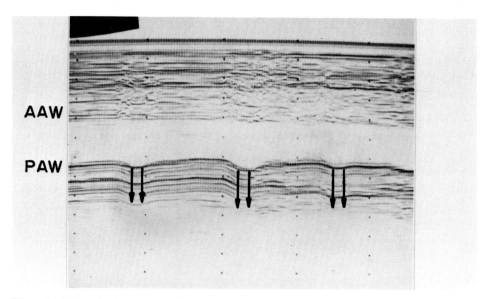

Figure 3.   TM-mode ultrasonogram shows exaggerated motion (arrows) of the posterior aortic wall (PAW) compared to the anterior aortic wall (AAW).

since the distance relationship of the transducer to the anterior wall will be maintained. Conversely, posterior wall motion will be accentuated since it is moving away from the transducer during systole (Figure 3). Thus, the transducer should be applied to the skin with only sufficient pressure to produce good acoustical coupling.

   If real-time sonography is not available, it may be difficult to begin scans in the longitudinal plane of section when the aorta is markedly tortuous since only short segments of the aorta will be recorded on individual parasagittal scans. To record the true longitudinal course of the aorta in such a situation it is best to chart the course of the aorta first by performing transverse scans. The transverse scans are obtained in the usual manner. The midplane of the aorta as determined on each transverse section is marked on the skin with a wax pencil. At the completion of the transverse B-scan examination, the dots are connected. The line thus formed is then used to obtain a true longitudinal ultrasonogram of the aorta. The patient is turned or the transducer arm is repositioned, depending on the type of ultrasonic arm used, to obtain the indicated longitudinal scan. If there is marked tortuosity of the vessel, several longitudinal or longitudinal oblique scans may be required in order to record the full length of the vessel. If there is any flexibility in the ultrasonic transducer arm, slight lateral displacement during the longitudinal movement of the transducer often will allow for the recording of a slightly tortuous vessel on a single ultrasonic tracing.

   Conventional Doppler equipment can be used to record flow patterns in the abdominal aorta (18). However, in the future, the use of combined B-scan and Doppler instrumentation (duplex systems) should result in improved assessment of aortic blood flow.

ADVANTAGES

Ultrasound is a rapid screening procedure and should be considered the modality of choice when a patient is suspected of having a pulsatile abdominal mass. Images obtained using B-scan ultrasound will clearly delineate the contour of the aorta as well as its dimensions. Thus, if the aortic size is seen to be within normal limits, there is no need for further studies.

Although the sonogram may have been preceeded by a lateral radiograph of the abdomen that showed sufficient calcification to confirm an aneurysm, in the majority of cases, the calcified portions of the aorta are incomplete preventing full evaluation of the entire vessel. Magnification is also a problem with radiography that is not encountered with ultrasonography. A nuclear scan that displays a relatively normal aortic lumen usually indicates a normal aorta; however, if a clot is present and the radionuclide does not enter portions of the clot, an aneurysm can be missed.

Contrast aortography requires catheterization of the vessel followed by the injection of iodinated material. While complications of aortography are low, the potential complications may be devastating to the patient. Contrast aortography is unnecessary to demonstrate the presence of an aneurysm, and in fact, if there is a significant clot within the aneurysm, the contrast-filled lumen may appear to be relatively normal in caliber. In this situation, secondary signs of the presence of an aneurysm may be present such as vessel draping around the aneurysm. However, in some instances, these secondary signs can be minimal and thus misinterpreted. Contrast aortography is necessary at the present time when it is clinically important to evaluate aortic branches such as the renal arteries. This topic will be discussed further in the section on aneurysms.

DISADVANTAGE

The only major disadvantage of the ultrasonic technique is that gas within the bowel interposed between the transducer and the aorta will prevent visualization (Figure 4). As discussed previously, barium has the same effect (19). Thus if the abdominal aorta cannot be visualized completely by ultrasonography, the possibility of aneurysm cannot be excluded. Interestingly, the presence of an aneurysm aids the ultrasonographer since

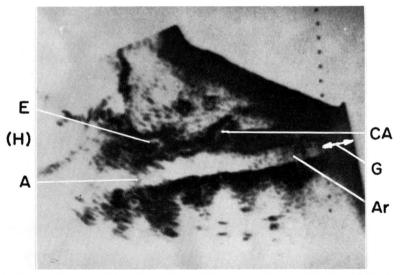

Figure 4. Longitudinal scan of the abdominal aorta (A) demonstrating the deleterious effects of bowel gas. Artifactual echoes (Ar) secondary to bowel gas reverberations are noted as well as inability to record the distal aorta because of a gas shadow (G) (H = head; E = esophagus; CA = celiac axis).

the bulk of the aneurysmal mass usually displaces interfering bowel loops that may prevent visualization.

THE ABNORMAL AORTA

Arteriosclerotic Changes

As individuals advance in age, atherosclerotic changes in the abdominal aorta become so ubiquitous that most older patients demonstrate changes. Generally, these changes are limited to plaque formation, mild dilatation, tortuosity, and calcification of the aortic wall. Small amounts of thrombotic material frequently are present.

With these pathologic changes, the aorta will present more irregular interfaces (Figure 5). Thus, when using routine B-scan ultrasonography, more sectoring may be required to record reflections from all portions of the aortic wall. The aorta may become quite tortuous and portions even may be found to the right rather than to the left of midline. As discussed in the technical section, the aorta may become so serpentine that it is difficult to obtain a single longitudinal sweep of the entire vessel. This situation will be apparent from the transverse scans. A series of longitudinal and/or oblique scans at short intervals will record segmentally the entire longitudinal extent of the diseased vessel.

If there is significant irregularity in the aortic contour, it usually can be demonstrated by B-scan sonography. It is generally impossible, even with gray scale equipment and high frequency transducers, to define clearly thrombotic or atherosclerotic plaques. Stenosis of the aortic lumen is discussed under a separate section.

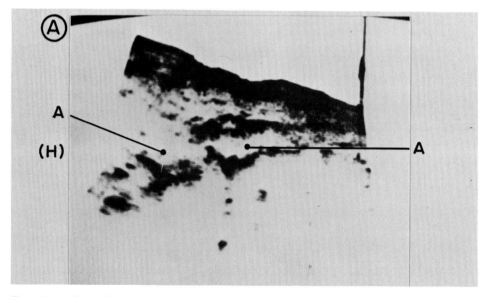

Figure 5. *A.* Longitudinal scan of an arteriosclerotic abdominal aorta (A). Marked contour irregularities are noted as well as high amplitude reflections from calcification of the wall. A stenotic area is seen proximal to the splenic vein (unlabeled). *B.* Limited cross-sectional scan demonstrating the irregular aortic wall distal to the origin of the superior mesenteric artery (SMA) (H = head; R = right). (*Continued on next page.*)

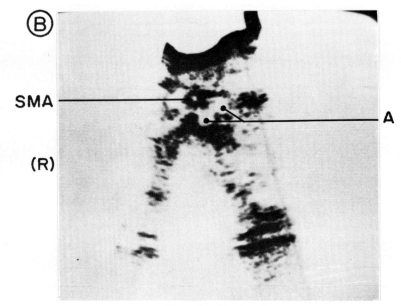

Figure 5.   (Continued)

Dilatation

Aortosonography is used most frequently to determine if there is significant dilatation of the abdominal aorta. The precise point at which ectasia becomes clinically significant or similarily becomes aneurysmal dilatation is not absolute (Figure 6). As a general rule, if the lumen of the aorta does not become gradually smaller in diameter as the aorta proceeds distally, this constitutes evidence of dilatation. A lumenal diameter that exceeds

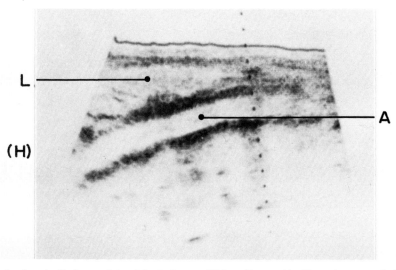

Figure 6.   Longitudinal scan of the abdominal aorta (A) in a 60-year-old white male suspected of having an aneurysm. The aorta demonstrates high amplitude reflections in its wall from calcification and does not demonstrate normal tapering. However, at no point does the aortic dimension exceed 3 cm. Thus, while ectatic, the patient's aorta could not be diagnosed as aneurysmal.

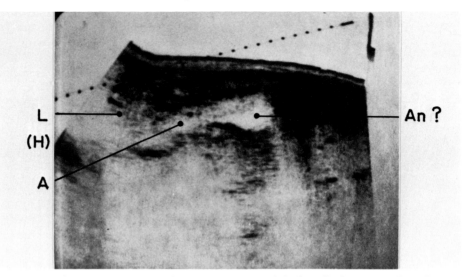

Figure 7. Longitudinal ultrasonogram demonstrating an aorta (A) whose distal segment is distinctly wider than the proximal segment, but the outer diameter is only 30 mm. This scan demonstrates the sensitivity of echoaortography. By one criteria this is aneurysmal dilatation (An ?) while by another it is not (H = head; L = liver).

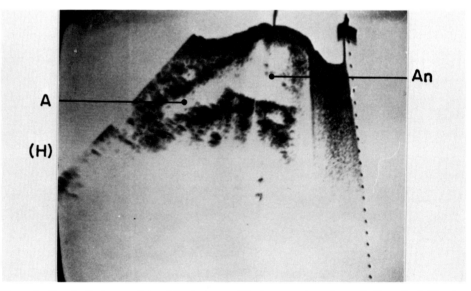

Figure 8. Longitudinal scan of the abdominal aorta (A) demonstrating a large, fusiform distal dilatation (An) typical of atherosclerotic aneurysms. Even large aneurysms such as this usually begin below the origins of the renal arteries.

30 mm is considered to be indicative of aneurysmal dilatation (20) (Figure 7). However, lumenal measurements are relative and, of course, normal values can vary from patient to patient, depending both on the size and age of the patient.

The point of maximum dilatation and its location in relationship to superficial structures such as the xyphoid or umbilicus can be determined readily. Lead markers can be placed on the skin for correlation with abdominal radiographs and contrast aortography. Also, if repeat ultrasonic examination is indicated, the localization x-ray can be useful for determining the exact points at which the initial sonographic measurements were obtained.

Aneurysm

Aneurysms of the abdominal aorta are usually atherosclerotic in etiology. Leutic aneurysms are essentially unheard of today in this country. Mycotic aneurysms are encountered occasionally, and dissecting aortic aneurysms may extend into the abdominal aorta.

The predominence of atherosclerotic aneurysms leads to similar pathologic findings in the vast majority of ultrasonograms performed on patients with aneurysms. Fusiform dilatation of the distal abdominal aorta is the most common presentation of atherosclerotic aneurysms. In 95 percent or more of patients the proximal extent of the dilatation begins below the origin of the renal arteries (9) (Figure 8). A distal abdominal aortic aneurysm rarely may be saccular, having only a small connection to the main portion of the aorta. In most cases there is sufficient area of communication to enable recognition of this type of aneurysm. However, if the communication to the main lumen of the aorta is small, this variety of aneurysm may be difficult to recognize. There have been cases in which large aneurysms of this type have become completely clotted resulting in no expansile motion (only transmitted motion). This further complicates the diagnosis of aneurysm by ultrasonic criteria. Of course, contrast aortography or radionuclide scans also would be unable to detect the true pathologic nature of the mass.

It has been shown that the prognosis of a patient with an abdominal aortic aneurysm is linked directly to the size of the aneurysm (9). Aneurysms less than 5 cm in maximum overall dimension rupture in 1 percent of cases while those that exceed 6 cm show a 40 percent chance of rupture. Aneurysms exceeding 7 cm rupture in 60–80 percent of cases. Thus, individuals with small aneurysms are more likely to succumb to other associated atheroslerotic problems such as coronary artery disease or cerebrovascular disease rather than as a result of the aneurysm itself. Conversely, patients with large aneurysms are at high risk for rupture.

Ultrasonography is unsurpassed by any other diagnostic modality in estimating the size of an abdominal aortic aneurysm (Figure 9). Radiographs of the abdomen must be corrected for magnification. However, since ultrasonography is unencumbered by problems of magnification, a simple and direct measurement of the aortic caliber can be obtained. Because laminated thrombus frequently is encountered in abdominal aortic aneurysms, aortography and radionuclide scans commonly will underestimate the size of the aneurysm; this is not true for ultrasonography.

A frequent question that arises in the evaluation of aneurysms is the relationship of the aneurysm to the origin of the renal arteries. In some instances ultrasonography can provide direct information as to the involvement or lack of involvement of the renal

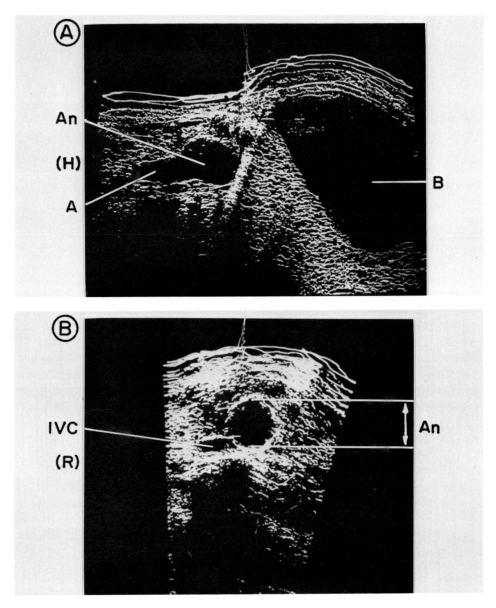

Figure 9. Some current gray scale units are equipped to do bistable sonography as well. Leading edge bi-stable sonograms generate crisp sharp lines that allow more precise measurements than the thicker, darker margins of gray scale sonograms. The longitudinal (*A.*) and cross-sectional (*B.*) sonograms of a fusiform distal aortic aneurysm demonstrate the sharply defined borders of the aneurysm (An). The dimensions may be precisely measured. The patient had bladder outlet obstruction (B) (R = right; H = head; A = aorta; IVC = inferior vena cava).

arteries by visualization of these vessels. In many other instances sonograms provide indirect information regarding the likelihood of renal artery involvement. Before considering these various methods, it is important to emphasize that only 5 percent or less of patients with abdominal aortic aneurysms will demonstrate renal artery involvement at surgery (9). Additionally, some surgeons do not require advanced knowledge about the relationship of the aneurysm to the renal arteries and will decide which type of graft to utilize by direct observation at laparotomy.

As discussed previously, renal arteries, particularly the right renal artery, occasionally can be visualized on ultrasonograms. A search for the renal arteries can be made by using the techniques described in the preceding chapter and, if visualized, a definitive statement can be made regarding the relationship of the renal vessels to the proximal portion of the aneurysm. A useful, indirect method of estimating renal artery involvement is to locate the more readily identifiable origin of the superior mesenteric artery (Figure 10A). Since the renal arteries usually originate at approximately the same level as the superior mesenteric artery one can state in general terms that aneurysms that do not extend proximally to the level of the SMA are unlikely to involve the renals. Obviously, the aneurysm that extends well into the proximal abdominal aorta is likely to involve the renals (Figure 10B).

Since the renal arteries usually originate between the first and second lumbar vertebrae, opaque lead markers can be placed on the skin indicating the proximal extent of the aneurysm. A roentgenogram then can be obtained to show the relationship of the dilatation to the lumbar vertebrae. When using this technique it is important to center the x-ray beam at the level of the lead markers in order to insure that beam divergence will not project the image of the markers at a higher or lower level. If the lead markers are seen to lie significantly below the junction of L-1 and L-2, then renal artery involvement is unlikely (1).

Transverse ultrasonograms usually demonstrate a characteristic feature of abdominal aortic aneurysms. In the majority of cases aneurysms are quite round (Figure 11A). Occasionally aneurysms may appear ovoid on cross-sectional scans (Figure 11B), but this seldom causes confusion. Uncommonly, aneurysms involve only the proximal abdominal aorta (Figure 12) or a predominantly distal abdominal aneurysm will extend into the proximal abdominal aorta (Figure 10B). More proximal abdominal aortic aneurysms often represent extentions of thoracic aneurysms below the diaphragm. Such aneurysms are frequently visible on PA and lateral chest roentgenograms. Aneurysms of the descending thoracic aorta occasionally can be measured ultrasonically by angling the transducer cephalad from a subxyphoid approach. If a thoracoabdominal aneurysm is large enough, it will displace the lung laterally and present against the posterior pleural surface to the left of the spine. In this situation, ultrasonograms can be obtained by positioning the transducer in the posterior thoracic intercostal spaces to the left of the spine. B-scan ultrasonograms may be recorded in both longitudinal and transverse views to outline the lumen (15, 21). Reverberations often will be recorded from the ribs. Such artifacts are generally easily identified by their scalloped appearance. Care should be taken not to misinterpret these artifacts as a thrombus. The overall contours of a descending thoracic aortic aneurysm are usually difficult to determine due to these reverberation echoes from the lungs and ribs. However, the internal diameter usually can be measured.

As previously mentioned, a laminated thrombus within an aneurysm is a frequent

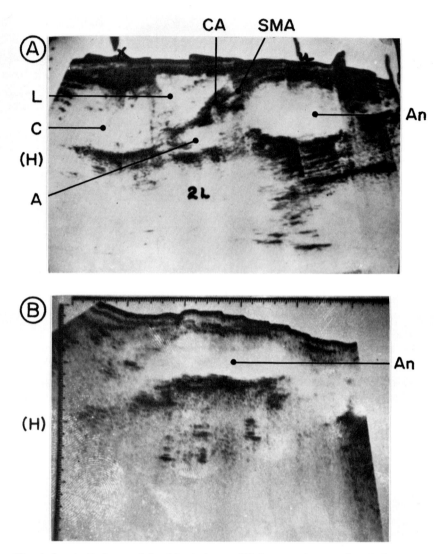

Figure 10. *A.* Longitudinal scan of the abdominal aorta (A) demonstrating a moderately large aneurysm (An). The distance from the proximal extent of the aneurysm to the origin of the superior mesenteric artery (SMA) can be estimated accurately. Also note that, although the aneurysm clearly extends distal to the umbilicus, no iliac aneurysms were present (H = head; C = cardiac area; L = liver; CA = celiac axis). *B.* Longitudinal scan of an abdominal aorta diffusely enlarged by aneurysm (An). While the distal aorta is more severely affected, the proximal aorta is also aneurysmal. Even though the superior mesenteric artery or renal arteries could not be demonstrated, one may state with assurance that they arise from an aneurysmal portion since virtually *all* the abdominal aorta is aneurysmal.

occurrence. Internal echoes may be produced by areas of the thrombus. Invariably, these echoes tend to be weaker than those produced by the walls of the aorta. As a result, if a medium or low sensitivity setting is used, these echoes may not have a sufficiently high amplitude to be recorded. Since gray scale B-scan equipment is generally run at a high receiver sensitivity, echoes from laminated thrombus are frequently recorded (Figure

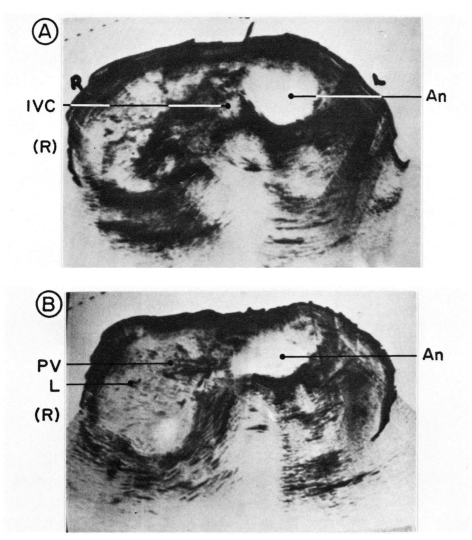

Figure 11. *A*. Transverse ultrasonogram in a patient with a large abdominal aortic aneurysm (An). Usually aneurysms appear as round, echo-free masses anterior to the left side of the spine (IVC = inferior vena cava). *B*. Occasionally aneurysms (An) appear ovoid on cross-sectional scans. In part, this is due to an oblique plane of section either by malpositioning the scanning arm or because the aorta is tortuous and a true trunkal transverse section does not "cut" the aneurysm perpendicular to its long axis. However, some aneurysms are ovoid (i.e., the transverse dimension is significantly greater than the anteroposterior dimension) (R = right; L = liver; PV = portal vein).

13). Such echoes are recorded as varying shades of gray. The outline of the aorta will not be lost. For the most part, the echoes produced will not conform completely to the full extent of the clot, especially if the thrombus is not well organized. Echoes that are persistent in more than one scan in the same location in both transverse and longitudinal directions should be considered as arising from a thrombus. Reverberations from the anterior wall of the aorta may masquerade as echoes from thrombus. Occasionally,

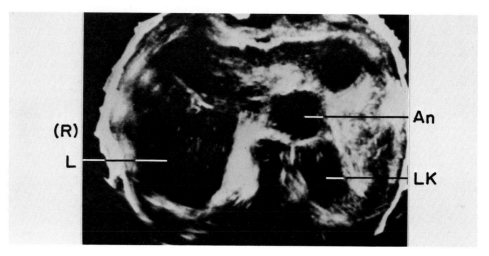

Figure 12.   Transverse ultrasonogram of the upper abdomen through the upper pole of the left kidney (LK) demonstrating a predominantly upper abdominal aortic aneurysm (An) (L = liver; R = right)

echoes may be depicted within the aortic lumen from structures adjacent to the aorta but recorded at the same depth due to poor lateral resolution of the ultrasonic beam. Artifactual echoes, in general, tend not to be persistent in their location, and with a slight change in the angle or position of the transducer, the echo pattern usually changes. These features are helpful in differentiating artifactual echoes from those produced by

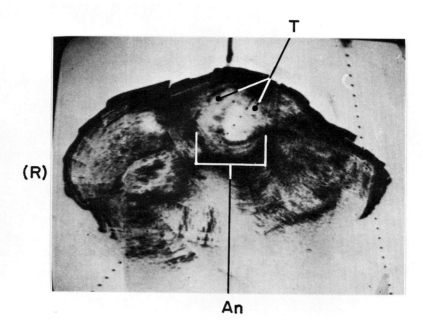

Figure 13.   Transverse echogram demonstrating a large amount of organized thrombus (T) in an aortic aneurysm (An) (R = right).

true intralumenal thrombus. There is variation in the reflective characteristics of thrombus depending on its degree of organization. A fresh clot that is completely jelled and uniform will tend to produce no echoes. A clot that has fissures or irregularities within it results in interfaces that will produce reflections. A thrombus that is organized and vascularized tends to generate many internal echoes.

Thrombi tend to be more extensive in distal than in proximal aortic aneurysms. Also, thrombus formation occurs more frequently along the anterior and lateral aspects of an aneurysm than along the posterior aspect.

In general, it is not worthwhile to spend a great deal of time attempting to demonstrate the full extent of the thrombus within an aneurysm. A thrombus does not buttress the aneurysm against rupture; thus, in this sense its demonstration does not affect the prognosis. Similarly, an organized thrombus is best demonstrated on sono-grams, and this variety of thrombotic material does not tend to embolize distally. Demonstration of a thick, laminated thrombus within the aneurysm tends only to con-firm that an aortogram or radionuclide scan would have misjudged the true dimensions of the aneurysm.

Aneurysms of the Aortic Branches

Aneurysms of the popliteal, femoral, and iliac vessels can be demonstrated by sonography. Common iliac artery aneurysms are usually seen in conjunction with aneurysms of the distal abdominal aorta (Figure 14). Iliac aneurysms are somewhat more difficult to visualize since bowel gas frequently overlies these vessels. Although the aorta usually bifurcates at the level of the umbilicus or slightly above, if an aneurysm appears to extend below the level of the umbilicus one cannot assume that the iliacs are involved since elongation of the aorta often accompanies aneurysm formation (Figure 10A).

Real-time ultrasonography has proved useful in evaluating for iliac artery dilatation. This modality aids in determining the proper obliquity for transducer alignment.

Aneurysms of the visceral branches occasionally are detected. Demonstration of an hepatic artery aneurysm has been reported (22). A renal artery aneurysm is seen in Figure 15. A saccular aneurysm at the origin of the superior mesenteric artery is depicted in Figure 16.

Stenosis and Occlusion

While current ultrasonographic instruments can detect aortic dilatation and aneurysm formation with a high degree of accuracy, there is difficulty in detecting areas of stenosis or occlusion. It is sometimes possible, employing gray scale B-scan equipment, to show irregularity of the aortic walls and actually to demonstrate point narrowing (Figure 5A). Obviously, the smaller the lumen the more difficult it is to resolve. Abnormal changes in the aortic wall usually are demonstrated in cases where there is some calcifi-cation of the wall resulting in strong reflecting interfaces.

Flow can be detected with a Doppler ultrasonic instrument. When flow is absent, no frequency shift will occur indicating aortic occlusion. In this situation, one must be sure that the ultrasonic beam has not been blocked by superimposed bowel gas or barium.

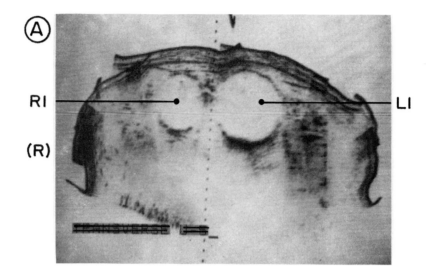

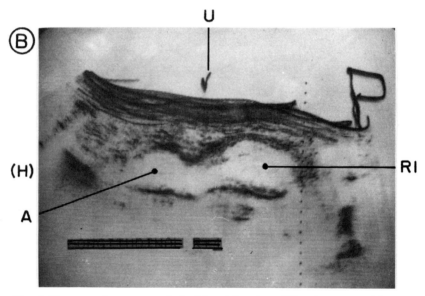

Figur 14. *A*. Transverse ultrasonogram obtained 5 cm below the umbilicus demonstrates bilateral giant iliac artery aneurysms (RI = right iliac; LI = left iliac). *B*. Right oblique longitudinal scan shows the connection between the dilated abdominal aorta (A) and right iliac artery aneurysm (RI) (U = umbilicus).

This can be confirmed by utilizing the B-scan that will demonstrate whether or not interference in penetration is present. A pulsed Doppler type of unit, which is able to analyze flow selectively within the aortic lumen, can be used to differentiate abnormalities in flow (23, 24). With stenosis, a degree of flow is always present, although the pitch will change dramatically through the area of narrowing signifying increased velocity. The pitch will change again distally as the blood leaves the region of narrowing.

Aortic Grafts

Aortic grafts can be detected readily by scanning techniques similar to those described for the abdominal aorta. The synthetic materials employed for the walls of the graft tend to generate high amplitude echoes. Additionally, the ultrasonographic appearance of graft material is often characteristic because of the ribbing employed in the graft wall, which may generate a series of bright echo dots conforming to the graft contour (Figure 17). Grafts in other areas also can be demonstrated ultrasonically (Figure 18).

Once surgery has been performed, the ultrasonographic evaluation of the para-aortic retroperitoneum becomes more difficult because of postoperative changes. This is particularly true if the original aneurysm was not resected but simply opened and the graft positioned within the bed of the aneurysm. Because of the peculiar ultra-sonographic appearance that may be created by such surgical intervention, it may be difficult to diagnose postoperative retroperitoneal hemorrhage or false aneurysm formation. Of course, a change in the appearance of the postoperative ultrasonograms may lead to a specific diagnosis.

Retroperitoneal Hemorrhage and False Aneurysm Formation

Detection of aortic wall thinning that could lead to rupture usually is not possible with present ultrasonic equipment. However, identification of localized fluid collections adjacent to an abdominal aortic aneurysm or an aortic graft in a patient with suspicious clinical symptomatology is highly suggestive of retroperitoneal hemorrhage (Figure 19). Similarly, detection of free intraabdominal fluid in association with an aneurysm also points toward a diagnosis of rupture (Figure 20). The documentation of either intra-abdominal or retroperitoneal extravasation is important in making such a definitive diagnosis.

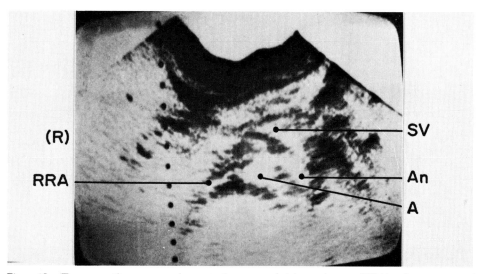

Figure 15.   Transverse ultrasonogram demonstrating a normal right renal artery (RRA) and an aneurysm of the left renal artery (An). One must exercise care since the segment of left renal vein lying to the left of the lateral aortic margin (A) may simulate a left renal artery aneurysm (R = right; SV = splenic vein).

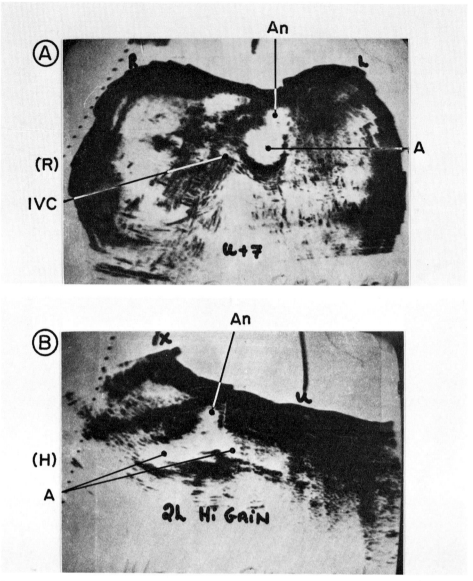

Figure 16. *A*. Cross-sectional ultrasonogram demonstrating a saccular aneurysm at the origin of the superior mesenteric artery (An). The aorta (A) is also ectatic and has high amplitude echoes from its wall indicating calcification (R = right; IVC = inferior vena cava). *B*. Longitudinal scan of same patient as in Figure 16*A* (H = head).

   The recording of incomplete aortic wall echoes does not indicate the presence of a rupture. The most likely explanation for the absence of a segment of wall echoes would be technical artifact; that is, improper angling or movement of the transducer and thus failure to record echoes from all portions of the aortic walls. Every attempt should be made to repeat the scan if this problem occurs since, with proper technique, a complete aortic wall echo pattern usually can be developed.

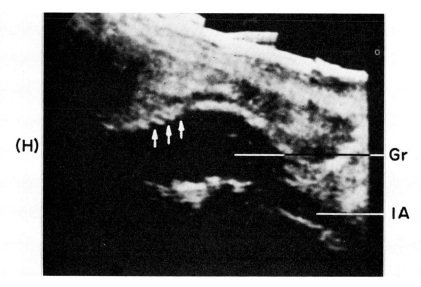

Figure 17. Longitudinal ultrasonogram of a large aortic graft (Gr) simulating an aneurysm. Individual echoes from the ribbing of the graft (arrows) are a clue to its true nature (H = head; IA = iliac vessel).

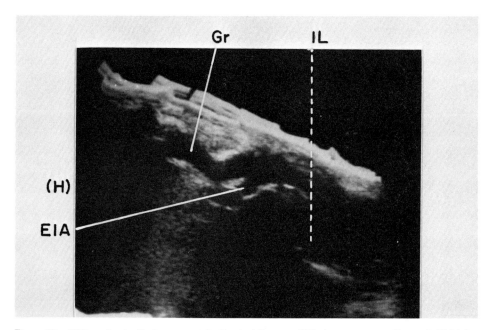

Figure 18. Oblique longitudinal scan near the inguinal ligament (IL). A tortuous aortoiliac graft (Gr) joins the native external iliac artery (EIA). A false aneurysm was suspected, but the slight distal dilatation with some thrombus formation demonstrated on the sonogram are equivocal findings. Postoperative areas are often difficult to evaluate.

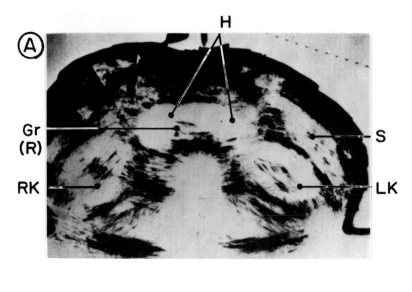

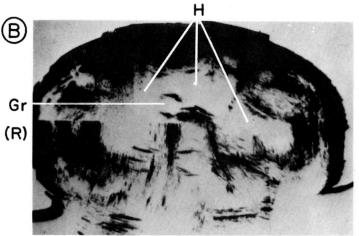

Figure 19. *A*. Transverse ultrasonogram at the level of the lower poles of the right (RK) and left (LK) kidneys in a patient with a recent aortic graft (Gr). The graft is displaced to the right by a large sonolucent retroperitoneal hemorrhage (H). Splenomegally (S) of undetermined etiology was present. *B*. More caudally, the hematoma (H) extends more laterally. Again, the displaced graft stands out in stark relief within the sonolucent hemorrhage (R = right).

False aneurysms of the abdominal aorta, which tend to occur at the surgical junction of the graft and the native vessel, can be detected ultrasonographically. As described previously postoperative changes in the retroperitoneum may cause confusion and considerable care should be exercised by the ultrasonographer before suggesting this diagnosis. False aneurysms may become quite large (Figure 21). In these situations, a strong clinical suspicion coupled with the ultrasonographic demonstration of a large pulsatile fluid-filled space is usually conclusive evidence for the diagnosis of false aneurysm formation.

Aortic Dissection

Aortic dissections that extend into the abdominal aorta can be detected ultra-sonographically. Dilatation of the abdominal aorta usually is noted, and a double lumen of the aorta may be demonstrated. These findings strongly suggest the possibility of a dissection (Figure 22). The most characteristic finding of aortic dissection, as visualized by ultrasonography, is the demonstration of an intimal flap within the diffusely dilated abdominal aorta. Real-time sonography or M-mode recordings of the intimal flap often will demonstrate a bizarre pattern of motion, quite dissimilar from the motion pattern of the aortic walls.

Serial Evaluation of the Abdominal Aorta

Ultrasound is the method of choice for serially evaluating the abdominal aorta. When an aneurysm or other abnormality is detected, and surgery is not contemplated for clinical or other reasons, ultrasound can be employed to detect changes in size. Serial evaluation has been especially useful in following aortic aneurysms in patients in the older age group who have medical contraindications to surgery. It also has proved useful in those cases where dilatation is minimal. Serial studies have shown that the increase in lumen size is generally minimal until the patient becomes symptomatic, at which time there may be significant dilatation. Surveying patients in the older, high incidence age group also has become feasible with ultrasound. These individuals can be followed at prede-termined intervals to assess for early dilatation and aneurysm formation (1).

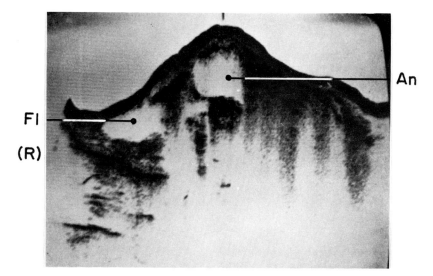

Figure 20.   Transverse ultrasonogram of a patient with a large aneurysm (An) demonstrating fluid (F1) in the right (R) flank. The left side of the abdomen is obscured by bowel gas. Peritoneal fluid in the presence of an aneurysm suggests leakage. Usually, this clinical diagnosis has been made prior to ultrasonography.

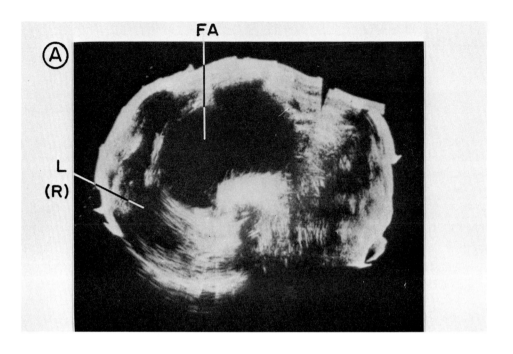

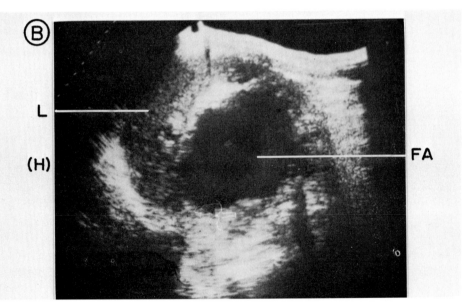

Figure 21. *A.* Transverse ultrasonogram of the upper abdomen of a patient with a pulsatile mass developing after aortic graft surgery. A huge false aneurysm (FA) is demonstrated. Note that the mass is not round or ovoid as the other aneurysms depicted in previous figures. This mass occupies the available space including the right renal fossa (the right kidney had been excised during the prior aortic graft surgery). *B.* Longitudinal scan through the right hepatic lobe (L) demonstrating the false aneurysm (FA). The patient did not survive corrective surgery (H = head; R = right).

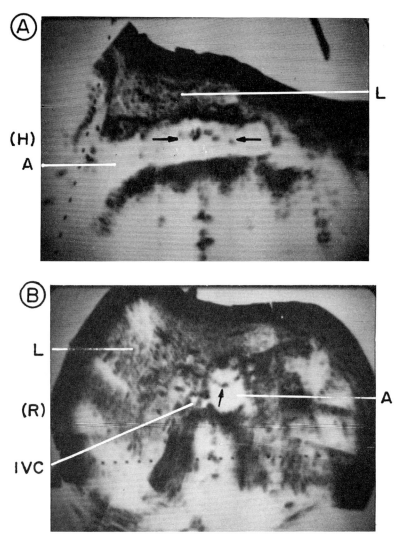

Figure 22.   *A*. Longitudinal sonogram of the aorta (A). There is diffuse dilatation of the entire aorta with persistant internal linear echoes (arrows), which on a real-time sonogram demonstrated a bizarre pattern of motion. *B*. A transverse section demonstrates the dissection (arrow) producing a "double-barrel" aortic lumen (A). The patient had a dissecting aortic aneurysm. (L = liver; IVC = inferior vena cava).

ABNORMALITIES OF THE ABDOMINAL VENOUS SYSTEM

The Inferior Vena Cava

As discussed in the preceeding chapter, the inferior vena cava (IVC) can be visualized throughout its entire length when interfering bowel gas or barium is not a problem. The proximal IVC can be seen through the substance of the liver in virtually all individuals. In normal persons, the IVC collapses during expiration and expands with inspiration.

Valsalva and Mueller maneuvers may have a dramatic effect on the caliber of the IVC (26).

Superimposed on the respiratory motion of the IVC is a transmitted pulsatile movement (27). This movement is seen only in the proximal segment. The origin of this pulsatile movement presumably arises from the right side of the heart or the aorta since it persists in the presence of inferior vena caval occlusion (28).

Recording of respiratory dynamics and pulsatile movements of the inferior vena cava is accomplished most easily with real-time sonographic equipment. However, M-mode recordings are adequate to demonstrate these changes. A more thorough discussion of techniques can be found in the chapter dealing with the normal inferior vena cava.

In a variety of pathologic conditions, the most frequent of which is right ventricular failure, the inferior vena cava distends and the respiratory kinetics disappear or become markedly dampened (28). Other causes of vena cava dilatation, are constrictive pericarditis, tricuspid stenosis or insufficiency, right atrial myxoma, and other central thoracic abnormalities. In one reported case, superior vena caval (SVC) obstruction demonstrated a similar picture since the SVC obstruction was relieved by collateral circulation developing through epigastric veins that drained into the inferior vena cava (27). Renal dialysis patients with arterial-venous shunts in the lower extremities also may have dilatation and decreased respiratory dynamics of the inferior vena cava.

Dilatation of the inferior vena cava may be one of the earliest findings in patients who have hepatomegaly and occult right ventricular failure (Figure 23). Usually, the hepatic veins will be dilated and the pressure from these veins will be transmitted through the sinusoids resulting in distention of the portal vessels (Figure 24). If the sinusoids are unable to transmit the pressure from the hepatic venous system because of severe cirrhosis, the portal vessels will not distend (Figure 25).

While it is conceivable that ultrasound can demonstrate abnormalities such as the absence of the vena cava with resultant dilatation of the azygous or hemiazygous vein, to date, ultrasonic visualization of such abnormalities has not been documented. The most widely observed abnormalities are those in which there is extrensic pressure on the vena cava. Retroperitoneal masses, including renal masses, pancreatic mass, and enlarged lymph nodes, as well as intraperitoneal mass such as hepatic neoplasms, may distort the vena cava. This will be discussed more fully later. Umbrellas within the IVC have been recorded on good quality gray scale sonograms (Figure 26).

Portal Venous System

Abnormalities of the portal venous system detectable ultrasonographically have been largely confined to the demonstration of portal venous dilatation (29) (Figure 27). The extrahepatic portal venous system may be dilated in cirrhosis or in such instances as right ventricular failure with transmitted back pressure through the hepatic sinusoids distending the portal system. The intraparenchymal hepatic tributaries of the portal venous system tend not to be dilated in cirrhosis, but maybe markedly dilated in patients with severe right ventricular failure. On rare occasions, a varix in the falciform ligament carrying hepatafugal blood toward the umbilicus may be demonstrated (30).

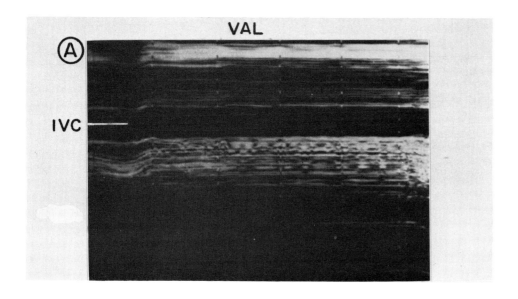

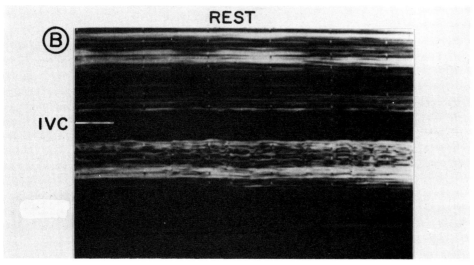

Figure 23. M-mode recording of the inferior vena cava (IVC) during (*A.*) Valsalva maneuver (VAL) and (*B.*) at rest (REST) in a patient with right heart failure and tricuspid insufficiency. The IVC is dilated, pulsations are dampened, and no respiratory variation is noted. Compare Figure 6 in the preceeding chapter.

Portacaval Shunts

Not only can ultrasound be used noninvasively to evaluate the portal vein and inferior vena cava but it also can be used to evaluate portacaval shunts. There are certain characteristic signs that are useful in determining whether a shunt is patent. Initial longitudinal scans are obtained starting from the umbilicus and moving up toward the xyphoid just slightly to the right of the midline in a plane of section through the IVC. The

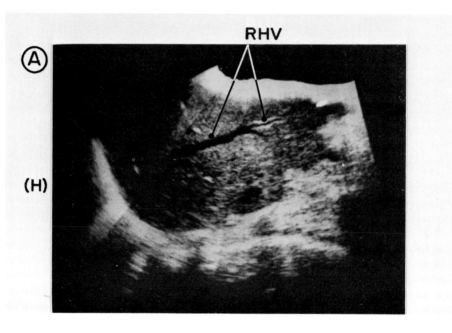

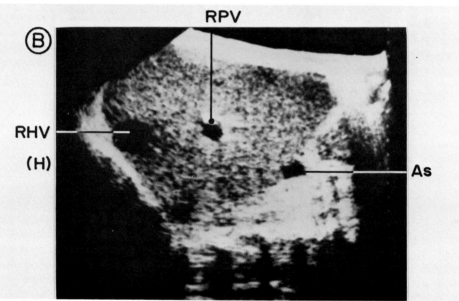

Figure 24. *A*. Parasagittal scan obtained in the lateral portion of the right hepatic lobe demonstrating grossly distended third and fourth order right hepatic veins in a patient with right ventricular failure. The liver is enlarged. *B*. More medially a major radicle of the right hepatic vein (RHV) is grossly distended as is the right portal vein (RPV). A small amount of ascites (As) is detected at the hepatorenal angle. *C*. Parasagittal scan of the inferior vena cava (IVC) demonstrates dilatation. The "middle" hepatic vein (MHV), and both left and main portal veins (L/MPV) are distended. A small amount of pericardial fluid (PE) is detected between the enlarged right atrium (RA) and the liver (H = head). *D*. Transverse limited sector scan near the xyphoid demonstrating gross distention of IVC and hepatic veins (HV). Compare the caliber of the aorta (A) to appreciate the dramatic venous dilatation depicted (R = right). (*Continued on next page.*)

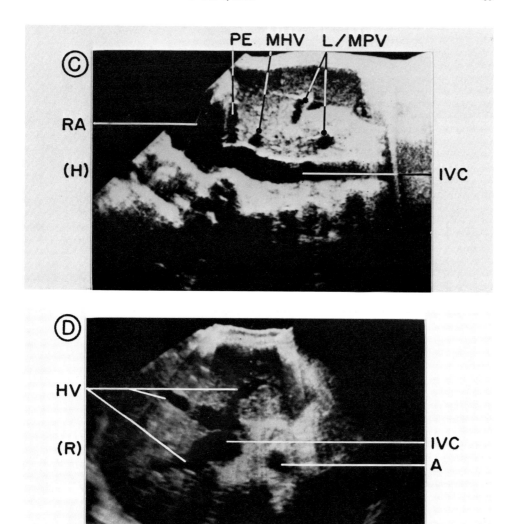

Figure 24.   (Continued)

portal vein should be seen in a position just anterior to the vena cava at the level of the porta hepatis.

In the case of a shunt, the vena cava usually will have its maximum diameter just cephalad to the area of portal vein entry due to the increased volume of blood flowing into the vena cava from the portal vein (Figure 28). Under normal circumstances, without a portacaval shunt or when the shunt is occluded, this distention will not be present. When a Valsalva maneuver is performed, there will be significant dilatation of the portal vein if the shunt is patent. In fact, in some cases the portal dilatation will be even greater than that of the IVC. This will not be true if there is occlusion.

Once the area of the portal vein and the inferior vena cava anastomosis is determined longitudinally, transverse scans are obtained in the area of interest. The actual opening of

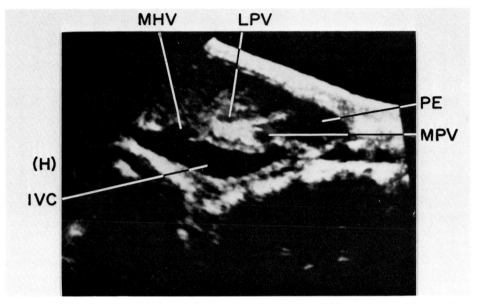

Figure 25. Parasagittal scan of the inferior vena cava in a patient with multiple complications from alcoholism including pancreatitis (PE) and cirrhosis. The inferior vena cava (IVC) is dilated at rest as well as being dramatically indented by the swollen pancreatic head. The middle hepatic vein (MHV) is dilated but the left (LPV) and main (MPV) portal veins are normal to small in caliber. Compare Figure 24C (H = head).

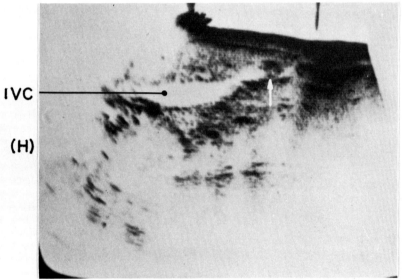

Figure 26. Longitudinal scan of the inferior vena cava (IVC) demonstrating a high amplitude reflection (arrow) from an umbrella. The etiology of the anterior displacement of the IVC is uncertain (H = head).

90

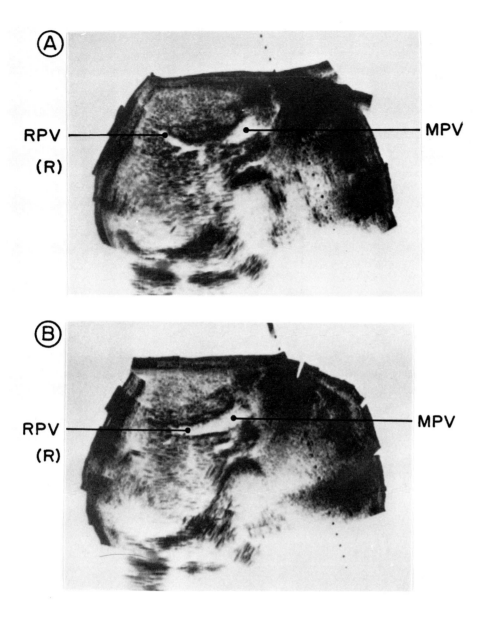

Figure 27. *A*. Transverse scan of a patient with well-documented cirrhosis. The intrahepatic right portal radicles (RPV) are not dilated as severely as the main portal vein (MPV). *B*. At the confluence of the main (MPV) and right (RPV) portal veins the striking dilatation of the extrahepatic portal system is apparent.

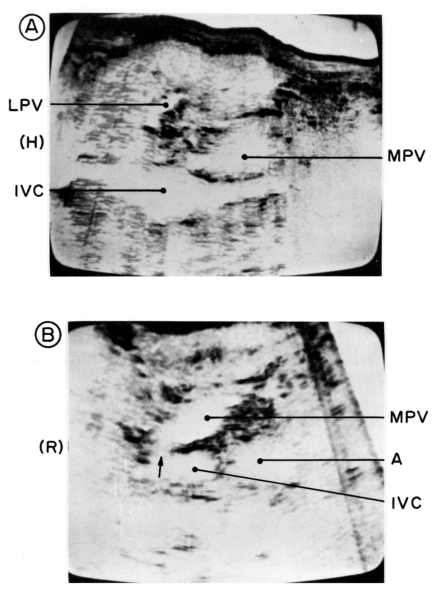

Figure 28. *A.* Longitudinal scan of the inferior vena cava (IVC) in a patient with a portacaval shunt. The left (LPV) and main (MPV) portal veins are dilated, as is the IVC cranial to the shunt. The MPV impresses the IVC. This finding is unusual in normal individuals but occasionally is seen. *B.* Transverse scan demonstrating the surgical shunt (arrow) between the main portal vein (MPV) and the inferior vena cava (IVC) (C = caudad; R = right; A = aorta).

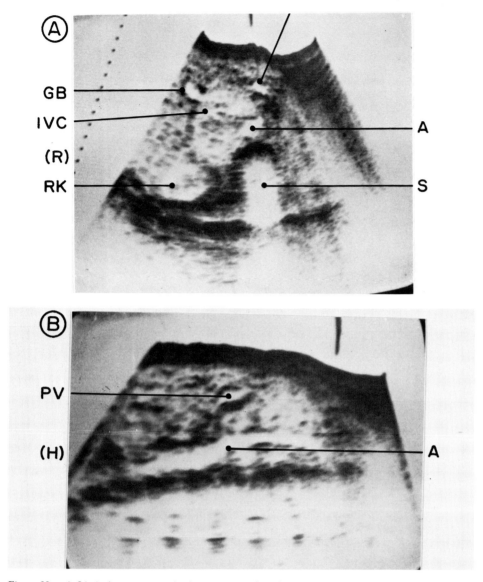

Figure 29.   *A.* Limited sector sweep in the transverse plane demonstrating a large retroperitoneal sarcoma encircling the inferior vena cava (IVC) and displacing the aorta (A). The portal vein (PV) is elevated (R = right; GB = gallbladder; S = spine, RK = right kidney). *B.* Longitudinal scan demonstrating encasement and elevation of the aorta (A) by the mass. The portal vessel (PV) is elevated (H = head). *C.* Longitudinal scan demonstrating displacement of the IVC (H = head; HV = hepatic vein). (*Continued on next page.*)

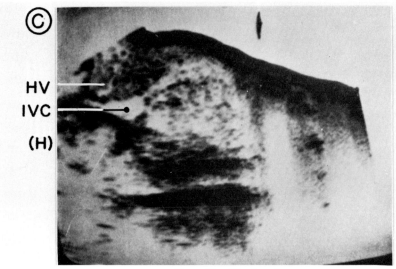

Figure 29.   (Continued)

the portal vein into the vena cava may be recorded. While no splenorenal shunts have
been demonstrated it has been possible to demonstrate mesocaval shunts.

OTHER VASCULAR ABNORMALITIES DEMONSTRABLE WITH ULTRASONOGRAPHY

The Effects of Neoplasms on the Major Abdominal Vessels

*Vascular Displacement and Compression of Major Abdominal Vessels by Neo-
plasms.*   As mentioned previously, the aorta and vena cava may be displaced or distorted by paravascular masses. In this regard, abnormalities of the aorta, which has a
rather firm wall, usually are restricted to displacement. On the other hand, the inferior
vena cava, in addition to displacement, also may show compression. A large number of
retroperitoneal masses may affect the great vessels including neoplasms of the adrenal
glands, kidneys, and pancreas. More commonly, retroperitoneal sarcomas (Figure 29)
or enlarged lymph nodes (Figure 30) tend to cause displacements of the aorta and vena
cava (31). Anteriorly located masses such as those in the region of the head of the
pancreas (Figure 31) (or even intraperitoneal masses such as hepatic masses or hydrops
of the gallbladder) may produce anterior extrinsic pressure effects resulting in
compression of the vena cava with distal distention (Figure 32). Posterior retroperitoneal
masses such as retrovascular lymph nodes tend to elevate the inferior vena cava and the
aorta. In the case of the vena cava, extrensic pressure defects can be made more visible by
the Valsalva maneuver which increases the overall vessel caliber.

   With bistable ultrasonography there was a potential for misinterpreting periaortic
lymph node enlargement as being part of the aorta that resulted in erroneous diagnosis
of aneurysm (32). This problem essentially has been negated with gray scale ultrasonography which tends to define the borders between the mass and the aorta with a
greater precision. Lymphomatous nodes tend to have a very sparse vascular supply and
a uniform tissue characteristic resulting in poor internal reflecting interfaces. Therefore,

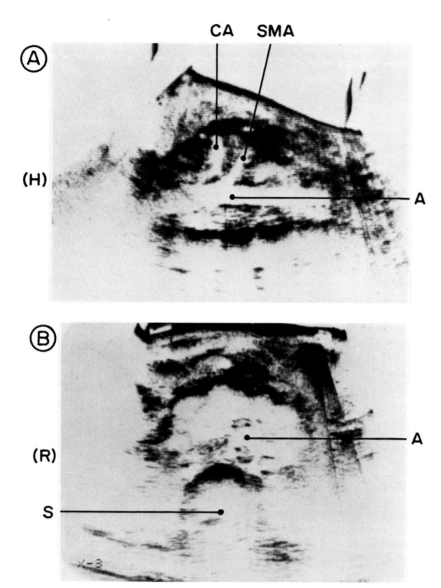

Figure 30. *A.* Parasagittal scan of the aorta (A). The aorta, celiac axis (CA), and superior mesenteric artery (SMA) are encased by enlarged retroperitoneal lymphomatous nodes. The aorta is displaced anteriorly from the spine. Note that the superior mesenteric artery–aortic angle is widened (H = head). *B.* In transverse sections the aorta (A) is encircled by enlarged lymph nodes. Note the lobulated contours of the mass which is typical to enlarged lymph nodes. Aneurysms do not demonstrate this mantlelike appearance or lobulated margins. (S = spine; R = right). (Sonograms courtesy of Carl Mani, M.D., 350 Parnassus Ave., San Francisco, California.)

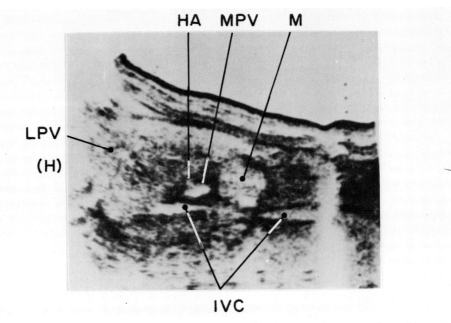

Figure 31. Longitudinal scan of the inferior vena cava (IVC) demonstrating compression and incomplete obstruction of the IVC (note the distal dilatation of the IVC) by a well-defined mass in the pancreatic head (M) (H = head; LPV = left portal vein; MPV = main portal vein; HA = hepatic artery).

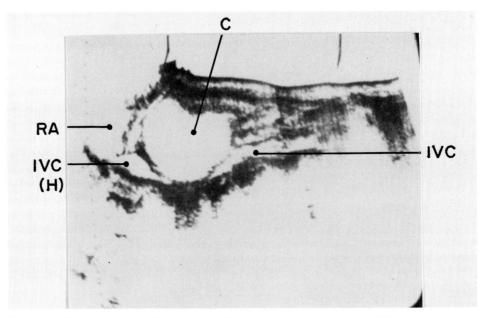

Figure 32. Even intraperitoneal masses may affect the retroperitoneal vessels. This parasagittal scan demonstrates a large hepatic cyst (C) impressing and partially obstructing the inferior vena cava (IVC). (H = head; RA = right atrium). (Courtesy of Department of Radiology, Allentown-Sacred Heart Hospital, Allentown, Pennsylvania.)

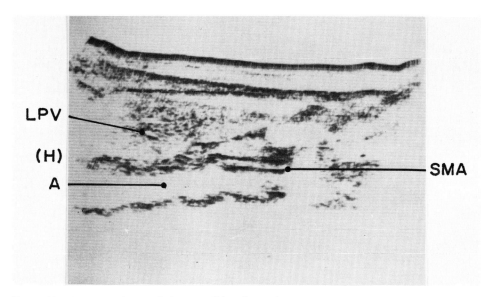

Figure 33.   Longitudinal scan of the aorta (A) and superior mesenteric artery (SMA) demonstrating an extremely narrow superior mesenteric artery angle (H = head; LPV = left portal vein).

the relatively echo-free zones produced may have an appearance similar to that of blood within the aorta. However, by obtaining ultrasonograms in both transverse and longitudinal directions, a typical mantle pattern of lymph nodes usually can be demonstrated, with the walls between the aorta and the lymph nodes being well defined (Figure 30).

Displacement of the superior mesenteric artery is also helpful in determining the site of origin of neoplastic masses. The aorto-mesenteric angle and distance can be determined readily. In most cases of enlarged periaortic lymph nodes, widening of this angle and distance can be demonstrated (Figure 30A). Serial examinations in patients undergoing treatment for abdominal lymphoma may be valuable in estimating decrease in node size. Downward displacement of the superior mesenteric artery by a retroperitoneal mass is seen most commonly with masses originating in the body of the pancreas.

Narrowing of the superior mesenteric artery angle has been demonstrated in some cases in which the vessel wall appears to be resting almost directly on top of the aorta (Figure 33). This has been thought to be one of the causes of compression of the duodenum resulting in duodenal ileus. However, a similar group of patients of the same age and body build had similarly small angles and distances. The mean normal measurements in a group of patients ranging in age from 20 to 84 years was 10 degrees for the angle and 8 mm for the distance (31). In the group in which there was widening, the angles were in excess of 30 degrees and the distance in excess of 20 mm. In the group in which there was narrowing, the mean angle measurement was 5 degrees and the distance 4 mm. There was no significant difference in the measurements of patients who had symptoms suggesting duodenal ileus when compared to a similar group of normals. A narrowed angle and distance was most prevalent in thin females.

Tumor Thrombus and Neoplasms of the Retroperitoneal Vessels.   Neoplasms of the retroperitoneal vessels, such as leiomyosarcomas of the inferior vena cava, are

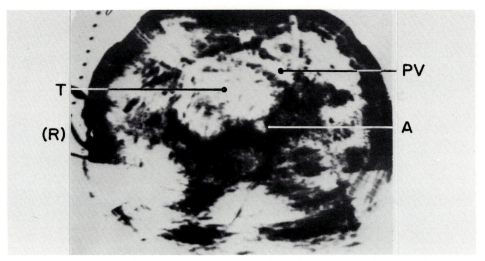

Figure 34. Transverse scan demonstrating a rare sarcoma of the inferior vena cava (T). A specific diagnosis cannot be made since the tumor resembles other retroperitoneal sarcomas (see Figure 29). (R = right; A = aorta; PV = displaced portal-splenic confluence).

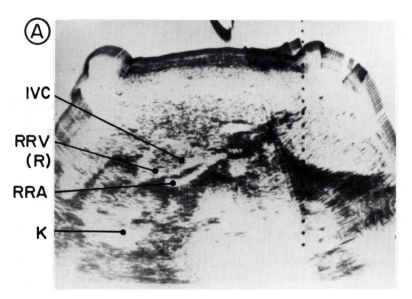

Figure 35. *A*. Supine transverse ultrasonogram shows tumor thrombus within the right renal vein (RRV) (RRA = right renal artery; K = kidney; L = liver). *B*. Supine longitudinal ultrasonogram obtained to the right of the vena cava demonstrates tumor thrombus within the right renal vein (RRV) as it enters the inferior vena cava (IVC) (L = liver). *C*. Supine longitudinal ultrasonogram delineates the inferior vena cava (IVC) with tumor thrombus (arrow). (Courtesy of Dr. R. Binder, Oakland, California.) (*Continued on next page.*)

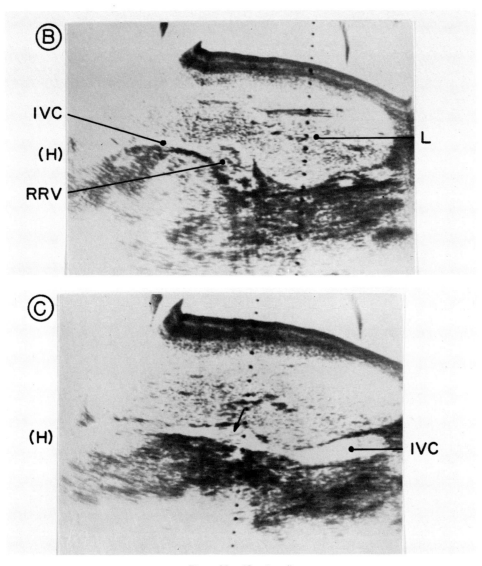

Figure 35.   (Continued)

exceedingly rare, but have been demonstrated on ultrasonograms. A specific diagnosis is, of course, impossible (Figure 34).

Tumor thrombus within the renal vein and the inferior vena cava from hypernephromas has been demonstrated by ultrasonography. When seen, the appearance may be very dramatic and highly diagnostic (Figure 35). Unfortunately, the inability to demonstrate tumor thrombus within the inferior vena cava by sonography does not constitute proof that the IVC has not been invaded. Tumor thrombus has been demonstrated within the right atrium by echocardiographic techniques and may be misinterpreted as a right atrial myxoma (Figure 36).

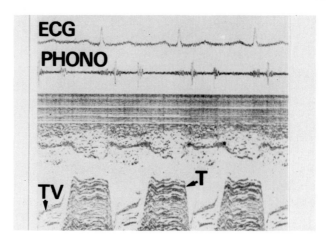

Figure 36.   M-mode recording of the tricuspid valve (TV) demonstrating a pattern usually associated with atrial myxoma. However, at surgery the tumor (T) was demonstrated to be an intraatrial extension of a hypernephroma that had extended into the inferior vena cava and had progressed cephalically into the atrium (ECG = electrocardiogram; PHONO = phonocardiogram). (Courtesy of Richard Popp, M.D., Department of Cardiology, Stanford University Medical Center, Stanford, California.)

Enlargement of Aortic Branches.   Enlargement of aortic branches, other than aneurysmal dilatations, has been demonstrated ultrasonographically. Usually, in these instances, the vessel has enlarged because of torrential flow through the vessel due to highly vascular malignant neoplasms (Figure 35). Nonmalignant arteriovenous fistulas may, of course, show similar findings, but in this circumstance a large echogenic solid mass would not be demonstrated.

SUMMARY

Advances in ultrasonic imaging techniques, particularly gray scale, real-time and pulsed Doppler ultrasonography, have made it possible to noninvasively image abdominal vascular abnormalities in an increasing number of patients. Particularly in the evaluation of aortic dilatation, ultrasonography has become an integral part of our medical diagnostic armamentarium and to a large extent has replaced other diagnostic modalities in the initial evaluation of abdominal aortic aneurysms. Abnormalities of the inferior vena cava more recently have come under study and some success has been demonstrated. Abnormalities of other abdominal vessels occasionally have been detected ultrasonographically. With progressive improvement in ultrasonic image resolution, ultrasonography should become more valuable as a noninvasive tool to assess smaller vascular abnormalities.

REFERENCES

1.   Goldberg BB, Ostrum BJ, Isard HJ: Ultrasonic aortography. *JAMA* **198:**4 353–358, October 1966.

2.   Holm HH, Kristensen JK, Mortensen T, Gammelgaard PA: Ultrasonic diagnosis of arterial aneurysms. *Scand J Thor Cardiovasc Surg* **2:**140–146, 1968.

3.   Laustela E, Tahti E: Echoaortography in abdominal aortic aneurysm. *Annales Chirurgiae et Gyn. Fenniae* **57:**506–509, 1968.

4. Leopold G: Ultrasonic abdominal aortography. *Radiology* **96**:9, 1970.

5. Kristensen JK, Holm HH, Rassmussen SN: Ultrasonic diagnosis of aortic aneurysms. *J Cardiovasc Surg* **13**:168–174, 1972.

6. Leopold G, Goldberger L, Bernstein E: Ultrasonic detection and evaluation of abdominal aortic aneurysms. *Surgery* **72**:939, 1972.

7. Hassani S, Bard R: Ultrasonic diagnosis of abdominal aortic aneurysms. *J of the National Med Assoc* **66**:298–299; 352, July 1974.

8. McGregor JC, Pollock JG, Anton HC: The value of ultrasonography in the diagnosis of abdominal aortic aneurysm. *Scot Med J* **20**:133–137, 1975.

9. Lee KR, Walls WJ, Martin NL, Templeton AW: A practical approach to the diagnosis of abdominal aortic aneurysms. *Surgery* **78**:195–201, August 1975.

10. Goldberg BB, Kotler MN, Ziskin MC, Waxham RD: *Diagnostic Uses of Ultrasound*. New York, Grune & Stratton, 1975.

11. Gosink BB, Leopold GR: Abdominal echography: *Seminars in Roent*. **10**:4 299–304, 1975.

12. Birnholz JC: Alternatives in the diagnosis of abdominal aortic aneurysm: combined use of isotope aortography and ultrasonography. *Am J Roent* **118**:809–813, August 73.

13. Wheeler WE, Beachley MC, Ranniger K: Angiography and ultrasonography. A comparative study of abdominal aortic aneurysms. *Am J Roent* **126**:95–100, January 1975.

14. Thomford NR: Echography: an advance in the diagnosis of abdominal aortic aneurysm. *The Ohio State Med J* 317–318, April 1971.

15. Goldberg BB, Lehman JS: Aortosonography: ultrasound measurement of the abdominal and thoracic aorta. *Arch Surg* **100**:652–655, June 1970.

16. Weill F, Kraehenbuhl JR, Ricatte JP, Aucant D, Gillet M, Makridis D: Le Diagnostic ultrasonore des dissections aortiques et des fissurations aneurismales. *Annales De Radiologie* **17**:49–54, 1974.

17. Winsberg F, Cole CM: Continuous ultrasound visualization of the pulsating abdominal aorta. *Radiology* **103**:455–457, May 1972.

18. Gosling RG, King DH: Arterial assessment by Doppler-Shift ultrasound *Proc Roy Soc Med* **67**:447–449, June 1974.

19. Leopold GR, Asher WM: Deleterious effects of gastrointestinal contrast material on abdominal echography. *Radiology* **98**:637–640, March 1971.

20. Leopold GR, Asher WM: *Fundamentals of Abdominal and Pelvic Ultrasonography*. Philadelphia, W. B. Saunders, 1975.

21. Tahti E, Laustela E, Tala P: Experiences with echoaortography in thoracic aortic aneurysms. *Annales Chirurgiae et Gyn. Fenniae* **57**:50–54, 1968.

22. Filly R, Freimanis AK: Thrombosed hepatic artery aneurysm. *Radiology* **97**:629–630, December 1970.

23. Mozersky DJ, Hokanson DE, Baker DW, Sumner DS, Strandness DE: Ultrasonic arteriography. *Arch Surg* **103**:663–667, December 1971.

24. Mozersky DJ, Hokanson DE, Baker DW, Strandness DE: Ultrasonic visualization of the arterial lumen. *Surgery* **77**:253–359, August 1972.

25. McGregor JC, Pollock JG, Anton HC: Ultrasonography and possible ruptured abdominal aortic aneurysms. *Brit Med J,* July 12, 1975, pp 78–79.

26. Filly RA, Carlsen EN: Newer ultrasonographic anatomy in the upper abdomen: II. The major systemic veins and arteries with a special note on localization of the pancreas. *J Clin Ultrasound* **4**:91–96, 1976.

27. Weill F, Maurat P: The sign of the vena cava: echotomographic illustration of right cardiac insufficiency. *J Clin Ultrasound* **2**:27–32, 1974.

28. Taylor KJW: Ultrasonic investigation of inferior vena-caval obstruction. *Brit J Radiol* **48**:1024–1026, 1975.

29. Carlsen EN, Filly RA: Newer ultrasonographic anatomy in the upper abdomen: I. The portal and hepatic venous anatomy. *J Clin Ultrasound* **4**:85–90, 1976.

30. Weill F: Ultrasonic visualization of an umbilical vein. *Radiology* **120**:159–160, July 1976.

31. Goldberg BB, Perlmutter G: Ultrasonic evaluation of the superior mesenteric artery. (Accepted for publication in the *Journal of Clinical Ultrasound*.)

5
Liver

Kenneth W. Albertson, M.D.
Assistant Professor of Radiology
University of California at San Diego

George R. Leopold, M.D.
Professor of Radiology
Head, Division of Ultrasound
University of California at San Diego

Although the liver is the largest organ in the body, it is one of the most difficult to evaluate. The potential of ultrasound as a noninvasive method to diagnose hepatic disorders is now well recognized. It is interesting to note the progress already made by comparing the older bistable and the newer gray scale scans (Figure 1). The recent introduction of real time ultrasound promises to add another dimension to hepatic imaging.

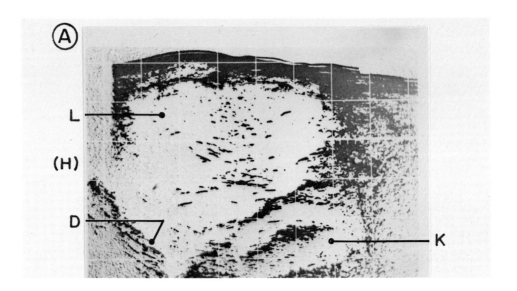

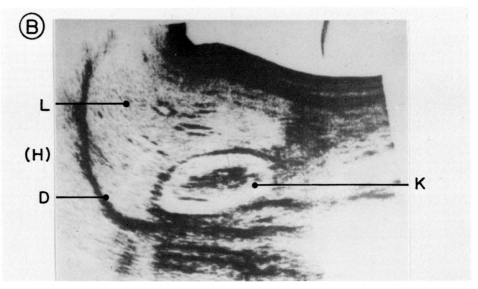

Figure 1.   *A.* Sagittal bistable scan of the right upper quadrant of the abdomen (L = liver; K = kidney; D = diaphragm). *B.* Sagittal gray scale scan of a different patient demonstrating the improved detail and resolution when gray scale is utilized.

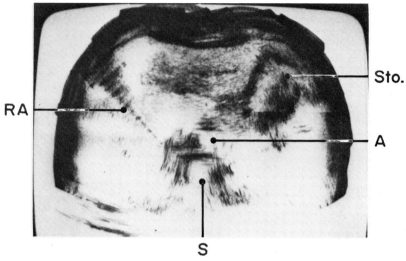

Figure 2. Transverse scan showing a prominent reverberation artifact (RA) from a rib projecting into the liver (A = aorta; S = spine; Sto. = stomach).

METHODS OF EXAMINATION

With the patient in the supine position the examination usually is initiated with transverse scans. The first scan is started at the level of the umbilicus. Scans are then made at 2 cm intervals progressing cephalad across the upper abdomen until the liver is demonstrated completely and the lower portion of the lung is reached. The lung is easily recognized by the poor penetration of the sonographic beam as it is completely reflected by the pleural-air interface. Occasionally, if the right lobe of the liver extends below the level of the umbilicus, additional transverse sections will be necessary. During the examination it is important to adjust the scanning arm so that the transducer makes adequate skin contact. This is most pertinent in patients with a scaphoid abdomen.

The type of transducer used for hepatic imaging depends on the size and cellular architecture of the liver. A 3.5 or if needed a 2.25 MHz transducer generally is satisfactory for most individuals. An obese patient or one with hepatocellular disease and marked hepatomegaly may require a transducer with a lower frequency to increase penetration. It should be realized there is some loss of resolution with the lower frequency transducer. Some adjustment of the gain setting may be necessary depending on the anterior-posterior thickness of the liver (1). With adequate penetration the examiner is able to obtain liver parenchymal echoes and demonstrate the right side of the spine.

Because a large portion of the anterior aspect of the liver is covered by the rib cage, transverse scans alone can never completely display the parenchyma. Also, reverberation echoes from the ribs frequently are seen (Figure 2). Scanning between, but parallel to, the ribs is sometimes helpful but interpretation of oblique sections is frequently difficult.

After completion of the transverse scans, the patient is positioned for the longitudinal (sagittal) scans. A midline section is used as the initial or reference plane. Parallel sections to this reference plane are then made on each side of midline. These scans are usually 2 cm apart. Two or three scans to the left of midline and five or six scans to the right of midline are generally necessary to demonstrate a normal liver completely. Additional sections may be necessary for certain abnormalities or a liver with an unusual shape or contour (2). Again it is important to maintain adequate skin contact with the transducer. This is particularly important along the lateral aspect of the abdominal wall where medial angulation may be necessary. Since the liver moves with the diaphragm, suspension of respiration during inspiration will enhance parenchymal detail. Also, with inspiration there is maximal. exposure of the liver beneath the rib cage and caudal displacement of gas-filled bowel.

Crossing the ribs with the transducer results in serious deterioration of the sagittal image. To alleviate this problem the following maneuver is usually helpful. The abdomen is scanned in a cephalad direction until the transducer touches the costochondral junction of the lower rib cage (Figure 3A). At this point the transducer is sectored toward the head so an arc is formed extending from the posterior aspect of the liver to the superior portion of the diaphragm (3) (Figure 3B). By slight depression of the skin beneath the costochondral junction, the examiner can sector nearly parallel to the chest wall and delineate the most superior aspect of the liver (Figure 3C). Otherwise, this portion of the liver may be obscured by interposed air in the anterior recess of the lung. Occasionally, conventional longitudinal sections may not fully delineate the liver because of intervening bowel gas or reverberation artifacts from the ribs. Oblique or subcostal scans may be helpful in these selected cases (4). Also, lesions in the extreme posterior portion of the liver may be indistinct because of decreased penetration through the liver. With the patient in the prone position, posterior scans can be obtained to depict these lesions better.

Real time sonography of the liver has proved extremely helpful. The easily maneuverable transducer lets the examiner determine the liver size, shape, and contour. Intrahepatic or adjacent structures, such as the gallbladder and porta hepatis also may be located quickly. Once the structures are identified by real time, conventional gray scale scans with improved resolution may be performed. The capability of real time sonography to appreciate motion of structures in the intrahepatic and perihepatic region becomes quickly evident. This is particularly true for the diaphragm, inferior vena cava, and larger hepatic vessels (Figure 4). Also, in difficult cases the anatomic course of a large vessel or duct can be traced with the real time instrument to determine its anatomic identity.

NORMAL ANATOMY

Transverse scans demonstrate the normal right lobe of the liver approximately 4 to 6 cm above the umbilicus as a crescent-shaped area in the right flank (Figure 5A). Since the liver is quite homogeneous only a few internal echoes are noted. The right kidney appears between the liver and the vertebral column. The left kidney also is seen frequently but may be obscured by overlying gas-filled bowel. With more cephalad sections the gallbladder also may be demonstrated (Figure 5B and C). The abdominal aorta and inferior vena cava frequently are shown as paired vessels, just anterior to the spine (Figure 5C and D). In the region of the porta hepatis numerous vascular structures are encountered. In Figure 6 the junction of the splenic and portal vein is seen. The superior mesenteric artery is noted end-on with the aorta below and the splenic vein above. Heavy echoes are demonstrated in the hilus of the liver depicting the portal venous radicles. Figure 7 is a section at a slightly different level. The portal vein as it

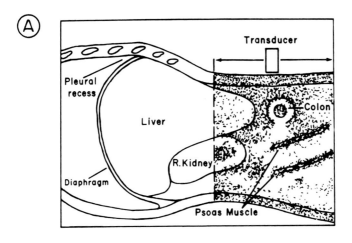

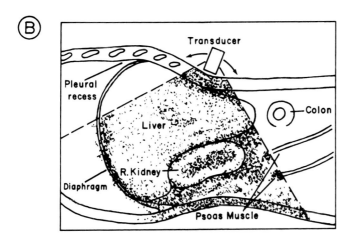

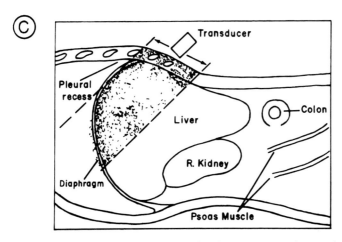

Figure 3.   Three diagrams of a sagittal scanning technique. Simple sector scans at the costochondral junction will demonstrate the dome of the liver.

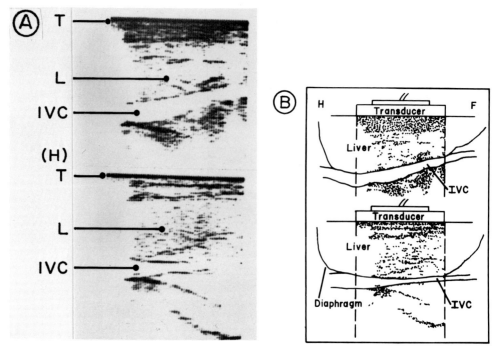

Figure 4. *A*. Sagittal real time scans demonstrating variable size of the inferior vena cava with normal inspiration (top) and expiration (bottom) (T = transducer-skin interface; L = liver; IVC = inferior vena cava). *B*. Diagrammatic representation showing transducer placement.

extends into the liver parenchyma is shown clearly. The identification of these vessels is frequently helpful for proper identification of the porta hepatis and adjacent anatomy (5, 6).

Sagittal sections through the inferior vena cava demonstrate the relationship of the portal vein, caudate lobe of the liver, and the pancreas (Figure 8). Unlike the aorta, the inferior vena cava varies in size with respiration and takes a gentle anterior course prior to entering the right atrium. Intrahepatic veins frequently can be seen in longitudinal sections of the liver and are sometimes noted joining the inferior vena cava (Figure 9). Sagittal sections through the right flank demonstrate the right kidney between the liver and the posterior abdominal wall (Figures 1 and 10). Change in position of the diaphragm can be documented by taking superimposed sections in inspiration and expiration (Figure 10). This usually eliminates the need for fluoroscopy of the diaphragm when a subdiaphragmatic abscess is suspected. Evaluating diaphragmatic motion may be easier with the real time apparatus, especially with the uncooperative patient. Paradoxical or other abnormal motion of the diaphragm also can be appreciated. Identification of the left hemidiaphragm and its motion may be more difficult because of frequent intervening air filled loops of bowel or stomach.

ANATOMIC VARIATIONS

As scanning experience increases the many anatomic variations of the liver become apparent. One of the most perplexing variations is the prominent caudate lobe. Care

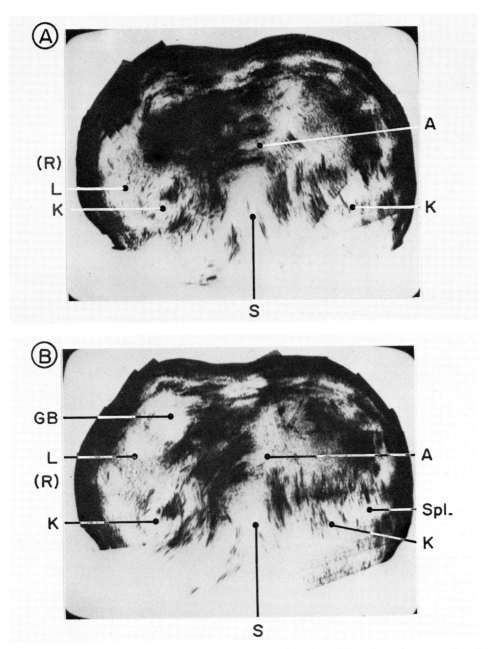

Figure 5. Transverse scans of a normal liver. *A.* Scan 4 cm above the umbilicus shows the crescent-shaped tip of the right lobe of the liver. (L = liver; A = aorta; K = kidney; S = spine). *B.* Scan 8 cm above the umbilicus demonstrates the liver (L), gallbladder (GB) and kidneys (K) (Spl. = spleen). *C.* Scan 12 cm above the umbilicus demonstrates more of the liver (L) as well as the neck of the gallbladder (GB). The spleen (Spl.) is demonstrated in the left flank. (IVC = inferior vena cava; A = aorta). *D.* Scan 14 cm above the umbilicus showing the right and left lobes of the liver (L). The superior pole of the spleen (Spl.) is seen (A = aorta; S = spine). (*Continued on next page.*)

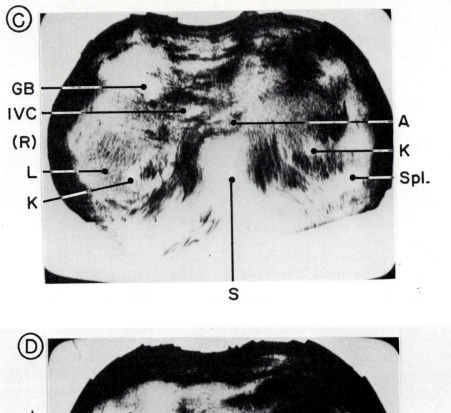

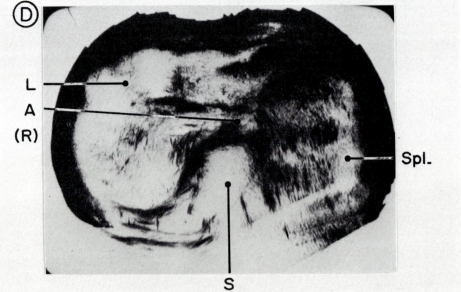

Figure 5. (Continued)

110

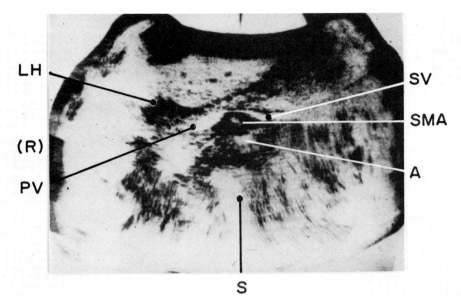

Figure 6. Transverse scan shows the splenic vein (SV) arching over the superior mesenteric artery (SMA) to join the portal vein (PV). A sonodense area from the liver hilus (LH) is seen.

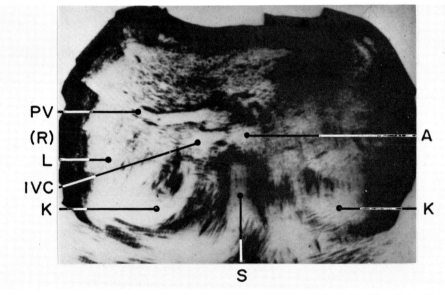

Figure 7. Transverse scan shows the portal vein (PV) extending into the liver (L). The relationship of the portal vein to the abdominal aorta (A) and inferior vena cava (IVC) is demonstrated (K = kidney).

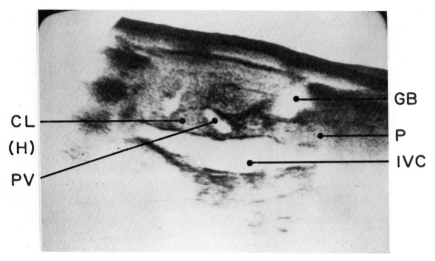

Figure 8. Sagittal scan of a section through a normal liver and inferior vena cava (IVC) demonstrates the relationship of the caudate lobe (CL), portal vein (PV), and pancreas (P), anterior to the inferior vena cava (IVC) (GB = gallbladder).

must be taken in delineating its margins so that it is not mistaken for a mass in the pancreatic head or enlarged nodes in the porta hepatis (Figure 11).

A long, narrow right lobe of the liver (Riedel's lobe) also may be confusing. The extreme caudal extent of this liver on the transverse scans may give the impression of hepatomegaly. However, the longitudinal sections will demonstrate the true narrow configuration of the right lobe of the liver (Figure 12).

A thin left lobe of the liver appears as a region of decreased uptake on the nuclear medicine scan. It is frequently mistaken for a lesion in or below the left lobe on the

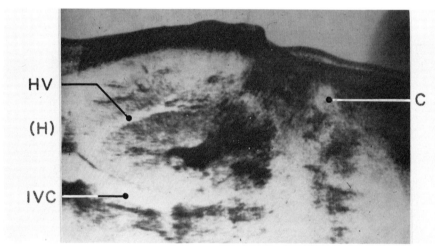

Figure 9. Sagittal scan obtained near the diaphragm shows a slightly dilated hepatic vein (HV) merging with the inferior vena cava (IVC) (C = colon).

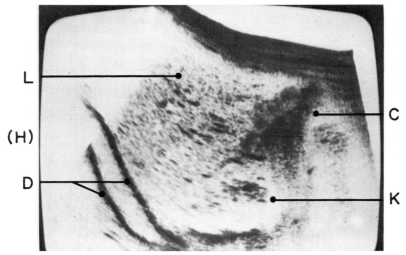

FIgure 10.   Sagittal scan demonstrates diaphragmatic motion (D). Superimposed scans were taken during peak inspiration and expiration (L = liver; K = kidney; C = colon).

isotope study. This normal variant can be demonstrated quickly on the ultrasound scan and preclude further evaluation (Figure 13).

A large left hepatic lobe frequently has a narrow waist separating it from the right lobe. On the more caudal transverse scans, the examiner could mistake this apparent separate left lobe for a mass. However, cephalad transverse scans will demonstrate the narrow waist connecting the right and left lobes of the liver and avoid this potential problem (Figure 14).

The body of the stomach is immediately adjacent to the left lobe of the liver on the transverse scans. It is important not to misinterpret the stomach as an abnormal mass of the left lobe or the tail of the pancreas. The stomach normally has a "C" shaped configuration with poor penetration of the sonographic beam because of gastric air (Figure 15).

PATHOLOGIC ANATOMY

Hepatocellular Disease

Fatty metamorphosis and fibrotic changes of the hepatic parenchyma may create distinctive changes in the sonographic pattern (7, 8). The changes are characterized by an increased number of fine parencymal echoes with a normal gain setting. There is also poor penetration of the sonographic beam due to increased absorption and scattering by the dense fibrotic liver. Therefore, the posterior aspect of the liver on the sagittal sections and the spine on the transverse sections are more difficult to demonstrate. Since the sonographic changes of hepatocellular disease are related to fibrotic replacement, these changes usually are seen only late in the course of the disease. Figure 16 demonstrates a sagittal section of a liver with advanced Laennec's cirrhosis. The liver is enlarged and has multiple fine internal echoes (9–12).

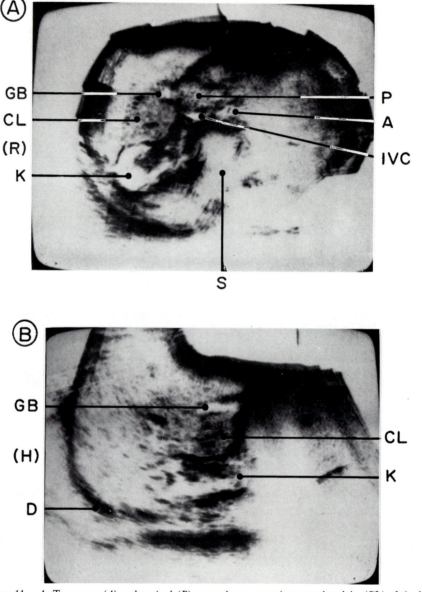

Figure 11.   *A*. Transverse (*A*) and sagittal (*B*) scans show a prominent caudate lobe (CL) of the liver (a normal variant). Note the enlarged pancreas (P) in this patient with pancreatitis (GB = gallbladder; A = aorta; IVC = inferior vena cava; K = kidney; S = spine; D = diaphragm).

Ascites frequently is associated with Laennec's cirrhosis and is easily detected by ultrasound (13–15). The transverse section shown in Figure 17*A* demonstrates the liver displaced medially from the abdominal wall. The gallbladder is floating in the ascitic fluid on the sagittal scan (Figure 17*B*). Ascitic fluid can collect just posterior to the liver as is shown in Figure 17*C*. However, care must be taken in interpreting a posterior fluid collection as ascites, especially in a patient with a right pleural effusion. A pleural

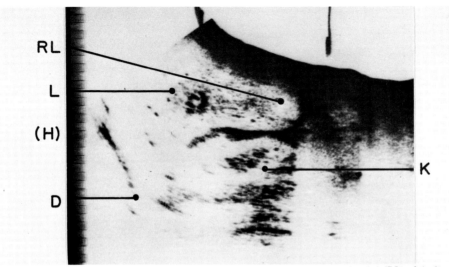

Figure 12. Sagittal scan demonstrates a narrow "tonguelike" right lobe (Riedel's lobe) (RL) of the liver (L) (D = diaphragm; K = kidney).

effusion collects in the posterior recess of the lung and will appear posterior to the liver as shown in Figure 17D. The sagittal scans will demonstrate that the true location of the fluid is supradiaphragmatic.

Regenerating nodules in a cirrhotic liver may be mistaken for other mass lesions. Figure 18A and B demonstrate a regenerating nodule with both bistable and gray scale scans. With the bistable study the regenerating nodule initially was confused with a pancreatic pseudocyst because of its sonolucent character and poorly defined borders.

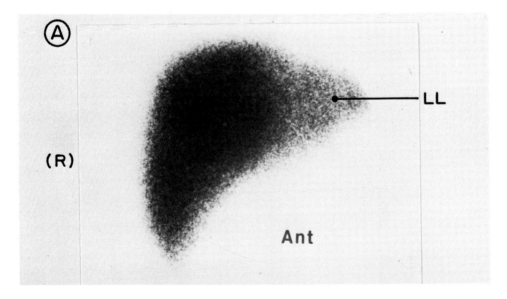

Figure 13. *A.* Isotope scintiphoto of the liver with diminished activity in the left lobe (LL). *B.* The transverse ultrasound scan demonstrates the diminished activity is from a thin left lobe (LL) and not an abnormality (L = liver; PV = portal vein; A = aorta; IVC = inferior vena cava; K = kidney; S = spine). (*Continued on next page*).

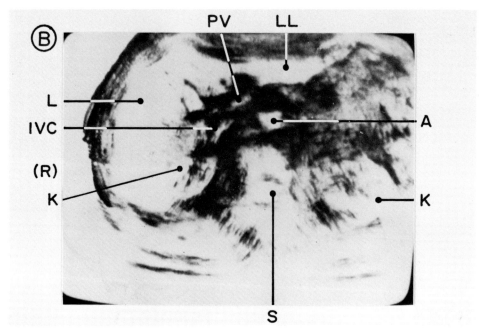

Figure 13. (Continued)

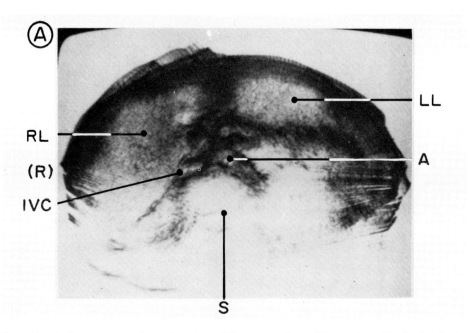

Figure 14. *A.* Transverse scan 8 cm above the umbilicus shows the caudal extension of the liver's left lobe (LL) giving the appearance of a separate mass (RL = right lobe; A = aorta; IVC = inferior vena cava; S = spine). *B.* Transverse scan 10 cm above the umbilicus demonstrates fusion of the right and left lobes of the liver (L). Note the fine echo pattern of hepatocellular disease.

116

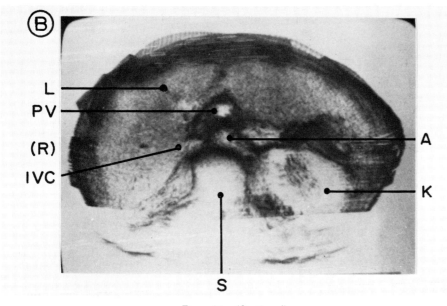

Figure 14. (Continued)

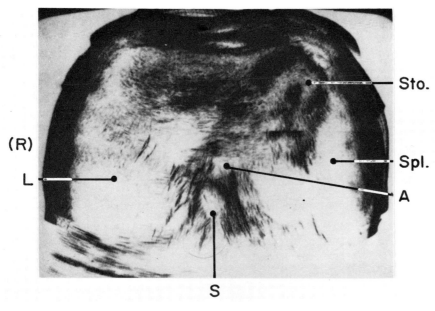

Figure 15. Transverse scan demonstrates the "C" shaped configuration of the gas-filled stomach (Sto) (Spl = spleen; L = liver; A = aorta; S = spine).

117

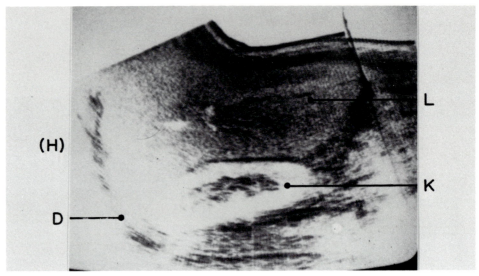

Figure 16. Sagittal scan of a patient with Laennec's cirrhosis. Multiple fine internal echoes and hepatomegaly are seen (L = liver; D = diaphragm; K = kidney).

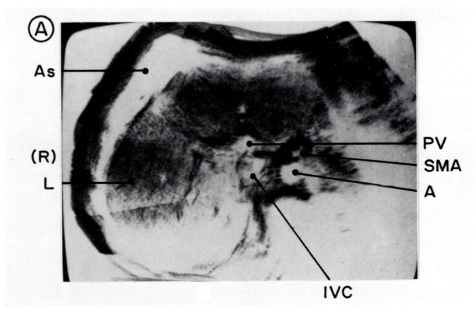

Figure 17. *A.* Transverse scan demonstrates an abnormal echo pattern within the liver (L). The liver is displaced away from the abdominal wall by ascites (As). *B.* Sagittal scan shows the gallbladder (GB) floating in ascitic fluid (As) in a patient with cirrhosis. *C.* Transverse scan shows the ascitic fluid (As) posterior to the liver (L) and separating it from the right kidney (K) Spl = spleen; PV = portal vein; K = kidney; GB = gallbladder; S = spine). *D.* Transverse scan demonstrates a right-sided pleural effusion (PE) that simulates ascites. (*Continued on next page.*)

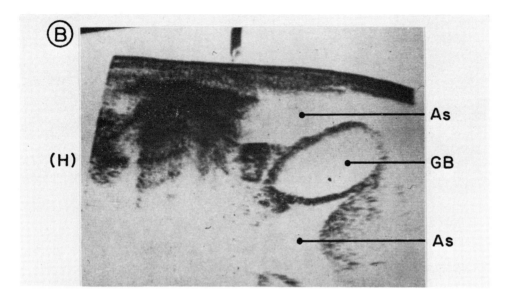

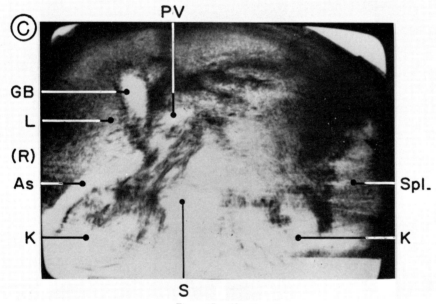

Figure 17.   (Continued)

However, the solid architecture of the nodule as well as its intrahepatic location is clearly shown with a later gray scale scan. Normal uptake on the isotope scan and other studies confirmed it as a regenerating nodule rather than a tumor mass (16, 17) (Figure 18C).

Biliary Obstruction

Dilated bile ducts may appear as multiple dense echoes in the liver and possibly be confused with metastatic disease. However, with suspension of respiration high detail

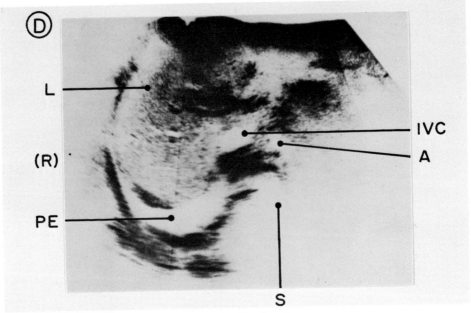

Figure 17. (Continued)

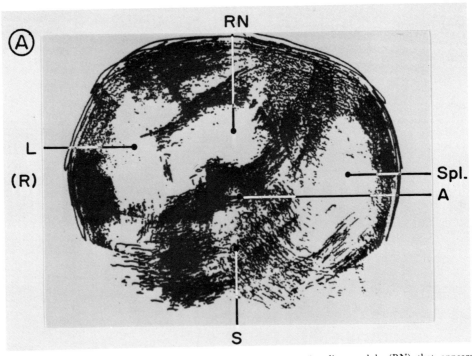

Figure 18. *A*. Bistable transverse scan reveals a large regenerating liver nodule (RN) that appears sonolucent and was confused with a pancreatic pseudocyst (L = liver; Spl = spleen; A = aorta; S = spine). *B*. Gray scale transverse scan clearly shows the intrahepatic location and solid character of the regenerating nodule (RN). *C*. Isotope scintiphoto. Unlike a metastasis, the regenerating nodule (RN) has nuclide uptake and activity similar to normal hepatic tissue (RtL = right lobe; LtL = left lobe). (*Continued on next page.*)

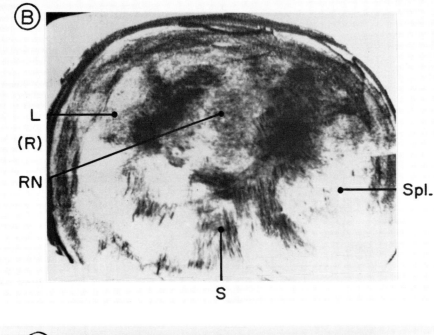

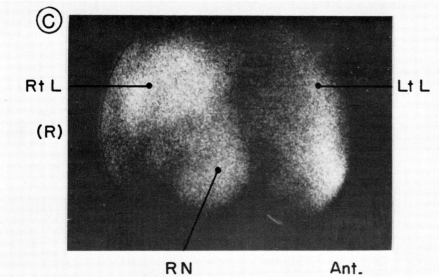

Figure 18. (Continued)

scans usually will demonstrate prominent tubular and branching structures. The clinical history and the demonstration of these abnormal ducts should confirm obstructing biliary disease (18–23) (Figure 19). The dilated common bile duct and the portal vein may have a similar appearance on the transverse scan (24, 25) (Figure 20). Real-time demonstration of the common duct as it descends posteriorly from the gallbladder and cystic duct usually will distinguish it from the portal vein. The latter usually courses anteriorly and is continuous with the splenic vein.

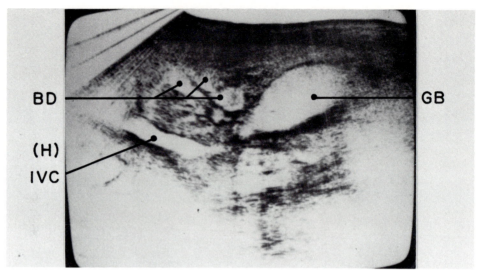

Figure 19. Sagittal scan demonstrates several dilated bile ducts (BD) and a large gallbladder (GB) in a patient with biliary obstruction (IVC = inferior vena cava).

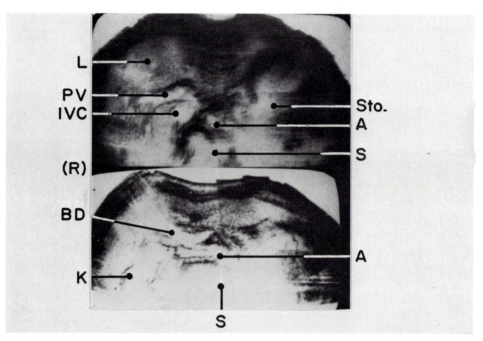

Figure 20. Transverse scans depict the marked similarity in appearance between the portal vein (PV) (top) and the dilated common bile duct (BD) (bottom) (Sto = stomach; L = liver; K = kidney; S = spine; A = aorta; IVC = inferior vena cava; PV = portal vein).

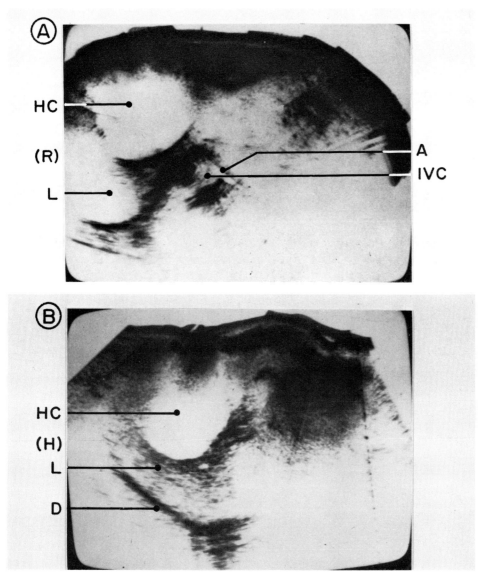

Figure 21. *A*. Transverse and (B) sagittal scans demonstrate a simple hepatic cyst (HC). The liver parenchyma (L) appears sonolucent in the transverse section because of a low gain setting (D = diaphragm).

Hepatic Cyst, Abscess, and Hematoma

Simple cysts of the liver have the same sonographic characteristics as cysts of other organs. Their sharp borders and good "through transmission" are usually diagnostic (26) (Figure 21). Ultrasound is more accurate in detecting small hepatic cysts than solid lesions of a comparable size, because the change in acoustic impedance between a cystic lesion and the adjacent tissue is greater than its solid counterpart (27–29).

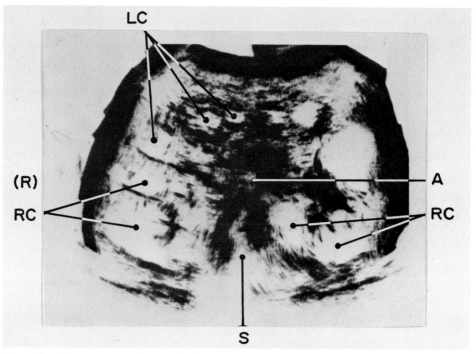

Figure 22. Transverse scan shows multiple intrahepatic (LC) and renal cysts (RC) in a patient with polycystic hepatic and renal disease (A = aorta; S = spine).

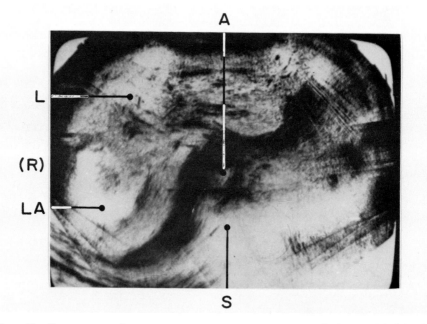

Figure 23. Transverse scan demonstrates a predominantly sonolucent area (LA) in the right lobe of the liver (L) that proved to be an amebic abscess (A = aorta; S = spine).

124

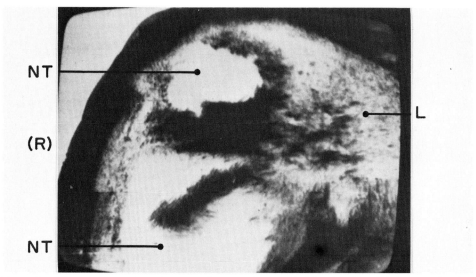

Figure 24. Transverse scan shows large echo-free areas in the right lobe of the liver (L) that were found to be necrotic metastatic tumors (NT) at surgery.

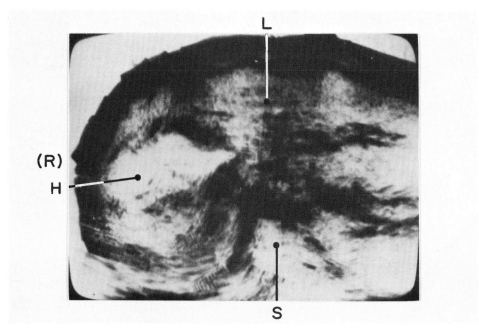

Figure 25. Transverse scan delineates a relatively sonolucent area in the right lobe of the liver (L) that proved to be an intrahepatic hematoma (H) (S = spine).

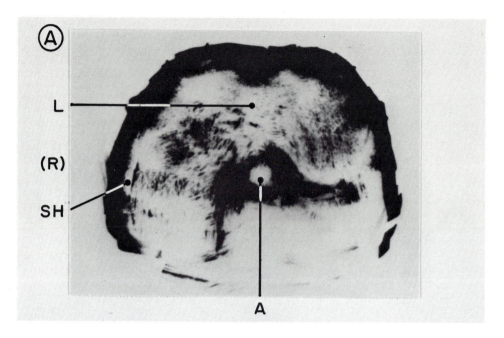

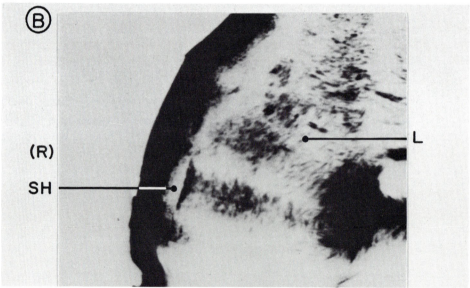

Figure 26.   Transverse (*A*) and coned-down (*B*) views of a hepatic subcapsular hematoma (SH) (L = liver; A = aorta).

Polycystic disease of the liver presents with numerous well-defined sonolucent areas (Figure 22). The size and shape of each cyst is variable because many are sectored obliquely with each scan. A kidney study made in the prone position also should be done to determine the presence or absence of associated polycystic renal disease.

An hepatic abscess is generally a sonolucent mass with an irregular border. The number of internal echoes is variable depending on the character and amount of cellular

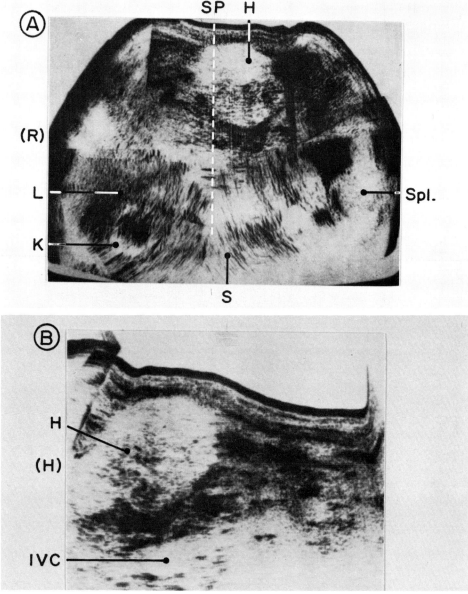

Figure 27. *A.* Transverse scan reveals a circumscribed mass in the left lobe of the liver proven to be a hematoma (H) (Spl = spleen; K = kidney; S = spine; SP = sagittal plane). *B.* The sagittal scan through the hepatoma (H) was made along the broken line noted on the transverse section (IVC = inferior vena cava).

debris within it. The typical liver abscess is a single fluid-filled mass (Figure 23). However, multiple fluid-filled pockets with pyogenic debris may be seen (30–33). Successful percutaneous aspiration of hepatic abscesses has been done after localization with ultrasound (35, 36). Differentiating an abscess from a necrotic tumor (Figure 24) or an intrahepatic hematoma (Figure 25) may not be possible by ultrasound. In most cases the clinical history is usually helpful in making this distinction.

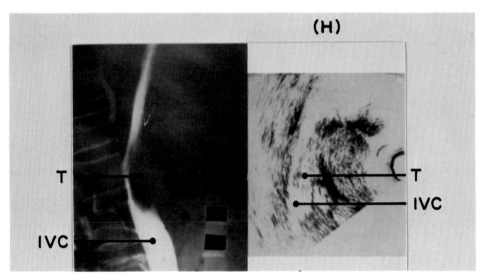

Figure 28. *Left.* The venogram demonstrates a hepatoma (T) invading the contrast-filled inferior vena cava (IVC). *Right.* The tumor mass (T) is shown within the inferior vena cava (IVC) on the ultrasound study. The ultrasonogram is oriented upright for better comparison with the roentgenogram.

The sonographic demonstration of a subcapsular hematoma may be difficult because of the numerous rib reverberation artifacts. Figures 26A and B show a subcapsular hematoma separating the hepatic capsule from the liver parenchyma.

Primary Liver Tumors

Primary tumors of the liver do not have a distinctive sonographic pattern with the present gray scale equipment. However, ultrasound usually can demonstrate the presence of a tumor mass and localize it for biopsy (37–40). Figures 27A and 27B demonstrate a well-marginated collection of echoes in the left lobe of the liver. A large hepatoma conforming to this mass was found at surgery. Figure 28 is another example of a hepatoma invading the inferior vena cava. There is excellent anatomic correlation between the ultrasound scan and the inferior vena cavagram.

Metastatic Tumors

The sonographic appearance of liver metastases is a spectrum from very sonolucent to very sonodense (41, 42). The character of the echoes is largely dependent on how homogeneous the mass or nodule is and if there is a necrotic center. Numerous metastatic nodules are noted in Figures 29A and B. The bull's-eye configuration may be created by a central area of necrosis within each nodule. Figures 30A and B show a large metastatic adenocarcinoma of the colon. The isotope study was done initially and interpreted as either a large cyst or a tumor. An obvious solid mass with necrotic center was demonstrated by ultrasound. A large colonic carcinoma was found on barium enema examination.

Lymphomas are very homogeneous and therefore quite sonolucent. Figure 31 is an example of partial hepatic replacement by a lymphosarcoma. Patients with known lymphoma also should have a careful ultrasonic examination for enlargement of extrahepatic and retroperitoneal nodes. Figures 32*A* and *B* are transverse and sagittal scans of

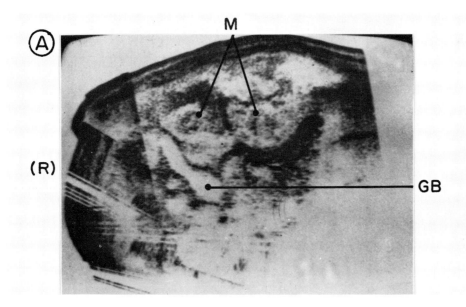

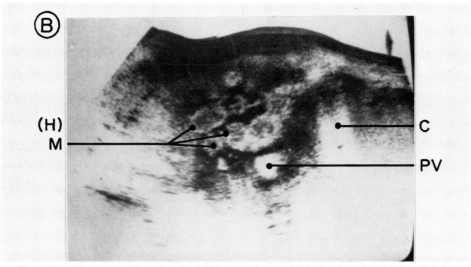

Figure 29. Transverse (*A*) and sagittal (*B*) scans show multiple intrahepatic "bull's-eye" lesions (M). Metastatic adenocarcinoma was found with biopsy (GB = gallbladder; PV = portal vein; C = colon).

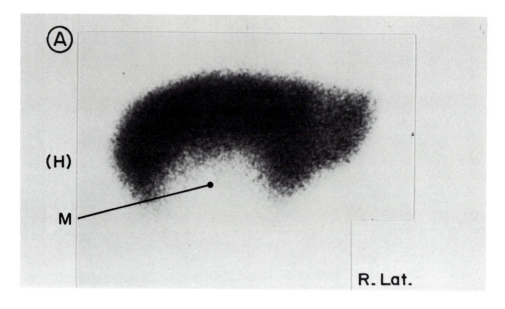

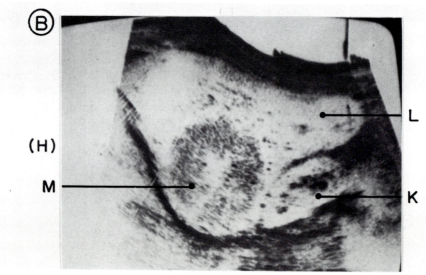

Figure 30. *A.* Right lateral scintiphoto demonstrates a large posterior defect (M) in the right lobe of the liver. The differential diagnosis was between a hepatic cyst or tumor. *B.* A sagittal ultrasonogram confirmed the presence of a necrotic tumor mass (M) which was secondary to metastatic adenocarcinoma of the colon (L = liver; K = kidney).

a patient with Hodgkin's disease. Large nodes impress on the inferior vena cava in the sagittal scan and displace the aorta anteriorly in the transverse scan (43).

Mixed cystic and solid metastatic lesions of the liver also occur. Figure 33 is a metastatic cystadenocarcinoma of the ovary. The mixed character of this lesion is quite apparent.

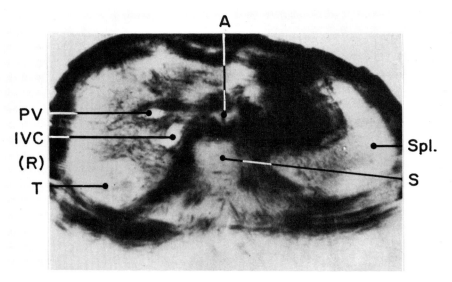

Figure 31. Transverse scan delineates a posterior hepatic lesion (T) with a few internal echoes. This lymphosarcoma demonstrates the typical sonolucent appearance of lymphomas. Associated splenomegaly (Spl.) is noted.

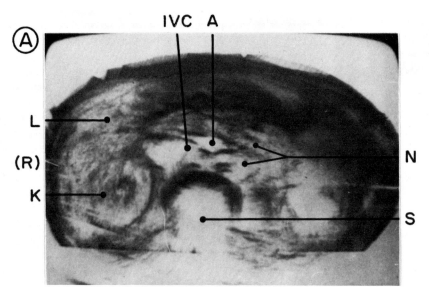

Figure 32. *A.* Transverse scan demonstrates anterior displacement of the abdominal aorta (A) by coalescent nodes (N). *B.* The sagittal scan shows that the nodes (N) are also compressing and displacing the inferior vena cava (IVC) (PV = portal vein; L = liver; K = kidney; S = spine). (*Continued on next page.*)

131

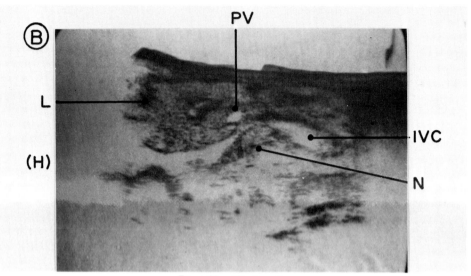

Figure 32.   (Continued)

Ultrasound is very useful in following the clinical response of hepatic tumors to various modes of therapy. Changes in the internal pattern of tumors treated with both chemotherapy and radiotherapy have been observed (44–46). A longitudinal and transverse scan of a metastatic undifferentiated carcinoma is shown in Figures 34A and B. The response to therapy is dramatically demonstrated in Figures 34C and D. The only residual tumor found was a small lucent area in the right lobe of the liver.

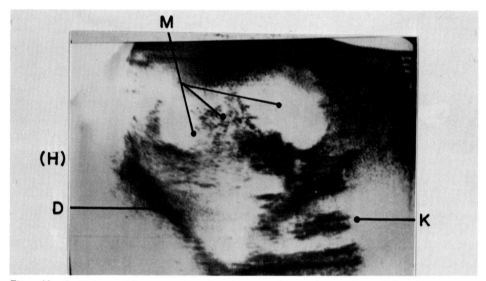

Figure 33.   Sagittal scan delineates an intraphepatic metastatic cyst-adenocarcinoma (M) of the ovary with both cystic and solid components. (D = diaphragm; K = kidney).

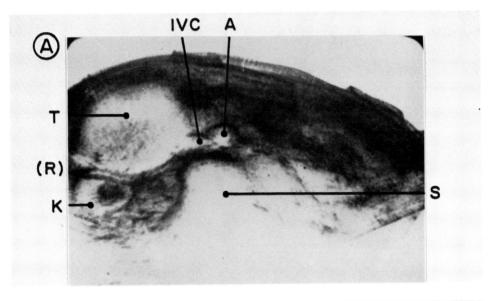

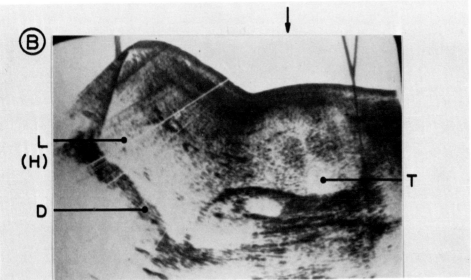

Figure 34. Transverse (A) and sagittal (B) scans show a metastatic undifferentiated cell carcinoma (T) (K = kidney; L = liver; D = diaphragm; A = aorta; IVC = inferior vena cava). Transverse (C) and sagittal (D) scans obtained after therapy demonstrating only a small residual tumor (T) remaining in the right lobe of the liver. (*Continued on next page.*)

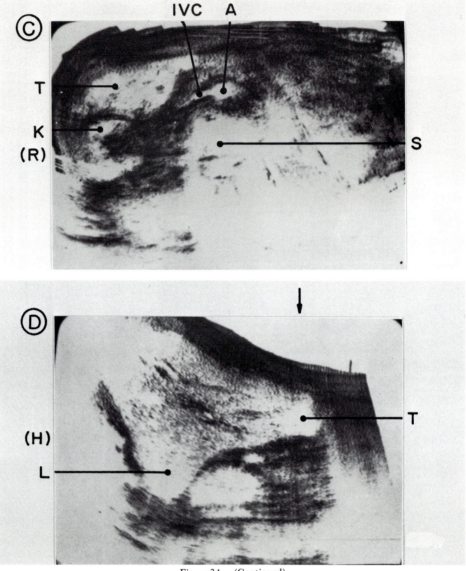

Figure 34.   (Continued)

The diagnostic value of ultrasound in hepatic disorders continues to expand. Each new development in the instrumentation adds a new dimension to the diagnosis of liver disease.

ACKNOWLEDGMENT

The authors would like to express their appreciation to Dr. Barbara Gosink for her valuable assistance and contribution of several cases from the Veterans Administration Hospital, La Jolla, California.

REFERENCES

1. Lehman JS: Ultrasound in the diagnosis of hepatobiliary disease. *Radiol Clin North Am* **4**:605, 1966.

2. Rasmussen SN, Nielsen SS, Stigsby B: Three-dimensional visualization of the liver by ultrasonic scanning. Presented at the 17th meeting of the Amer Inst Ultrasound Med, Philadelphia, Oct 31-Nov 2, 1972.

3. Taylor KJW, Hill CR: Scanning techniques in grey-scale ultrasonography. *Br J Radiol* **48**:918, 1975.

4. McCarthy CF, Davies ER, Wells PNT, Ross FGM, Follett DH, Muir KM, Read AE: A comparison of ultrasonic and isotope scanning in the diagnosis of liver disease. *Br J Radiol* **43**:100, 1970.

5. Leopold GR: Gray-scale ultrasonic angiography of the upper abdomen. *Radiology* **117**:665, 1975.

6. Taylor KJW, Carpenter DA: The anatomy and pathology of the porta hepatis demonstrated by gray-scale ultrasonography. *J Clin Ultrasound* **3**:117, 1975.

7. Duncan JG: The diagnostic value of ultrasound in hepatomegaly and upper abdominal masses. *J R Coll Surg Edinb* **20**:107, 1975.

8. Mountford RA, Wells PNT: Ultrasonic liver scanning: the A-scan in the normal and cirrhosis. *Phys Med Biol* **17**:261, 1972.

9. Kaude JV, DeLand F: Hepatomegaly. *Med Clin North Am* **59**:121, 1975.

10. Kardel T, Holm HH, Rasmussen SN, Mortensen T: Ultrasonic determination of liver and spleen volumes. *Scand J Clin Lab Invest* **27**:123, 1971.

11. Rasmussen SN, Kardel T, Jörgensen BJ: Liver volume estimated by ultrasonic scanning before and after portal decompression surgery. *Scand J Gastroenterol* **10**:25, 1975.

12. Rasmussen SN: Liver volume determination by ultrasonic scanning. *Br J Radiol* **45**:579, 1972.

13. Goldberg BB, Clearfield HR, Goodman GA, Morales JO: Ultrasonic determination of ascites. *Arch Intern Med* **131**:217, 1973.

14. Goldberg BB, Goodman GA, Clearfield, HR: Evaluation of ascites by ultrasound. *Radiology* **96**:15, 1970.

15. Hünig R, Kinser J: The diagnosis of ascites by ultrasonic tomography (B-scan). *Br J Radiol* **46**:325, 1973.

16. Leyton B, Halpern S, Leopold G, Hagen S: Correlation of ultrasound and colloid scintiscan studies of the normal and diseased liver. *J Nucl Med* **14**:27, 1973.

17. Pritchard JH, Winston MA, Berger HG, Blahd WH: Diagnosis of focal hepatic lesions. Combined radioisotope and ultrasound techniques. *JAMA* **229**:1463, 1974.

18. Ferrucci JT, Eaton SB: Radiologic evaluation of obstructive jaundice. *Surg Clin North Am* **54**:573, 1974.

19. Goldberg BB: Ultrasonic cholangiography: grey-scale B-scan evaluation of the common bile duct. *Radiology* **118**:401, 1976.

20. Hawkins IF, MacGregor AM, Freimanis A: Radiologic approach to obstructive jaundice and pancreatic disease. *Med Clin North Am* **59**:121, 1975.

21. Leopold GR, Sokoloff J: Ultrasonic scanning in the diagnosis of biliary disease. *Surg Clin North Am* **53**:1043, 1973.

22. Sherlock S: *Diseases of the Liver and Biliary System,* ed 4. Philadelphia, Davis, 1968.

23. Taylor KJW, Carpenter DA: Letter: Grey-scale ultrasonography in the investigation of obstructive jaundice. *Lancet* **2**:586, 1974.

24. Taylor KJW, Carpenter DA, McCready VR: Ultrasound and scintigraphy in the differential diagnosis of obstructive jaundice. *J Clin Ultrasound* **2**:105, 1974.

25. Weill F, Eisenscher A, Aucant D, Bourgoin A, Gallinet D: Ultrasonic study of venous patterns in the right hypochondrium: an anatomical approach to differential diagnosis of obstructive jaundice. *J Clin Ultrasound* **3**:23, 1975.

26. Birnholz JC: Sonic differentiation of cysts and homogeneous solid masses. *Radiology* **108**:699, 1973.

27. Gilday DL, Brown R, MacPherson RI: Choledochal cyst—a case diagnosed by radiographic and ultrasonic collaboration. *J Can Assoc Radiol* **20**:25, 1969.

28. McCarthy CF, Wells PNT, Ross FGM, Read AE: The use of ultrasound in the diagnosis of cystic lesions of the liver and upper abdomen and in the detection of ascites. *Gut* 10:904, 1969.

29. Suruga K: Clinical and pathological study on choledochocyst. *Jpn J Surg* 3:199, 1973.

30. King DL: Ultrasonography of echinococcal cyst. *J Clin Ultrasound* 1:64, 1973.

31. Lydon SB, Dodds WJ: Amebic hepatic abscess. *Am J Gastroenterol* 62:71, 1974.

32. Matthews AW, Gough KR, Davies ER, Ross FGM, Hinchliffe A: The use of combined ultrasonic and isotope scanning in the diagnosis of amoebic liver disease. *Gut* 14:50, 1973.

33. Monroe LS, Leopold GR, Brown JW, Smith JL: The ultrasonic scan in the management of amebic hepatic abscess. *Am J Dig Dis* 16:523, 1971.

34. Wang HF, Wang CE, Chang CP, Kao J, Yu L, Chiang Y: The application and value of ultrasonic diagnosis of liver abscess. A report of 218 cases. *Chin Med J* 83:133, 1964.

35. Friday RO, Barriga P, Crummy AB: Detection and localization of intra-abdominal abscesses by diagnostic ultrasound. *Arch Surg* 110:335, 1975.

36. Smith EH, Bartrum RJ: Ultrasonically guided percutaneous aspiration of abscesses. *Am J Roentgenol Radium Ther Nucl Med* 122:308, 1974.

37. Burcharth F, Rasmussen SN: Localization of the porta hepatis by ultrasonic scanning prior to percutaneous transhepatic portography. *Br J Radiol* 47:598, 1974.

38. Holm HH: Ultrasonically guided percutaneous puncture technique. *J Clin Ultrasound,* 1:27, 1973.

39. Lutz H, Weidenhiller S, Rettenmaier G: Ultrasonically guided fine-needle biopsy of the liver. *Schweiz Med Wochenschr* 103:1030, 1973.

40. Rasmussen SN, Holm HH, Kristensen JK, Barlebo H: Ultrasonically-guided liver biopsy. *Br Med J* 2:500, 1972.

41. Damascelli B, Fossati F, Livraghi T, Severini A: B-scan ultrasound exploration of neoplastic disease. *Am J Roentgenol Radium Ther Nucl Med* 105:428, 1969.

42. Melki G: Ultrasonic patterns of tumors of the liver. *J Clin Ultrasound* 1:306, 1973.

43. Taylor, KJW: Ultrasonic investigation of inferior vena-caval obstruction. *Br J Radiol* 48:1024, 1975.

44. Gilby ED, Taylor KJW: Ultrasound monitoring of hepatic metastases during chemotherapy. *Br Med J* 1:371, 1975.

45. Kobayashi T, Takatani O, Hattori N, Kimura K: Echographic evaluation of abdominal tumor regression during antineoplastic treatment. *J Clin Ultrasound* 2:131, 1974.

46. Tolbert DD, Zagzebski JA, Banjavic RA, Wiley AL: Quantitation of tumor volumes and response to therapy with ultrasound B-scans. *Radiology* 113:705, 1974.

6

Gallbladder and Bile Ducts

Barry B. Goldberg, M.D.
Professor of Radiology
Director, Division of Diagnostic Ultrasound
Thomas Jefferson University Hospital
Philadelphia, Pennsylvania

Although the gallbladder is normally located anteriorly in the right upper quadrant of the abdomen beneath the inferior edge of the liver, its position can vary significantly. There is also much variability in its size and shape. When possible, ultrasonic examination of the gallbladder should be performed with the patient in a fasting state, similar to the conditions required for obtaining a roentgenographic oral cholecystogram. This insures maximum physiologic distention of the gallbladder. In general, the larger the gallbladder, the better the ultrasonic delineation. In emergency situations, nevertheless, an examination may be performed at any time, since fasting will not alter the size of the gallbladder if there is an obstruction.

TECHNIQUE

The patient is placed in the supine position. Scanning may be initiated either in the longitudinal or transverse direction (Figure 1). The initial longitudinal scan usually is obtained in the midline, and scanning is continued at 1-cm intervals toward the right. Since respiration can produce significant movement of the liver and gallbladder, each sweep of the transducer should be made during a suspended respiration in order to obtain maximum detail. Each longitudinal sweep usually is started from the region of the umbilicus with the transducer moved upward in a cephalad direction toward the costal margin. When the transducer comes in contact with the costal margin, it usually is angled steeply up under the rib cage so the ultrasonic beam is projected in a cephalad direction, rather than moving the transducer in a linear fashion over the ribs (Figure 2). This technique will avoid echo artifacts produced by rib absorption and reverberation. Scanning is continued until the gallbladder is located and completely outlined in the longitudinal plane. Marks can be placed on the skin indicating the margins of the gallbladder, information that will be useful during the transverse scanning sequence. If the gallbladder is found to be located high up under the costal margin, scanning at the end of a deep inspiration often will prove to be helpful by inferiorly displacing the liver and gallbladder out from under the rib cage. This technique is helpful both for transverse and longitudinal scanning since interference from the rib cage can be a problem with either approach.

Transverse scanning usually is started at the level of the umbilicus unless the longitudinal ultrasonograms demonstrate an unusually low-lying gallbladder. The transducer is moved at set intervals (usually 1 cm) upward toward and, if necessary, beyond the costal margin. Since the axis of the gallbladder may not lie in an exact longitudinal or transverse plane, the true axis can be determined by placing marks on the skin that designate the maximum transverse diameter of the gallbladder obtained at each level. A line, which will indicate the path for obtaining the maximum longitudinal or oblique lumen diameter, can then be drawn through these dots. It is important during the final scanning sequence, particularly if looking for abnormalities within the gallbladder (i.e., stones) that the increments between sweeps be no more than a 0.5 cm. With this technique, the possibility of missing small stones (i.e., those in the 3-mm range) will be reduced. Real-time B-scan ultrasound is being used with increasing frequency to locate the gallbladder rapidly and to determine its axis prior to obtaining gray scale B-scan ultrasonograms (Figure 3).

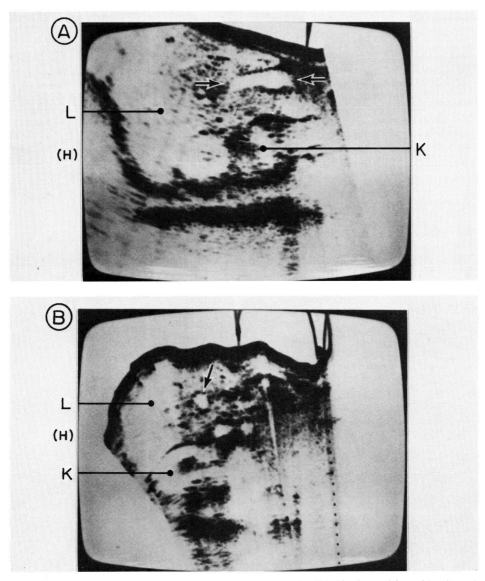

Figure 1. *A*. Longitudinal ultrasonogram demonstrating a normal gallbladder (arrows) located just beneath the inferior edge of the liver (L = liver; K = kidney). *B*. Transverse ultrasonogram showing gallbladder (arrow) obtained from same patient as Figure 1*A* (L = liver; K = kidney).

FUNCTIONAL EVALUATION

The gallbladder, once it is identified and evaluated with respect to its size, shape, and internal contents, also can be studied for its function. This can be accomplished by giving a fatty meal as is done for oral cholecystographic function studies. As in x-ray studies, maximum contraction usually will occur in 20 to 30 minutes, at which time a

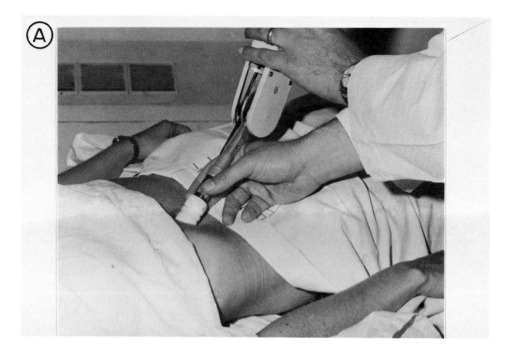

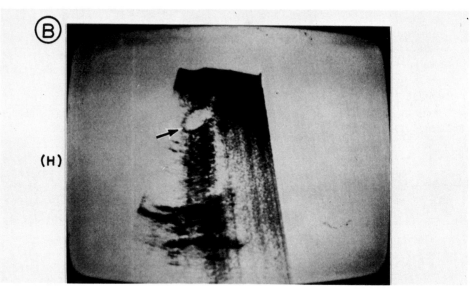

Figure 2. *A.* Ultrasonic transducer is seen being angled steeply up under the rib cage. *B.* Longitudinal ultrasonogram obtained by angling transducer under the rib cage showing a normal gallbladder (arrow).

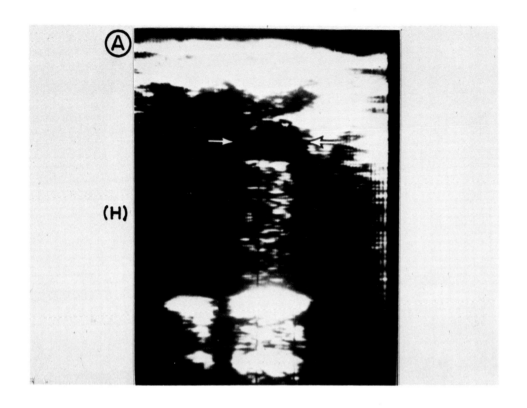

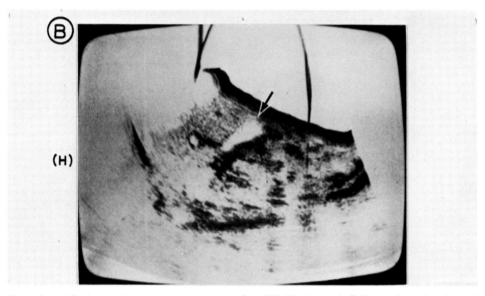

Figure 3. *A*. Real-time ultrasonogram demonstrates the gallbladder (arrows). *B*. From information obtained using real-time imaging as to the axis of the gallbladder, this gray scale ultrasonogram was obtained. The resolution of the gallbladder (arrows) is seen to be better with present gray scale ultrasonic equipment compared to available real-time equipment.

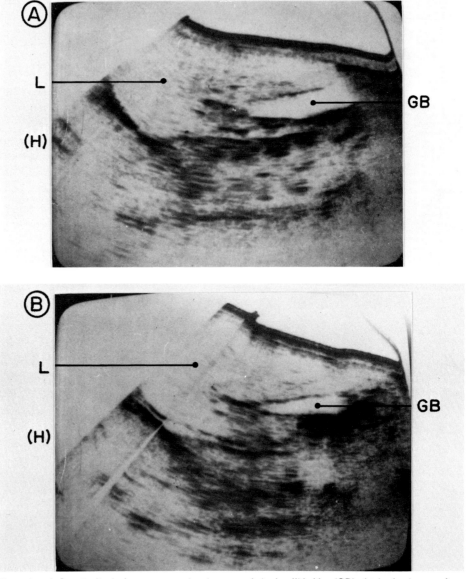

Figure 4. *A.* Longitudinal ultrasonogram showing normal-sized gallbladder (GB) obtained prior to a fatty meal (L = liver). *B.* Longitudinal ultrasonogram obtained after fatty meal showing normal contraction of the gallbladder (GB).

repeat ultrasonogram is obtained. The change in size due to contraction can be readily demonstrated ultrasonically, and results compare favorably with roentgenographic studies (1). The contraindications for a functional examination are similar to those for oral cholecystography (Figure 4).

POSITIONAL EVALUATION

In addition to evaluating the gallbladder in the supine position, changes in its position as well as shifting of stones can be demonstrated by having the patient sit or stand erect. When the patient cannot stand, a decubitus view is often successful in showing gravitational shifting of gallstones.

CYSTIC AND COMMON BILE DUCTS

Portions of the cystic and common bile ducts sometimes may be recorded (2). For localization, the most medial part of the gallbladder should be determined and a mark placed on the skin surface. A series of longitudinal and longitudinal-oblique scans are obtained in an area just medial to the mark. Scanning should be performed during suspended respiration for optimal detail. The cystic duct, if located, usually will have an irregular contour as opposed to the more linear appearance of the common bile duct. Normally, the common bile duct measures 8 mm in diameter and usually angles downward from the gallbladder as it courses toward the duodenum. For obvious reasons, the larger the ducts, the easier they are to record (Figure 5).

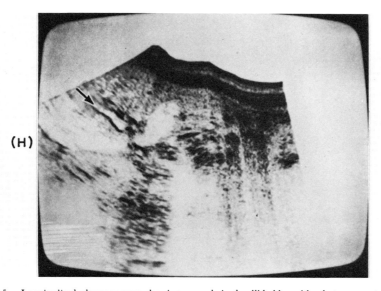

(H)

Figure 5.   Longitudinal ultrasonogram showing normal-sized gallbladder with what appears to be a ductlike structure emanating from its superior aspect. From its location this probably represents a portion of the cystic and biliary duct (arrow).

GALLBLADDER POSITION

As stated previously, there can be considerable variation in the position of the gallbladder, and it is not always found in the right upper quadrant of the abdomen. For
instance, it has been known to herniate through the foramen of Winslow into the lesser
peritoneal sac presenting to the left of the midline. With significant hepatomegaly, as
would be expected, it may be displaced both inferiorly and medially. In severe cases, the
gallbladder even may be displaced downward into the pelvis. With upward rotation of the
right kidney, the gallbladder actually may drape over the anterior renal surface (Figure
6). In these situations, inflammation of the gallbladder could produce symptoms that are
renal in nature. Ultrasound can be helpful in establishing the proper diagnosis. Gallbladders, moreover, may be intrahepatic or at least may appear to be intrahepatic on routine
oral cholecystography. Ultrasound is able to demonstrate whether the gallbladder actually
lies within the liver parenchyma, which is a rare phenomena, or is just projected in such a
way on the x-ray film.

GALLBLADDER SIZE

As is well known, the size of the gallbladder can vary significantly, due either to normal
physiologic differences or to pathologic causes. The normal gallbladder is approximately
2.5 cm in diameter and up to 8 cm in length. However, this figure is essentially mean-
ingless due to the great variation in size and shape of normal gallbladders.

Ultrasound can determine accurately the dimensions of the gallbladder. With multiple
sections and the use of a planimeter or computer, volume measurements can be made.
The ultrasonic approach appears to be the method of choice since there are no magnification factors, as is the case with oral cholecystography, and since visualization is not

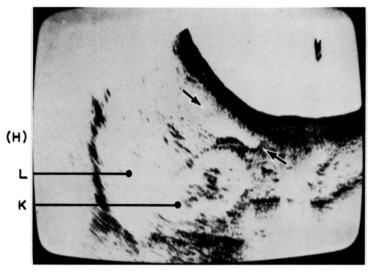

Figure 6.   Longitudinal ultrasonogram shows the normal-sized gallbladder (arrows) draped over a rotated
kidney (K) (L = liver).

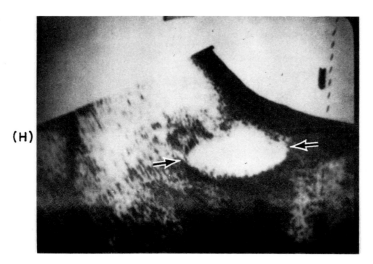

Figure 7.   Longitudinal ultrasonogram shows an enlarged gallbladder (arrows) that did not decrease in size after a fatty meal. This is consistent with the clinically suspected diagnosis of hydrops.

function dependent. Gross enlargement, i.e., hydrops, can be demonstrated easily (Figure 7). However, the size can vary dramatically. The width tends to have less variation than the length. In general, when lumen width, i.e., the shortest diameter, is greater than 3.5 to 4 cm, a diagnosis of dilatation can be suggested. It is important to remember that a person who has been on intravenous feedings and has not had any food by mouth often will have a physiologically distended gallbladder. A fatty meal or an injection of cholecystokinin, if it can be tolerated, should produce contraction, proving that the apparent dilatation is in fact nonpathologic.

Gallbladders were examined ultrasonically and correlated with oral cholecystography measurements. After correcting for x-ray magnification factors, no significant difference in gallbladder size as determined by ultrasound and x-ray was found. Of course, ultrasound was the only method that could be used when oral cholecystography failed to visualize the gallbladder. In these cases, the gallbladder diameters tended on the average to be larger, which is not unexpected since obstruction of the cystic duct is one of the common causes for such findings. Of course there can be other causes for dilatation, such as bile duct obstruction due to pancreatic carcinoma, known as a Courvoisier's gallbladder. The finding of a small or normal-sized gallbladder does not in itself exclude the possibility of bile duct obstruction due to pancreatic tumor or other causes.

In general, the larger the gallbladder, the easier it is to obtain an ultrasonic image. In fact, ultrasound should be considered as the procedure of choice for rapidly determining the presence of a dilated gallbladder since the method is not function dependent. If the gallbladder cannot be visualized ultrasonically, this usually means that it is either empty or at least too small to be differentiated ultrasonically, i.e., less than 1 to 2 cm in diameter. As emphasized previously, the entire abdomen should be examined in order to be sure that the gallbladder is not merely in an abnormal location. The next step would be to repeat the ultrasonic examination after fasting, preferably in the morning before breakfast. If the gallbladder is still not visualized, such a finding is highly suggestive of a diseased gallbladder. The accuracy of this prediction is similar to that for a nonvisualized gallbladder on x-ray studies after two doses of oral contrast material. Failure to visualize the gallbladder usually indicates that it is severely contracted and/or filled with stones to such an extent that the fluid content is insufficient for the ultrasonic beam to detect (3).

In conclusion, ultrasound has been found to be a reliable method of determining gallbladder size. Volume measurements compare favorably with corrected roentgenographic measurements. Physiologic evaluation is possible either by ingestion of a fatty meal or cholecystokinin injection in order to demonstrate contraction or by fasting to evaluate for further distention. Failure to delineate a gallbladder after fasting often means that it is severely diseased and contracted and/or filled with stones, with relatively little fluid content.

VARIATIONS

The gallbladder can vary not only in size but also in shape and even number, i.e., a double gallbladder (Figure 8). These variations can be diagnosed ultrasonically. Care should be taken in the differential diagnosis to be sure that a gallbladder bent on itself or a septated (Phrygian cap) gallbladder is not misinterpreted as a double gallbladder (Figure 9). Two distinct gallbladders should be identified in several planes, with ultrasonograms recording the major longitudinal axis of each and then a transverse ultrasonogram transecting both gallbladders.

Another variation is the absence of the gallbladder. The missing gallbladder is a more difficult problem since nonvisualization of the gallbladder also can mean that it is either so filled with stones that very little fluid is present or it is severely contracted. Neverthe-

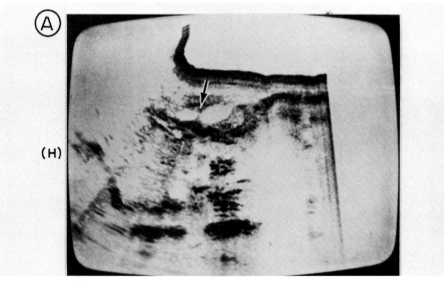

Figure 8. *A*. Longitudinal ultrasonogram demonstrates a double gallbladder with arrow denoting the echoes indicating the separation between the two structures. *B*. Transverse ultrasonogram obtained from the more cephaladly located smaller gallbladder (arrows) (K = kidney). *C*. Transverse ultrasonogram obtained from the more caudad larger gallbladder (arrows). (*Continued on next page*.)

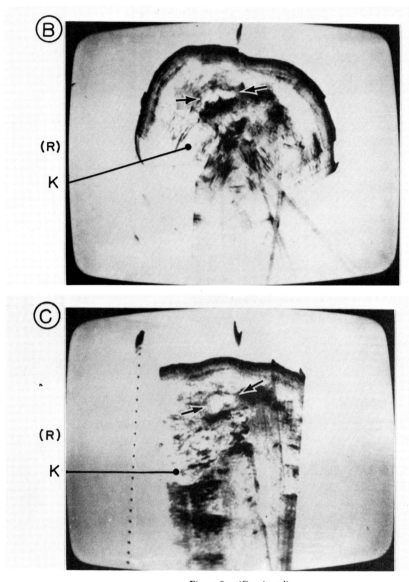

Figure 8. (Continued)

less, ultrasound is useful during the newborn period to evaluate for biliary atresia in which there is congenital atresia of the bile ducts and, in severe cases, of the gallbladder. If ultrasound is able to demonstrate the presence of a gallbladder, it is then often possible to do a life-saving bypass operation by which the bile can be drained from the liver into the gallbladder and then into the bowel. However, if no gallbladder is present, an operation is usually not successful.

GALLSTONES

In evaluating for the presence of gallstones, ultrasound has lower overall accuracy than does oral cholecystography. Thus, if a patient is able to ingest oral contrast agents, x-

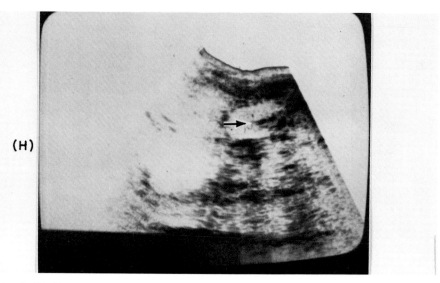

Figure 9. Gallbladder bent on itself producing echoes having the appearance of a septation (arrow). This should not be confused with the diagnosis of a double gallbladder.

ray examination usually is performed first. However, if the gallbladder does not visualize after a single dose, then an ultrasonic study should be performed. Also, in those patients in whom oral cholecystography is not feasible, ultrasound becomes the primary method.

There are many situations in which x-ray examination is not feasible, most important of these being significant jaundice or the inability to take or assimilate an oral contrast agent. Moreover, when an immediate evaluation of the gallbladder is needed, as might be the case when there is a history suggesting acute cholecystitis, ultrasound is the procedure of choice. The ultrasonic examination technique is the same as that previously described for obtaining the size of the gallbladder. Stones will produce internal echoes within the normally echo-free lumen of the gallbladder. The echo patterns recorded can vary depending on the size and type of stones present as well as their location. These variations will be described in the following sections.

Gallstone Patterns

In order to perform a satisfactory ultrasonic examination for gallstones, the entire gallbladder must be surveyed. It is convenient to use a real-time B-scan ultrasonic instrument, which will easily determine the major axes of the gallbladder, for the initial examination. Then, for optimal definition of internal detail, gray scale B-scan imaging is utilized. Each sweep should be linear or sector in nature with no compounding. The patient should hold his breath during each sweep. Final scanning should be limited to the region of the gallbladder in order to obtain optimal detail. While a linear motion is used below the level of the rib cage, a sector sweep is usually needed when the gallbladder is up under the costal margin. A sustained deep inspiration often will displace the gallbladder inferiorly out from under the ribs. With a single linear or sector sweep,

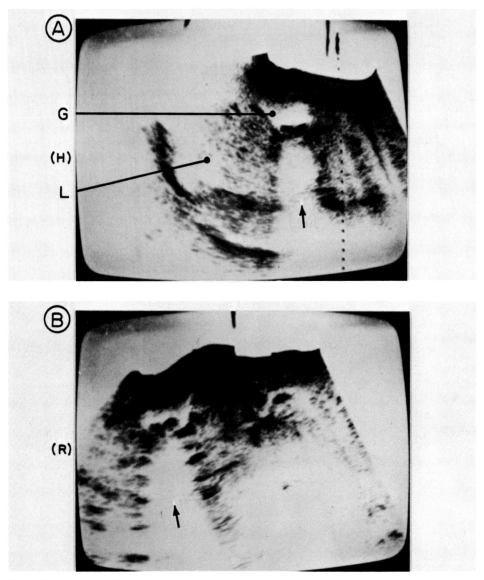

Figure 10. *A.* Longitudinal ultrasonogram reveals strong echoes coming from the inferior aspect of the gall-bladder with acoustic shadow distally (arrow) (G = gallbladder; L = liver). *B.* Transverse ultrasonogram again shows the gallstones that are producing strong echoes and absorption of the ultrasonic beam resulting in an acoustic shadow distally (arrow).

sound reflection and absorption by a stone almost always will result in a decrease in echoes distal to the stone, producing an acoustic shadow (Figure 10). This phenomenon is very helpful in making a definitive diagnosis of gallstones. On occasion, some stones, especially those of high cholesterol and low calcium content as well as those that are very small, will not produce a significant shadow effect. To make a definitive diagnosis in these cases, persistent echoes arising from within the lumen must be demonstrated in several views (Figure 11). To confirm the identification of stone echoes, it is also important to demonstrate shifting of the echo patterns thought to represent gallstones by changing the position of the patient. Scanning is repeated with the patient either decubitus or standing erect and the examiner observes whether the intralumenal echoes shift according to gravitational influences (Figure 12). The best results usually are obtained in the erect position. In the sitting position, any significant subcutaneous fat will produce skin folds that will make it difficult to maintain proper skin contact.

Gallstones usually will gravitate to the most dependent portion of the gallbladder. Also, it is not uncommon for gallstones to layer within the bile assuming a linear pattern parallel to the table top. Changing the patient's position will produce a shift in this layering. If the gallstones are multiple and layer along the entire bottom of the gallbladder in a linear fashion, the novice ultrasonographer might not appreciate their presence (Figure 13). As with any fluid-solid interface, the backwall echoes will be very strong. The correct diagnosis can be made by evaluating the echo pattern distal to the gallbladder. If stones are present, there will be an acoustic shadow. An acoustic shadow often can be better appreciated by looking at the echoes on either side of the gallbladder. These lateral echoes will be stronger and more multiple than the echoes produced after the sound beam has passed through the gallbladder and stones.

Naturally, it is possible to demonstrate not only the presence of multiple stones but also single stones. To date, with present gray scale B-scan equipment, the smallest single stone that has been detected has had a diameter of 3 mm (Figure 14). If the entire gallbladder is not surveyed ultrasonically, small stones can be missed easily. It must be remembered that any significant compounding or retracing over the area of interest can easily obliterate the distal shadow effect. It is often possible to differentiate between a single stone and multiple stones that are in close contract with each other. A single stone usually will produce a curvilinear echo pattern representing its curved anterior surface.

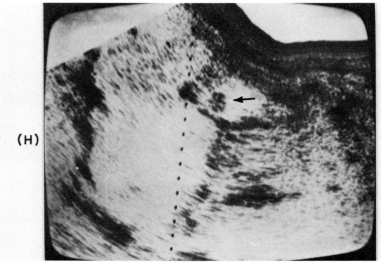

Figure 11.   Longitudinal ultrasonogram shows a gallstone (arrow) that has produced only minimal absorption of the ultrasonic beam distal to it. Note the visualization of its internal structure which is not seen with stones of a more reflective and absorptive character.

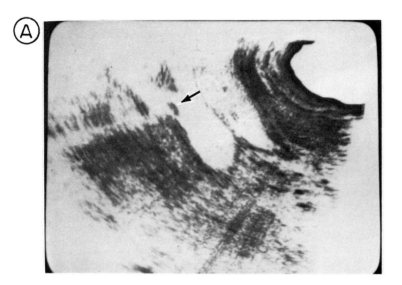

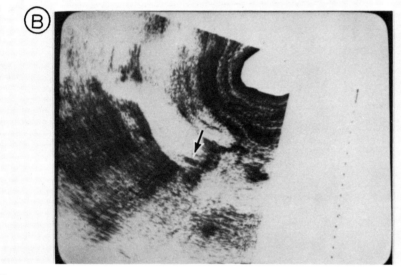

Figure 12. *A.* Initial erect longitudinal ultrasonogram shows gallstone (arrow) located within the upper portion of the gallbladder. *B.* Repeat erect longitudinal ultrasonogram obtained several minutes after the first
examination shows that the stone (arrow) has fallen under gravitational effects to the most dependent portion
of the gallbladder.

In fact, it is possible with a large stone to extend the curve into a complete circle and, in
this way, obtain an estimate of its size. Multiple stones, particularly when relatively
small, will tend to layer in a linear configuration dependent on the effects of gravity.

In general, gallstones are best demonstrated when surrounded on at least three sides
by bile. If the gallbladder is contracted or is so filled with stones that there is very little
fluid present, its outline will be poorly defined. In this situation, the only evidence of
gallstones may be the previously described shadow effect just distal to a group of strong

echoes. The acoustic shadow often will be curvilinear in shape, arising from the anterior stone surface(s) (Figure 15). It may be difficult to differentiate this pattern from acoustic shadows caused by other sound absorbing substances such as bowel gas. If confusion with bowel gas shadows is a concern, the examination should be repeated the next morning after fasting. If the pattern, i.e., strong echoes and a distal shadow effect, remains unchanged in position, it is unlikely that bowel gas could be responsible. In

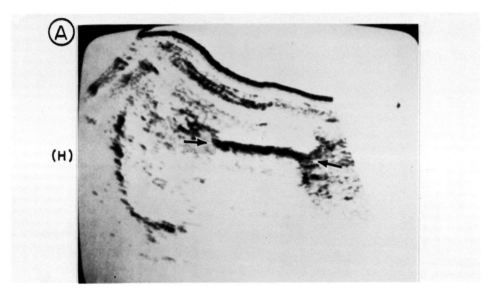

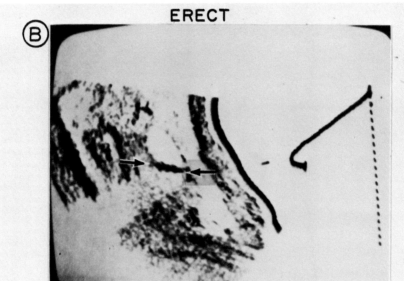

Figure 13. *A.* Supine longitudinal ultrasonogram demonstrates multiple gallstones (arrows) layering along the bottom of the gallbladder. *B.* Erect longitudinal ultrasonogram shows shifting of the layering gallstones (arrows) due to gravitational effects. Note the distal acoustic shadow that also is helpful in making the appropriate diagnosis.

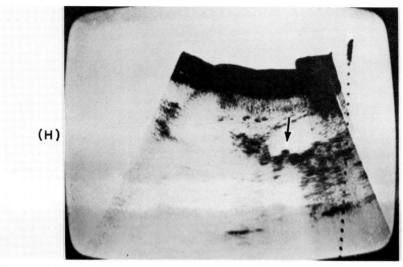

Figure 14.   Longitudinal ultrasonogram reveals a 3-mm gallstone (arrow) within a normal-sized gallbladder.

summary, a persistent pattern in the right upper quadrant in the region of the bed of the gallbladder is highly suggestive of a stone-filled gallbladder.

Most of the studies evaluating the accuracy of ultrasound in diagnosing gallstones have been performed utilizing units not equipped with a gray scale display. The reported accuracy has varied from 100 percent to as low as 50 percent (1, 4–12). With gray scale B-scan techniques, the accuracy in stone detection has been found to be approximately 92 percent. These results are still slightly less than the accuracy of oral cholecystography. False negative results occur most commonly when: (a) there are very small stones, (b) the gallbladder is large (since it is more likely that a thorough examination will not be carried out), and (c) when a stone is impacted in the cystic duct. A cystic duct stone represents essentially the same diagnostic problem as does a stone-filled contracted gallbladder. Due to the lack of fluid surrounding the stone, it is often difficult to identify a cystic duct stone. However, it is sometimes possible to suggest the presence of a cystic duct stone by eliciting a typical stone shadow effect in the region where the cystic duct would normally be located. Of course, if there is associated gallbladder distension or stones in the main portion of the gallbladder, these conditions increase the probability of such an abnormality.

In conclusion, while ultrasonic gallstone evaluation is not the primary study of choice if x-ray can visualize the gallbladder, it is useful either when there is nonvisualization after oral cholecystography or when an x-ray examination cannot be performed due to many different causes. Also, ultrasound should be considered as the primary method of study whenever an immediate evaluation is clinically indicated.

INFLAMMATION OF THE GALLBLADDER

While it is not routinely possible even with gray scale B-scan ultrasound to define the presence of minimal thickening of the walls, thickening can be demonstrated in advanced cases. Using standard ultrasonic techniques as previously described, a double-rim effect will be produced due to reflections from both the inner and outer walls of the diseased gallbladder (Figure 16). This pattern appears to be seen most commonly with chronic rather than acute thickening. Of course, repeated bouts of inflammation usually will result in a contracted gallbladder that is difficult to visualize ultrasonically. With an acute process, there can be perforation and abscess formation. Ultrasound is able to demonstrate the presence of an abscess. However, if the walls are smooth and a separate

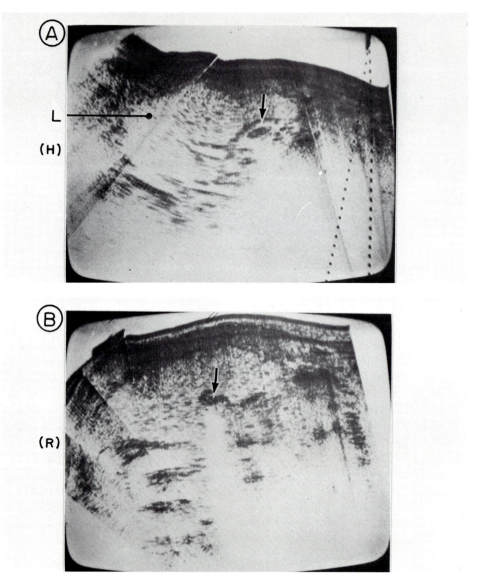

Figure 15. *A.* Longitudinal ultrasonogram demonstrates strong echoes from within the region where the gallbladder normally is located thought to represent gallstones (arrow). Note distal shadow effect (L = liver). *B.* Transverse ultrasonogram obtained from the same patient again shows strong echoes thought to represent gallstones (arrow), producing a distal shadow effect. For confirmation a repeat examination the following day showed no change in this pattern.

gallbladder cannot be identified, differentiating an abscess from a dilated gallbladder (i.e., hydrops) sometimes may be impossible. Obviously, there can be other causes for the presence of predominantly cystic or complex masses in the right upper quadrant, such as pancreatic pseudocyst, hydronephrosis and subhepatic abscess. Thus, the history and other clinical findings are important in helping to arrive at a specific diagnosis.

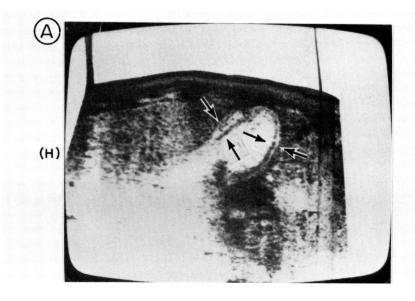

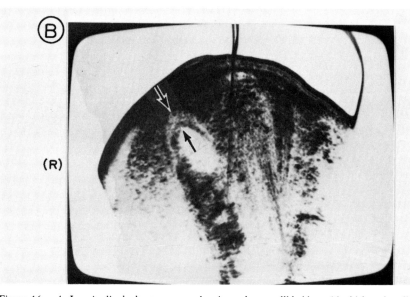

Figure 16.   *A.* Longitudinal ultrasonogram showing a large gallbladder with thickened walls shown by a double-rim effect of echoes (arrows). *B.* Transverse ultrasonogram from the same patient again shows the thickening of the gallbladder walls (arrows).

In addition to a localized abscess, a ruptured gallbladder also may produce peritoneal irritation with development of ascitic fluid, which also can be evaluated ultrasonically. The ultrasonic transducer initially is positioned to examine the most dependent parts of the abdomen, where free fluid will normally tend to collect. If a positive cystic ultrasonic pattern is obtained, the patient is moved to the opposite decubitus position without changing the transducer-skin relationship. The transducer will then be at a point furthest away from the table. The fluid, if free, will gravitate away from the transducer with disappearance of the cystic ultrasonic pattern. The exception is loculated collections that will show no significant pattern change.

In conclusion, although it is possible to demonstrate thickening of the walls produced by inflammation, this is not a consistent finding. Thickened wall echo patterns have been recorded most frequently with chronic rather than acute gallbladder disease. As is true in any examination site, if there is gas within the walls, as can occur from severe infection, there would be poor ultrasonic definition. Ultrasound can demonstrate successfully secondary signs of acute inflammation, such as abscess formation or ascitic fluid due to peritoneal irritation by bile. Of course, ascites and cholelithiasis can occur independently (Figure 17). Other cystic or complex masses can also occur in the right upper quadrant making it difficult to determine a specific diagnosis without additional clinical information.

GALLBLADDER SLUDGE

In obtaining ultrasonograms of the gallbladder, internal echoes not due to stones occasionally may be demonstrated in the most dependent portions. This type of echo is not accompanied by significant sound absorption resulting in distal shadow effects as would be the case with almost all stones (Figure 18). At surgery it has been found that these echoes are produced by sludge, that is, thick secretions and granules resting on the bottom of the gallbladder. The echoes arising from sludge are normally weaker than those produced from the surface of stones. Sludge-type echoes are seen most commonly in gallbladders that have not emptied over a prolonged period, such as can occur when a patient is obstructed. When a patient is turned into a decubitus position or stood erect, the sludge-type echoes tend to shift at a much slower rate than do stones. This can be helpful in making the proper diagnosis.

CARCINOMA OF THE GALLBLADDER

To date, polyps or other types of masses have not been detected ultrasonically within the gallbladder. Carcinoma usually is seen in an advanced state, and often there is complete involvement of the gallbladder so that a differential diagnosis of right upper quadrant solid mass must include the possibility of carcinoma (Figure 19). There may be associated jaundice due to involvement of the common bile duct resulting in dilatation of the proximally located bile ducts. Nodes also may be visualized in the region of the porta hepatis. As is well known, other tumors can project into the right upper quadrant, i.e., renal and pancreatic tumors, resulting in compression of the gallbladder. Thus, a high degree of suspicion must be maintained if the diagnosis of carcinoma of the gallbladder is to be made ultrasonically.

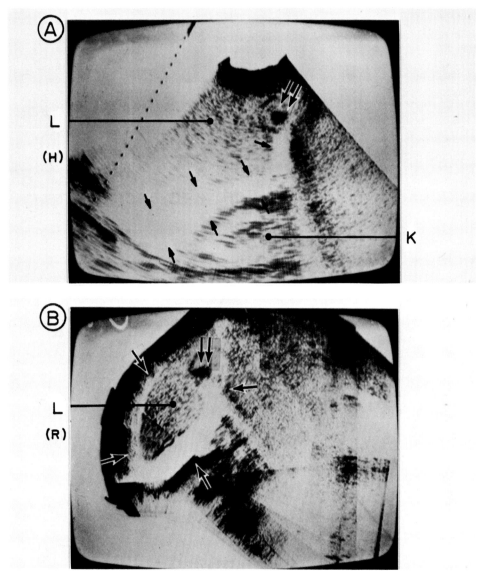

Figure 17. *A*. Longitudinal ultrasonogram demonstrates a gallstone (double arrow) producing acoustic shadow effect. Echo-free areas around liver represent ascites (arrows) (L = liver; K = kidney). *B*. Transverse ultrasonogram of the same patient shows the gallstone (double arrow) and echo-free zones around liver representing ascites (arrows) (L = liver).

BILE DUCTS

As noted earlier in the discussion of examination techniques, it is possible to record portions of the bile ducts, especially when dilated, using gray scale B-scan ultrasound (13). Not only can the intrahepatic ducts be visualized but also portions of the common bile duct. The ducts tend to be seen as linear tubular structures when normal. In order to record the common bile duct, the gallbladder is first visualized. Longitudinal scans are

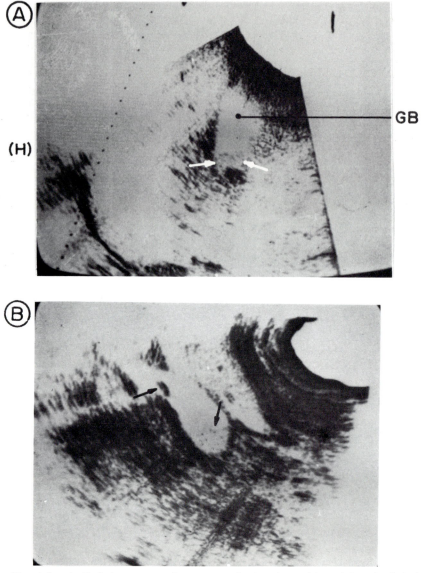

Figure 18.   *A*. Longitudinal ultrasonogram shows very weak echoes (arrows) located dependently in the gallbladder (GB) producing no significant shadow effect. This is consistent with the diagnosis of sludge. *B*. Longitudinal ultrasonogram shows the very weak echoes (lower arrow) due to sludge in contrast to the superiorly
located stone (upper arrow) that is producing a distal shadow effect.

then started at a point just medial to the gallbladder. Linear sweeps are obtained during
suspended respiration at small intervals, usually 0.5 cm, since the common bile duct is
normally less than 1 cm in diameter. If the duct is not located, longitudinal oblique
scans then are obtained in varying degrees of obliquity, since the duct often does not
have a true longitudinal course. Real-time B-scan ultrasound may be helpful in locating
the correct pathway. However, it should be noted that in the vast majority of cases it is
impossible to detect any significant portion of a normal common bile duct.

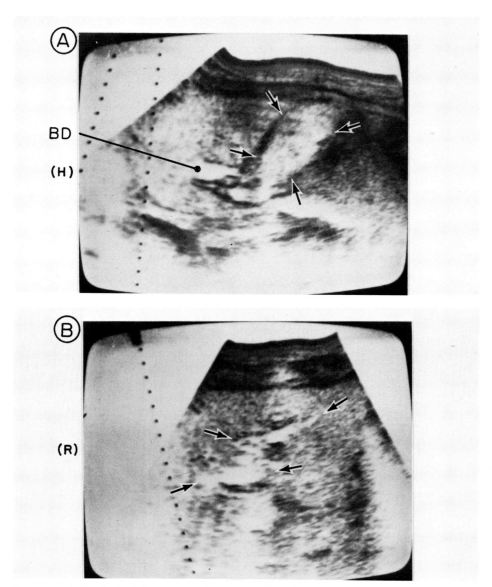

Figure 19. *A*. Longitudinal ultrasonogram shows faint outline of what appears to be an enlarged gallbladder with multiple internal echoes (arrows). This is consistent with the diagnosis of carcinoma of the gallbladder. Note proximal echo-free area representing a dilated bile duct (BD). *B*. Transverse ultrasonogram obtained just proximal to the region of the gallbladder carcinoma showing multiple dilated bile ducts (arrows).

As the bile ducts dilate they become much easier to visualize ultrasonically. The intra-hepatic portions become more tortuous and can be recorded in both longitudinal and transverse scans (Figure 20). It is usually not difficult to differentiate them from the hepatic veins that can be seen near the diaphragm usually extending in a vertical direction and entering the inferior vena cava. If there is any question, a Valsalva maneuver will produce venous distention helping to make the correct diagnosis. However, there may be some initial difficulty in differentiating the intrahepatic bile ducts from the portal veins. The best approach is to demonstrate a communication between the intrahepatic dilated structures and their extrahepatic components, that is, either the common bile duct or portal vein. Real-time B-scan ultrasound is helpful in locating and following these structures (14, 15). The common bile duct tends to run with its long axis predominantly longitudinal, whereas the extrahepatic portion of the portal system tends to run with its major axis transverse. Also, the portal system can be seen to cross the midline. This does not occur with the common bile duct. As with the hepatic veins, the portal veins usually will distend in response to a Valsalva maneuver, helping to make

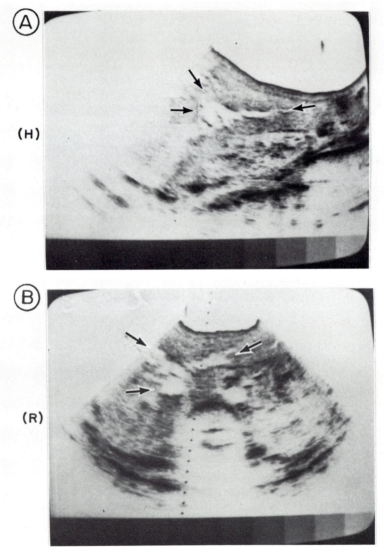

Figure 20. *A*. Longitudinal ultrasonogram shows multiple dilated intrahepatic bile ducts (arrows). *B*. Transverse ultrasonogram shows multiple intrahepatic dilated bile ducts (arrows). *C*. Longitudinal ultrasonogram obtained just medial to the gallbladder shows a portion of the dilated common bile duct. Branching can be seen near its cephaled portion (arrows). (*Continued on next page.*)

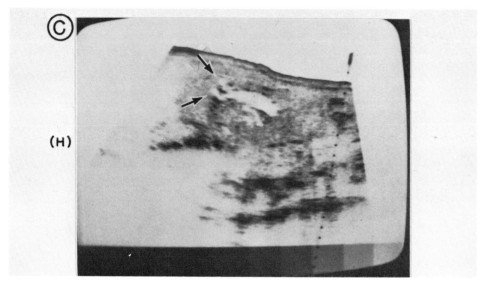

Figure 20. (Continued)

the correct differential diagnosis. By careful scanning and deductive reasoning, it is usually possible to decide whether the dilated intrahepatic structures are bile ducts or portal veins. Of course, it is possible to have both occurring in the same patient. The bile ducts are located anatomically anterior to the portal veins. On occasion both may be visualized, especially with bile duct dilatation. The common bile duct passes anterior to the main portal vein as the duct courses downward towards the pancreas.

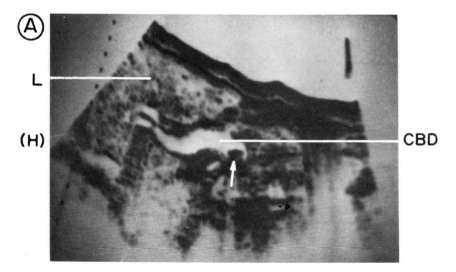

Figure 21. *A*. Longitudinal ultrasonogram shows a dilated common bile duct (CBD) with proximal branching. Near the distal end are strong internal echoes consistent with the diagnosis of a common duct stone (arrow). *B*. Transverse ultrasonogram obtained at the level of the suspected common bile duct stone on the previous longitudinal ultrasonogram shows strong echoes within the dilated duct consistent with the diagnosis of a stone (arrow). Note distal shadow effect. In this patient the gallbladder had been previously removed.

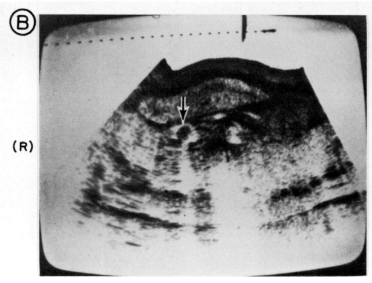

Figure 21.   (Continued)

Ultrasound is able to differentiate jaundice that is due to intrahepatic disease from jaundice due to extrahepatic obstruction (16–19). If careful scanning of the liver reveals no dilated ducts, the jaundice is due to a nonobstructive cause, most likely intrahepatic in nature such as hepatitis or severe cirrhosis. On the other hand, if there is evidence of dilated ducts, this indicates an extrahepatic obstructive cause for the jaundice. If a dilated common bile duct can be demonstrated, then the obstruction must be distal to the porta hepatis and is most likely due to either choledocholithiasis or pancreatic carcinoma. If a dilated common bile duct cannot be recorded, the possibility that the obstruction is in the region of the porta hepatis must be considered. Obstruction in this region is most commonly due to metastatic nodes or perhaps carcinoma of the gallbladder and/or bile ducts. Of course with acute obstruction, the bile ducts may not yet have dilated.

Secondary signs are often helpful in arriving at an appropriate diagnosis. Thus, in the presence of jaundice, ultrasonograms of the pancreas always should be obtained to check for indications of enlargement that would suggest carcinoma. It must be remembered that chronic pancreatitis may also cause pancreatic enlargement and even produce jaundice by stricture formation. The presence of painless jaundice, pancreatic enlargement (especially of its head, associated with a dilated gallbladder without stones known as a Courvoisier's gallbladder) is strongly suggestive of pancreatic carcinoma. The presence of stones within the gallbladder without evidence of pancreatic enlargement would indicate that choledocholithiasis is a more likely cause for the presence of dilated bile ducts. It is possible to demonstrate the presence of internal echoes within the common bile duct indicating the presence of stones (Figure 21). If a linear scan has been obtained, a distal shadow effect can often be demonstrated beneath the stones. Even if a cause for the dilated bile ducts cannot be detected, the usefulness of the ultrasonic examination is not impaired, since the presence of a dilated common bile duct usually indicates a need for surgery. As a result of the ultrasonic technique, there has been a definite decrease in the need for transhepatic cholangiography or other invasive methods to establish a cause for jaundice. The overall accuracy of ultrasound in its ability to differentiate obstructive

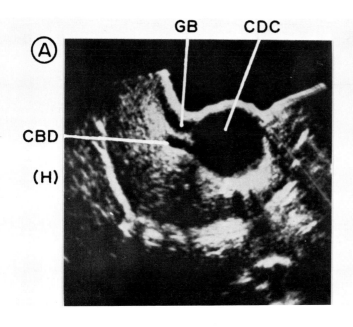

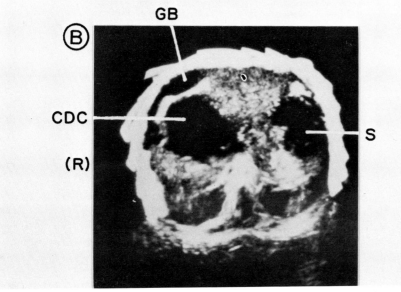

Figure 22. *A.* Longitudinal ultrasonogram demonstrates the choledochal cyst (CDC). A portion of the common bile duct (CBD) can be seen to enter the choledochal cyst. The gallbladder (GB) is located anterior and superior to the area of interest. *B.* Transverse ultrasonogram shows the choledochal cyst (CDC) with its relationship clearly defined to the gallbladder (GB) which is located to the right and superiorly (S = spleen). (Courtesy of Filly RA, Carlsen EN: *J Clin Ultrasound* **4**:7–10, 1976. Reproduced from *Journal Clinical Ultrasound* with permission.)

from nonobstructive jaundice has been reported to be as high as 97 percent, better than for any other noninvasive method (20). Thus, ultrasound should be considered as the primary study of choice in any patient with jaundice.

Finally, a congenital cystic dilatation of the common bile duct, although uncommon, may occur. This is known as a choledochal cyst. It may be difficult to differentiate initially from other cystic structures that can be found in the right upper quadrant such as a markedly dilated gallbladder or pancreatic pseudocyst. However, there are certain characteristics that can be helpful. One of the most important is the establishment ultrasonically of the cystic or common bile duct entering the choledochal cyst (21). Also, an attempt should be made to demonstrate the presence of the gallbladder and its relationship to the cystic structure (Figure 22). While oral cholecystography can make the diagnosis of choledochal cyst, if jaundice is present, which is not uncommon, ultrasound certainly becomes the initial procedure of choice.

REFERENCES

1. Goldberg BB, Harris K, Broocker W: Ultrasonic and radiographic cholecystography. *Radiology* **111**:405–409, May 1974.

2. Carlsen EN: Liver, gallbladder and spleen. *Radiology Clinics of N Amer* **13**:543–555, December 1975.

3. Leopold GR, Sokoloff J: Ultrasonic scanning in the diagnosis of biliary disease. *Surg Clin N Amer* **53**:1043, 1973.

4. Hublitz UF, Kahn PC, Sell LA: Cholecystosonography: an approach to the nonvisualized gallbladder. *Radiology* **103**:645–649, June 1972.

5. Inada G, Ishizaki M: Comparative studies on roentgenologic and ultrasonic diagnosis of gallstone patients. *Nagoya Med J* **14**:145–149, October 1968.

6. Mastriukov VA, Shpinela EA: Ultrasonic study in cholecystitis. *Nov Med Priborostr* **1**:118–126, 1970.

7. Matsukara S, Shirota A, Miki M, et al: A new ultrasonic diagnostic recording apparatus for cholelithiasis: the supersonogram. *Int Surg* **50**:381–398, October 1968.

8. Smoldas J: Impulse reflection passage ultrasonic method in the diagnosis of bile stones. *Rev Czech Med* **14** (2):73–78, 1968.

9. Smoldas J: Some problems of the ultrasonic diagnosis of bile stones. *Digestion* **3**:65–72, 1970.

10. Tala P, Lieto J, Kerminen T, et al: Ultrasonic diagnosis of cholelithiasis. *Ann Chir Gynaec Fenn* **55**:124–128, 1966.

11. Zobkov VV, Gaisinskii BE: Ultrasound echography of the gallbladder. *Urach delo* **2**:8–10, February 1967.

12. Doust BD, Malsad NF: Ultrasonic B-mode examination of the gallbladder, technique and criteria for diagnosis of gallstones. *Radiology* **110**:643–647, 1974.

13. Taylor KJW, Carpenter DA: The anatomy and pathology of the porta hepatis demonstrated by grey scale ultrasonography. *J Clin Ultrasound* **3**:117–119, 1975.

14. Weill F, Bourgoin A, Aucant D, Eisencher A, Faivre M, Gillet M: L'exploration tomo-echographique des dilatations de la voie biliarire principale. *Arch Fr Mal App Dig* **63**:453–472, 1974.

15. Weill F, Eisenscher A, Aucant D, Bourgoin A, Gallinet D: Ultrasonic study of venous patterns in the right hypochondrium: an anatomical approach to differential diagnosis of obstructive jaundice. *J Clin Ultrasound* **3**:23–28, 1975.

16. Fukada M, Natori H, Matsumura M, Urushizaki I: Sensitivity graded ultrasonotomography on bile duct disorders. *Med Ultrason* **11**:19–21, 1973.

17. Taylor KJW, Carpenter DA, McCready VR: Ultrasound and scintigraphy in the differential diagnosis of obstructive jaundice. *J Clin Ultrasound* **2**:105–116, June 1974.

18. Stone SB, Ferrucci JT, Jr, Warshaw AL, Wittenberg J, Slutsky M: Gray scale ultrasound diagnosis of obstructive biliary disease. *Am J Roentgenol* **125:**47–50, September 1975.

19. Goldberg BB: Ultrasonic cholangiography. *Radiology* **118:**401–404, February 1976.

20. Taylor, KJW, Glees JP, Smith IA, Carpenter DA: Accuracy of grey-scale ultrasonic examination of the liver, in White DN, Barnes RW (eds): *Ultrasound in Medicine,* vol 2. New York, Plenum Press, 1976, pp 173–197.

21. Filly RA, Carlsen EN: Choledochal cyst: report of a case with specific ultrasonographic findings. J Clin Ultrasound **4:**7–10, 1976.

7
Pancreas

Gordon S. Perlmutter, M.D.
Clinical Associate Professor of Radiology
Temple University Health Sciences Center
Philadelphia, Pennsylvania

Director, Ultrasound Section
The Reading Hospital
West Reading, Pennsylvania

In spite of all attempts to evaluate it, the pancreas continues to be an elusive organ from the standpoint of diagnosis. This generalization applies not only to indirect methods of visualizing the pancreas but also to direct inspection and palpation at laparotomy.

Each new modality for imaging the pancreas and related structures has generated much initial enthusiasm in the belief that a reliable diagnostic tool finally has been found. However, with increasing clinical experience, each modality has been found to be of less value than first anticipated.

Barium contrast studies of the upper gastrointestinal tract can provide only indirect evidence of pancreatic disease consisting of changes in the stomach and duodenum secondary to extrinsic pressure or direct invasion by diseases of the pancreas. This information, however, is usually only the tip of the iceberg barely revealing far advanced, and all too often incurable, disease of the pancreas, if at all. This inadequacy is reflected in the relatively low accuracy rate of 50–60 percent reported for upper gastrointestinal series (1, 2). Even with hypotonic studies, the accuracy of an upper gastrointestinal series is only 78 percent, including one series reporting 40 percent of patients with known pancreatic disease as having a normal study (3).

Nuclear medicine generated renewed interest in the pancreas as the result of the initial discovery that the pancreas could be visualized with selenomethionine Se 75 and, in more recent times, with gallium citrate Ga 67. After the initial flurry of investigations with these agents, it became clear that the pancreas again had eluded all but gross detection. The procedure is not only costly and time consuming, but also has a disappointingly low accuracy rate of 50 percent for patients with abnormal scans. A radionuclide scan, if normal, may be useful in ruling out pancreatic disease with an accuracy of 90 percent in patients where other tests yield equivocal results (4).

Angiography provided an additional tool in evaluating the pancreas via its blood supply. Investigators have gone to great length detailing the angiographic signs of various diseases of the pancreas. To be sure, specific pancreatic tumors such as islet cell carcinomas can be detected by angiography with an accuracy rate in the 90 percent range. Yet the differentiation of pancreatitis, particularly chronic focal pancreatitis, from a relatively avascular tumor can be exceedingly difficult if not impossible by angiography even with selective and pharmacoangiographic techniques. Angiography remains the method of choice in diagnosing small islet cell tumors and in determining the extent of tumor invasion and metastasis (1, 5, 6). Because of the cost and invasiveness of the procedure, it usually is performed only on those patients who are highly suspect of having pancreatic carcinoma and on whom the other screening tests are negative. It also may be performed as a preoperative planning procedure on patients with known carcinoma.

Endoscopic retrograde cannulation of the pancreatic duct is a relatively new method of pancreatic evaluation. This procedure is time consuming, costly, prone to a high failure rate, and not without complication. The accuracy rate is poor in diagnosing acute pancreatitis but good (87–90 percent) in diagnosing chronic pancreatitis and neoplasm. Retrograde filling of pancreatic pseudocysts has been achieved in several cases (7).

Computerized axial tomography, from early reports, appears to offer yet another means of imaging the pancreas. While it appears that it will be a relatively effective way of detecting enlargement of and masses in the pancreas, the degree of specificity remains to be investigated. Because of equipment costs, this procedure will not be widely available for some time to come. Where available, it will be costly and probably invasive in that contrast enhancement most likely will have to be used.

Ultrasound provides a noninvasive method of evaluating the pancreas which, unlike the other modalities already mentioned, is free of ionizing radiation. The earliest investigations conducted with A-mode equipment were able to evaluate only masses large enough to be localized by palpation or by correlative radiographs. Cystic and solid masses could be differentiated if large enough, but the normal pancreas could not be seen. Bistable B-mode scans of the pancreas offered a new dimension in imaging the pancreas. Masses 3 cm or greater as well as generalized pancreatic enlargement often could be visualized. Accuracy rates of 85–90 percent have been reported (8, 9). The criteria developed for differentiating the various types of pancreatic disease using these bistable displays have proved reliable and remain essentially unchallenged in spite of the many articles that have been written on this topic in the recent literature (1, 5, 8, 10–14). Despite claims to the contrary, it continues to be difficult if not impossible to visualize the normal pancreas with commercially available bistable scanners. Articles purporting to demonstrate the normal pancreas on bistable units must be taken with reservation since in several cases the structures identified were the splenic vein, duodenum, or a pathologically enlarged pancreas (5).

The development of gray scale ultrasound units has resulted in a dramatic improvement in ultrasound imaging. The improved resolution and dynamic range of commercially available gray scale units permits visualization not only of the normal and abnormal pancreas but also of the contiguous vascular structures and biliary tract (15, 16). Examples of the normal pancreas and its relationship to surrounding retroperitoneal structures will be shown in the following section. With this newer modality, subtle differences in pancreatic structure can be shown and improved accuracy, probably in the 90–95 percent range, is to be expected although statistics are as yet unpublished.

Not only is it possible to evaluate the pancreas directly but it is also possible with gray scale ultrasound to evaluate adjacent structures such as the common bile duct, intrahepatic biliary radicles, and the gallbladder. The interrelationship of the biliary tract and the pancreas often result in associated changes in both areas that together provide valuable clues to a diagnosis (17–22). An example of this would be the demonstration of a dilated stone-filled gallbladder in a patient with pancreatitis. In evaluating the pancreas it is therefore mandatory also to evaluate the biliary tract thoroughly.

Ultrasound is a cheap, rapid, noninvasive, and relatively accurate means of evaluating the pancreas. In institutions where it is available, ultrasound is used either as an initial screening study or is performed in conjunction with an upper gastrointestinal series (23). If both studies are negative and the clinical suspicion of pancreatic disease is weak, further evaluation of the pancreas is not indicated. Radionuclide scans are the next step in the evaluation when there is strong clinical indication of pancreatic disease but inconclusive or discrepant findings on the barium and ultrasound studies. If both the upper gastrointestinal series and the ultrasound studies are positive and the ultrasound scans demonstrate the presence of acute pancreatitis or pancreatic pseudocyst with good clinical correlation, the work-up is considered completed (1). Solid masses documented on ultrasound examination probably will be evaluated further preoperatively with angiography, endoscopic retrograde pancreatography, and needle aspiration biopsy depending on the clinical setting and the availability of these studies. It is envisioned that computerized axial tomography will probably be of greatest value where ultrasound is unable to yield an adequate diagnostic study.

Techniques for performing ultrasound scans and the ultrasound manifestations of various disease processes of the pancreas will be presented in detail in the following sections.

TECHNIQUE

Ultrasound scans of the pancreas are performed on commercially available gray scale scanning units. A standard 2.25 MHz 19-mm diameter scanning transducer focused at 10 cm is used in most cases. Occasionally it is helpful to substitute a 1.6 MHz transducer for obese patients in whom depth penetration is limited. The use of focused transducers is critical for the lateral resolution needed in pancreatic scanning. It is also important for the scanning arm to be in good alignment and to track accurately.

Scans are first performed transversely on the supine patient beginning at the level of the xiphoid process and proceeding caudally at 2-cm steps to approximately the level of the umbilicus. These scans are performed at 3 cm per graticule magnification, but as the pancreatic region comes into view, additional scans at higher magnification, usually 2 cm per graticule, are obtained.

The pancreas is recognized as an echo-producing structure 2–3 cm thick paralleling but slightly anterior and inferior to the splenic vein (5, 15) (Figure 1). The splenic vein usually can be recognized even if the pancreas at first eludes detection (Figure 2). As these structures are located, marks are made on the skin surface corresponding to them. These marks indicate an oblique plane of scanning that parallels the long axis of the pancreas and is quite variable from patient to patient. Additional scans are then performed in this plane of obliquity at 1-cm steps (Figure 3). A technique has been described wherein the transducer also is angled approximately 20 degrees cephalad, but this method has proved successful only in patients with a low rib cage and narrow xiphoid angle (1).

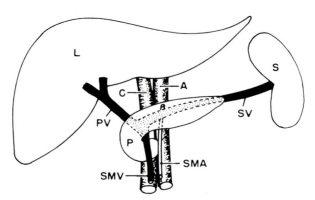

Figure 1.   Frontal view of the upper abdominal anatomy (C = inferior vena cava; A = aorta; P = pancreas; PV = portal vein; SV = splenic vein; SMV = superior mesenteric vein; SMA = superior mesenteric artery).

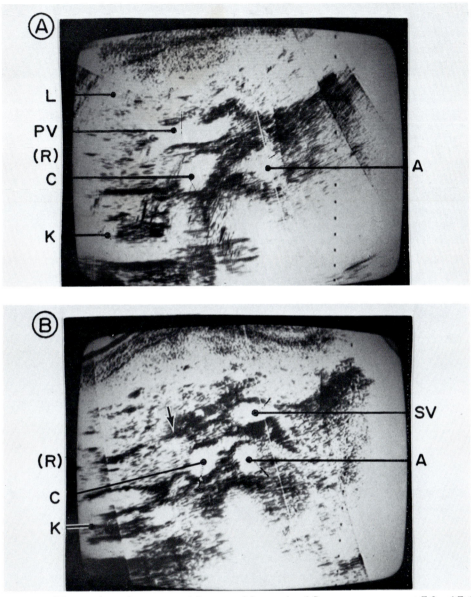

Figure 2.   Ultrasound vascular anatomy of the upper abdomen. *A* and *B* are transverse scans at Z-2 and Z-4 respectively. (R) = right side on all transverse scans. Arrow in *B* indicates caudate lobe of liver, not to be confused with the pancreas (K = kidney; L = liver).

Finally, a series of longitudinal or sagittal scans at 2-cm intervals across the abdomen are performed with the patient supine. Additional scans in various obliquities also are performed when necessary to help clarify the course and orientation of structures such as the gallbladder, portal vein, and common bile duct. Although some investigators perform the longitudinal scans first, this is purely a matter of personal preference since adequate scans can be obtained either way (14, 24).

At times, the conventional methods of scanning fail to image the pancreas satisfactorily. When this occurs, the head of the pancreas frequently can be rendered accessible to the ultrasonic beam by turning the patient in the right decubitus position. This is due to movement of the liver and transverse colon antero-inferiorly displacing the bowel gas out of the area of interest. The displaced liver serves as an acoustic window. In this posi-

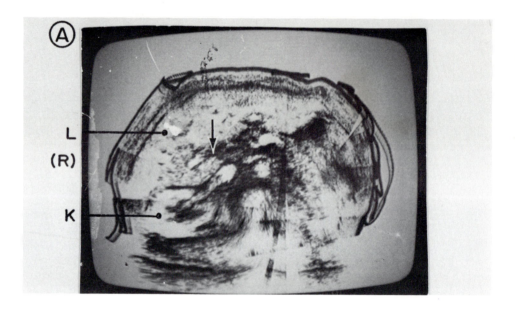

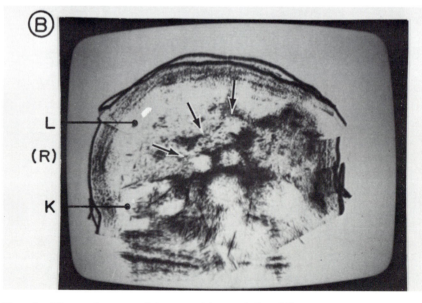

Figure 3.   Ultrasound anatomy of the upper abdomen. *A, B,* and *C* are transverse scans at Z-4, Z-5, and Z-6 respectively. Arrow in *A* indicates caudate lobe of liver. Arrows in *B* and *C* indicate the pancreas. (*Continued on next page.*)

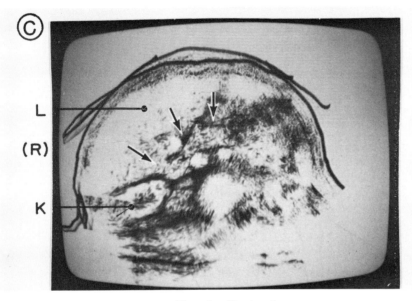

Figure 3.   (Continued)

tion, fluid, rather than air, occupies the second portion of the duodenum which one should not mistake for a cystic mass. The tail of the pancreas often can be visualized, when not otherwise seen, by scanning over the left kidney with the patient in the prone position.

All scans are performed by a single sweep technique with the patient in suspended respiration insofar as possible. A suspended deep inspiration or Valsalva maneuver often is helpful in distending the inferior vena cava and portal vessels rendering them more obvious (5).

Scans are performed on fasting patients insofar as scheduling permits. Patients are not scheduled following barium studies because of the deleterious effects of barium on scan quality (25). Scheduling after meals also is avoided since air in the stomach and upper intestine also interferes with sound penetration.

The best scans are obtained on thin patients and patients with hepatomegaly since the enlarged liver covers the pancreas displacing the loops of bowel away from the area of interest. The opposite is true for obese patients with protuberant abdomens and normal or small livers. The technique of applying gentle pressure to the abdominal wall with the scanning transducer is often helpful in displacing interfering bowel gas.

The bowel gas problem turns out to be one of the most serious impediments to obtaining adequate ultrasound scans. A scan is not considered adequate for pancreatic imaging unless the aorta, inferior vena cava, and anterior border of the spine are seen in the plane of the pancreas (14). Occasionally passing a nasogastric tube may be of some help in aspirating air from the stomach. Distending the stomach with fluid has not been helpful unless air, which is inevitably swallowed along with the fluid, can be aspirated (5, 15). Attempts to reduce the bowel gas content by administering a simethicone preparation starting 2–3 days prior to the examination has met with some success in elective cases (26).

NORMAL PANCREAS

The normal pancreas is a uniformly echo-producing structure with coarse internal echoes as strong or stronger than the echoes seen within the liver. The normal pancreas measures 3 cm in thickness (AP dimension) at its head and 2 cm in thickness in the body and tail (Figure 4). The body of the pancreas is located anterior, inferior, and in close

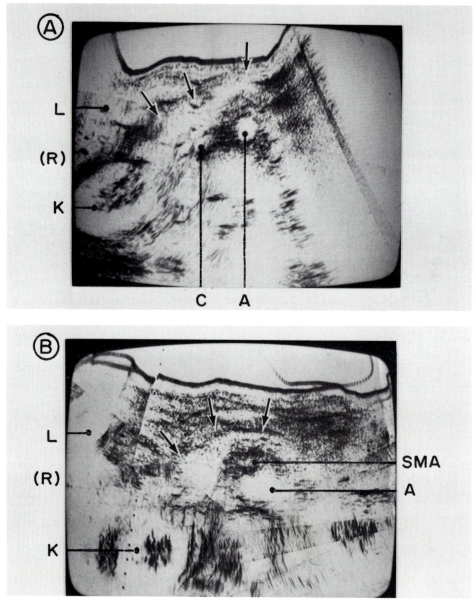

Figure 4.   Normal ultrasound anatomy of the pancreas in three different patients. All scans are transverse at Z-4 to Z-6. (*Continued on next page.*)

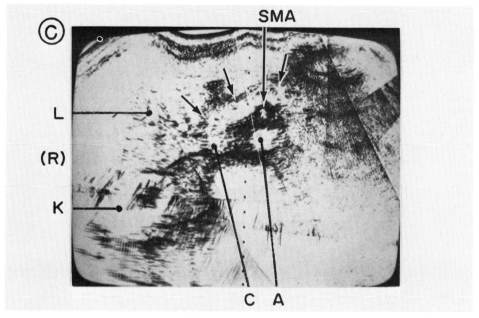

Figure 4.   (Continued)

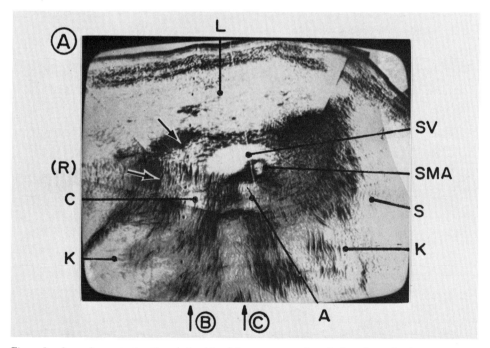

Figure 5.   Scans demonstrating the relationship of the pancreas to the splenic and portal veins. Arrows in *A* and *B* indicate the head of the pancreas. Arrows below transverse scan *A* indicate plane of longitudinal scans *B* and *C*. (R) = right on all transverse scans. (H) = cephalad on all longitudinal scans.

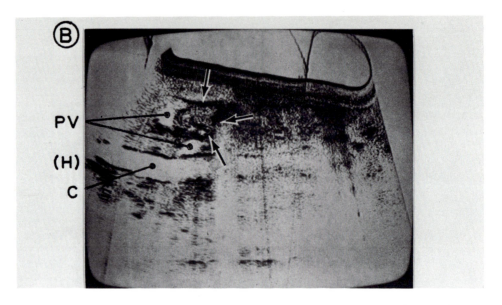

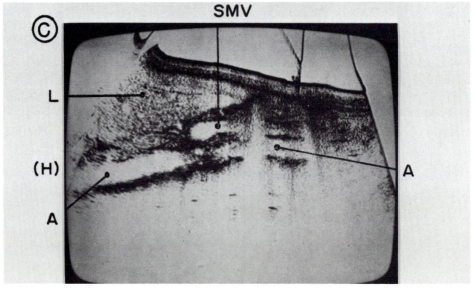

Figure 5. (Continued)

proximity to the splenic vein (14) (Figure 5). The neck of the pancreas is at the confluence of the splenic and superior mesenteric veins with the portal vein (27, 28). The pancreatic head is immediately anterior to the inferior vena cava. The pancreas is anterior to the aorta and superior mesenteric artery (except for an occasionally prominent uncinate process that may be interposed between these two arteries) and posterior only to the left lobe of the liver, the gallbladder, and the stomach. Although a retroperitoneal structure, the pancreas is located surprisingly close to the anterior abdominal wall, particularly in the thin patient (29).

A clear border should be visible between the liver and the pancreas. Care should be taken not to confuse a prominent caudate lobe of the liver for the head of the pancreas (Figure 3). A tubular echo-free or nearly echo-free structure measuring 0.6–1.2 cm in diameter coursing transversely across the abdomen anterior to the origin of the superior mesenteric artery all too frequently has been identified erroneously as the pancreas. It is not the pancreas, but the splenic vein with which the pancreas is intimately related (Figure 5). The identity of the splenic vein can be established by demonstrating its

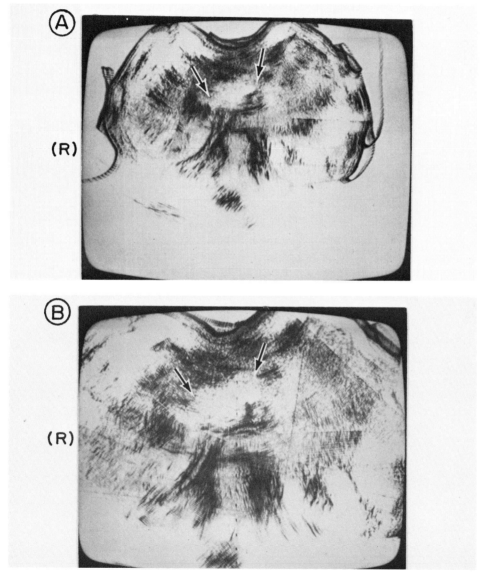

Figure 6.   Acute pancreatitis. Diffuse pancreatic enlargement and decreased echogenicity are demonstrated (arrows). *B* is a magnified view of *A*. (*Continued on next page.*)

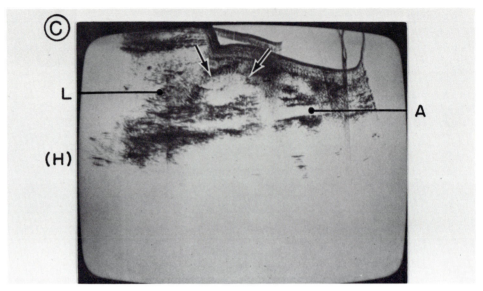

Figure 6.   (Continued)

confluence with the portal vein and by observing changes in caliber of both these vessels as the result of a Valsalva maneuver. Occasionally the pancreas is confused with the third and fourth portions of the duodenum which, unlike the pancreas, lie posterior and inferior to the origin of the superior mesenteric artery.

The normal pancreas is visible on commercially available gray scale units in over 70 percent of cases (30). The thinner the patient, the easier it is to image the pancreas. Thin patients with prominent livers and portal vessels yield the most optimal scans of the normal pancreas.

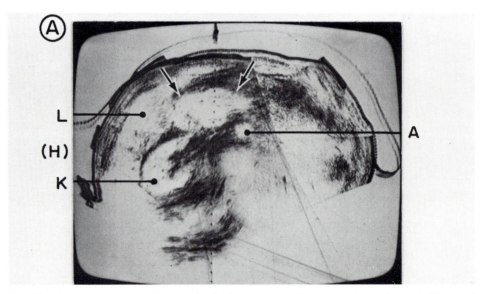

Figure 7.   Acute pancreatitis manifesting as localized enlargement of the pancreatic head (arrows). (*Continued on next page.*)

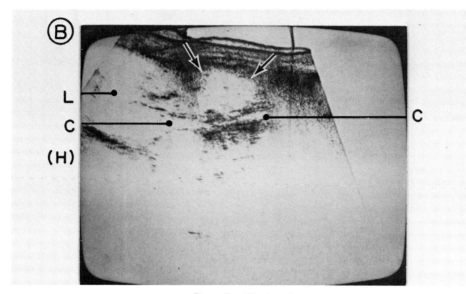

Figure 7.   (Continued)

ACUTE PANCREATITIS

Acute pancreatitis most commonly presents as generalized enlargement of the gland
(5, 8) (Figure 6). This, however, is not always the case. Sometimes enlargement is
confined predominently to the head and neck of the gland with relative sparing of the
body and tail (Figure 7). In such cases, pancreatitis and carcinoma are both likely diag-

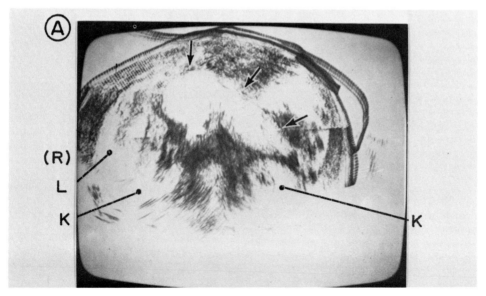

Figure 8.   Acute pancreatitis. Note marked pancreatic enlargement (arrows). The edematous pancreas has
increased transsonicity and decreased echogenicity. *B* is a magnified view of *A*. Arrow above *B* indicates plane
of longitudinal scan *C*. (*Continued on next page.*)

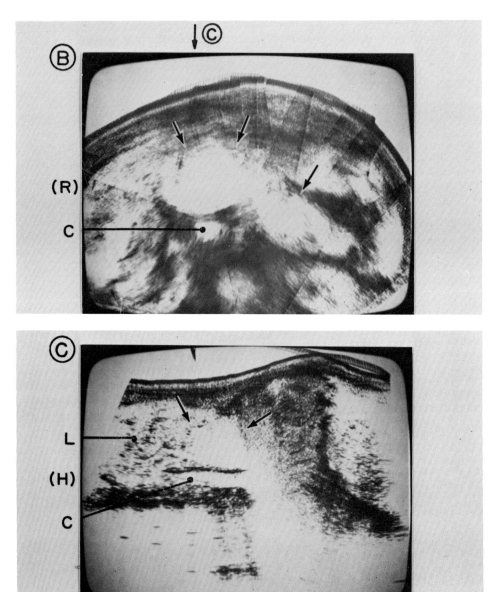

Figure 8.   (Continued)

nostic possibilities usually differentiated by correlating the ultrasound findings with the patient's clinical and laboratory data. On the other hand, when enlargement is localized in the body and tail of the gland with sparing of the head of the pancreas, malignancy is the most likely diagnosis since inflammatory disease rarely spares the pancreatic head (14).

In acute pancreatitis the pancreas becomes less echo-producing or more sonolucent as it becomes more edematous. Sound transmission is enhanced and a stronger back wall of the pancreas is seen. At times, the pancreas may become so edematous that no internal echoes can be detected (Figure 8). Except for its size and irregular borders, a pancreas in this state can mimic and obscure the splenic vein (5). A lymphoma can have a strikingly similar picture but must be considered a less likely etiologic possibility in the absence of demonstrable paraaortic and retroperitoneal nodes (Figure 9). Occasionally pockets of fluid, which various authors ascribe to edema or small pseudocysts, are seen in the acutely inflammed pancreas (1, 12, 24) (Figure 10).

It is possible for pancreatitis to occur in association with a tumor obstructing the

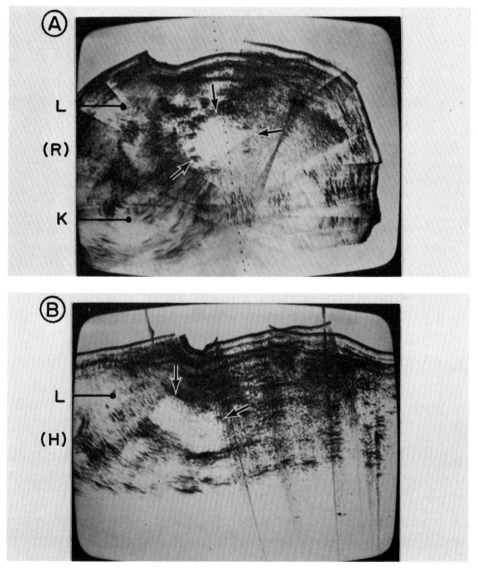

Figure 9.   Lymphoma simulating an edematous pancreatic head.

pancreatic duct. If the tumor is small enough, the only ultrasound findings may be those of pancreatitis.

The changes of acute pancreatitis are evanescent and change often occurs within a matter of days (Figures 11 and 12). Clinical and laboratory changes often parallel the changes seen on ultrasound scans, but this is not always the case (24).

Patients with acute pancreatitis often have ileus in the vicinity of the pancreas. This can result in a failure to visualize the pancreas. A nonvisualized pancreas does not rule out disease (14).

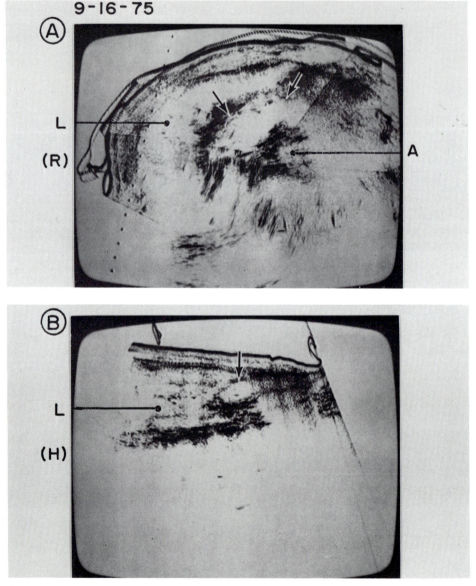

Figure 10. Acute pancreatitis. Initial scans demonstrate fluid collections within the gland. Later scans demonstrate interval resolution. Arrows indicate pancreas. (*Continued on next page.*)

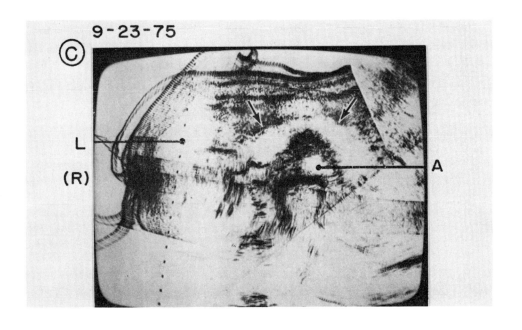

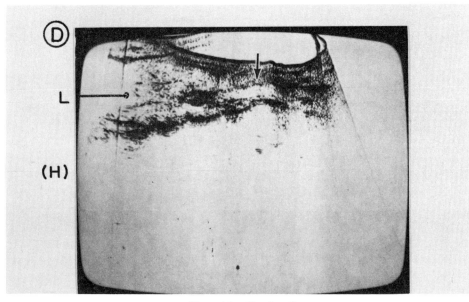

Figure 10. (Continued)

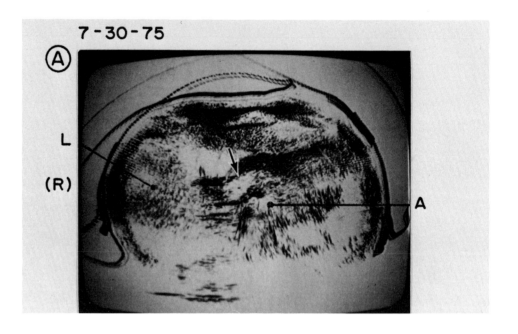

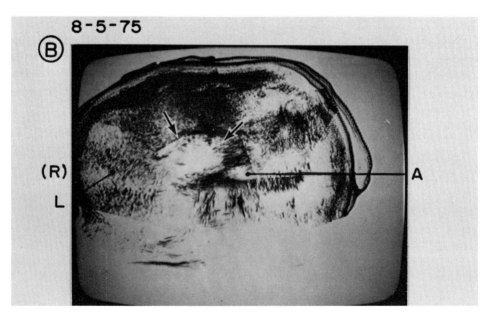

Figure 11.   Acute pancreatitis. Repeat scans demonstrate rapidly evolving changes of acute pancreatitis. In *A*, the pancreas appears normal; in *B*, an edematous pancreatic head is identified; and in *C*, a pseudocyst of the head of the pancreas has developed. (*Continued on next page.*)

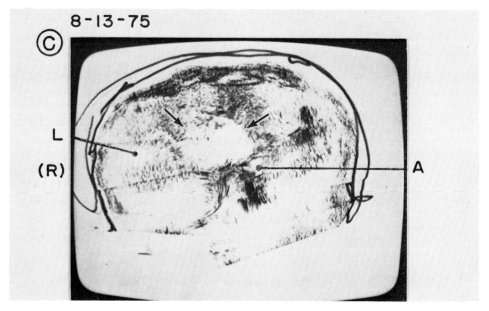

Figure 11. (Continued)

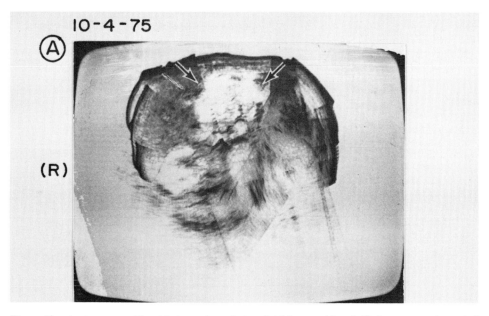

Figure 12. Acute pancreatitis with interval resolution. Initial scans (*A* and *B*) demonstrate the typical changes of acute pancreatitis (arrows). Subsequent scans (*C* and *D*) demonstrate considerable interval improvement in the extent of pancreatic enlargement and edema. (*Continued on next page.*)

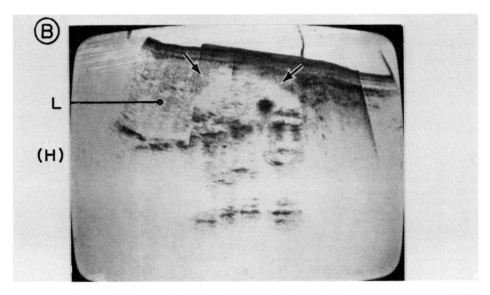

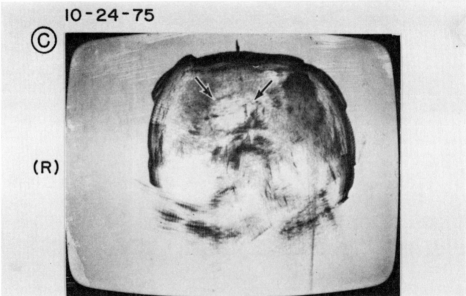

Figure 12. (Continued)

CHRONIC PANCREATITIS AND PANCREATIC PSEUDOCYST

The changes of chronic pancreatitis are similar to those of acute pancreatitis except that the time base is much longer (12). The pancreas often takes on a lobulated or lumpy appearance due to interspersed areas of inflammation and fibrosis (5). Generally the internal echoes in the gland are nonhomogeneous and of the same or decreased intensity

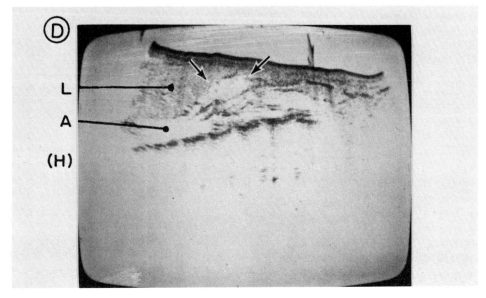

Figure 12. (Continued)

compared to the normal pancreas (Figure 13). An exception to this is chronic calcific pancreatitis in which stronger than normal clusters of echoes are seen with decreased sound transmission or acoustic shadowing corresponding to the calcifications within the gland (Figure 14).

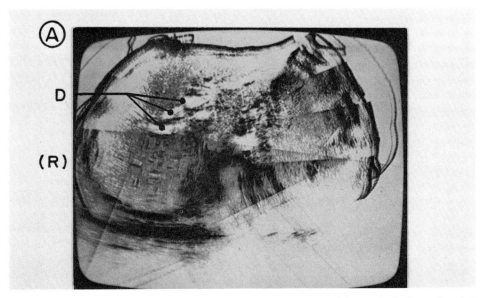

Figure 13. Biliary obstruction and chronic pancreatitis from recurrent biliary calculi. Scans *A* and *D* demonstrate multiple dilated biliary ducts (D). Arrows in *B* indicate an enlarged irregular pancreas with nonhomogeneous internal echoes typical of chronic pancreatitis. Arrows in *C* and *D* indicate a layer of multiple small calculi in the gall bladder. (*Continued on next page.*)

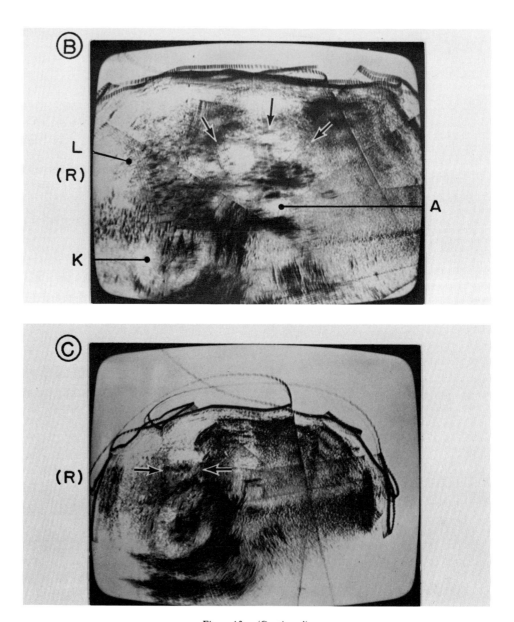

Figure 13.   (Continued)

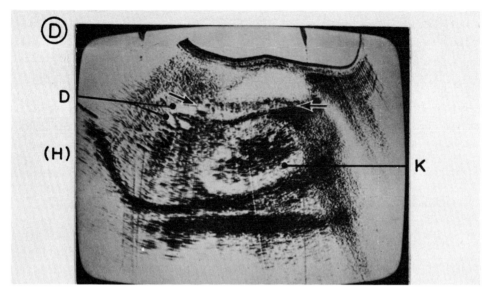

Figure 13. (Continued)

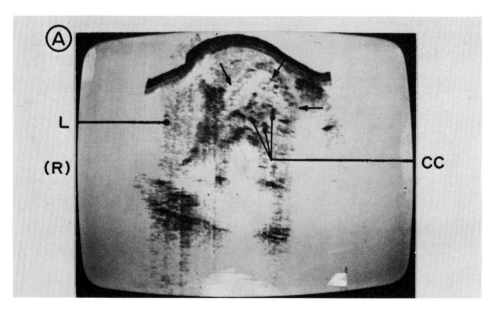

Figure 14. Chronic calcific pancreatitis. *A* is a transverse and *B*, a longitudinal scan. The pancreas is enlarged and contains areas of both decreased and increased echo production (arrows). Clusters of strong echoes with associated decreased transsonicity (acoustic shadowing) represent calcifications within the gland (CC = calcific clusters). (*Continued on next page.*)

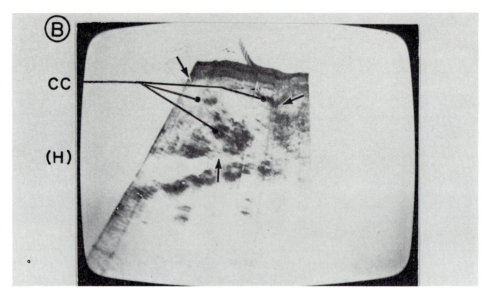

Figure 14. (Continued)

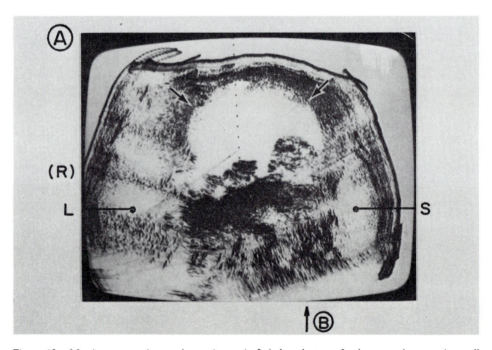

Figure 15. Massive pancreatic pseudocyst (arrows). Lobular clusters of echoes on the posterior wall represent entrapped loops of bowel and semidigested debris. The debris is seen to shift in position (C) when the patient assumes a lateral decubitus position. Arrow below A indicates longitudinal plane of scan B. (*Continued on next page.*)

190

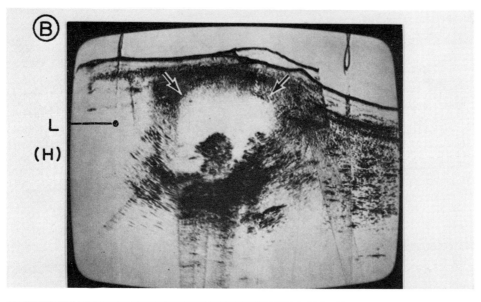

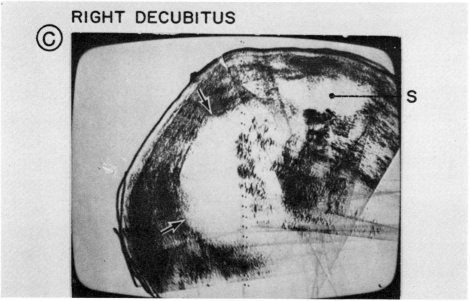

Figure 15.   (Continued)

A localized echo-free expansion of the pancreas in a patient with chronic pancreatitis most likely reflects the development of a pseudocyst. Pseudocysts can involve any portion of the pancreas and can grow to massive size (Figure 15). Their growth rate is often dramatic, growing to huge proportions in a matter of days (31). Similarly, a pseudocyst may just as suddenly, or more gradually, disappear by spontaneously decompressing into a patent pancreatic duct or hollow viscus without clinical complication, or into the peritoneal cavity with a high risk of shock and death (31, 32) (Figure 16). More commonly, pseudocysts are seen to resolve following surgical marsupialization (Figure 17).

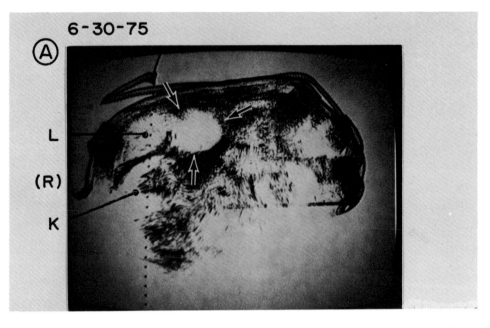

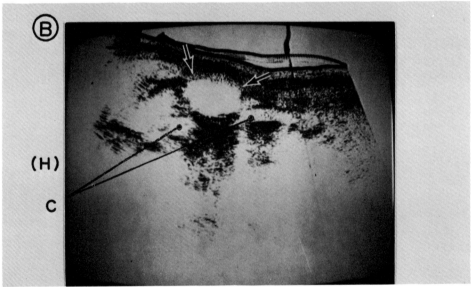

Figure 16. Pancreatic pseudocyst demonstrating spontaneous resolution after several weeks of observation. Arrows in *A* and *B* indicate the pseudocyst. Arrows in *C* and *D* indicate residual thickening of the pancreatic head at the site of pseudocyst (*Continued on next page.*)

192

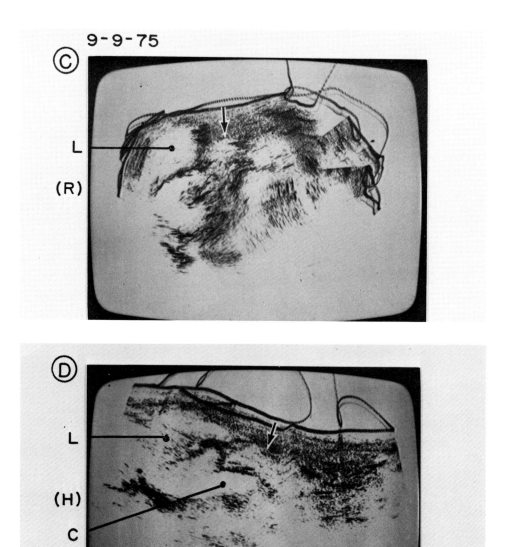

Figure 16. (Continued)

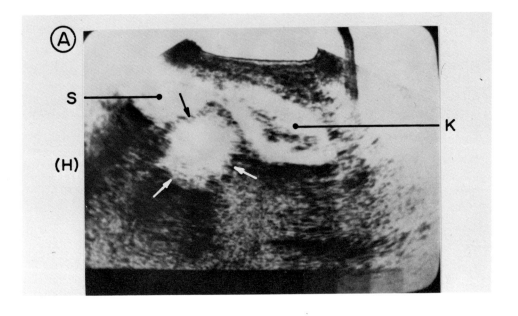

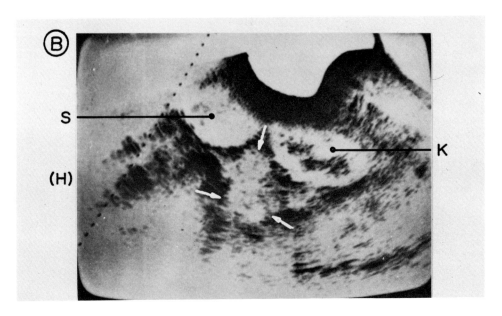

Figure 17. Pancreatic pseudocyst demonstrating resolution following surgical marsupialization (arrows). *A* shows pseudocyst prior to surgery. In *B* residual pancreatic edema is seen in the tail of the pancreas following surgery. The lesion in the tail of the pancreas was best demonstrated by scanning over the left kidney (K) with the patient in the prone position. The normal spleen (S) is seen superiorly.

Pseudocysts of 1 cm or greater are detected easily on gray scale scans. Unlike a true cyst, pseudocysts do not have a cyst wall. Consequently, they tend to grow around and incorporate surrounding structures. Loops of bowel often can be seen included within a pseudocyst. The typically strong back wall echoes of a true cyst are sometimes less obvious in a pseudocyst because of the irregularities of the posterior wall. Semidigested debris also can be demonstrated within the most dependent portions of the pseudocyst and can be seen to shift position when the patient is turned (5, 33) (Figure 15).

Evanescent fluid collections, which may represent a forme fruste of a pseudocyst, can form within a portion of the pancreas involved with acute pancreatitis. Pseudocysts also may be posttraumatic in etiology (34). Unless a pseudocyst is itself border forming and expansile, care must be taken not to rule out the possibility of a tumor with a central necrotic core (10). A lymphomatous mass at the root of the mesentery may be indistinguishable from a pancreatic pseudocyst except for the presence of other areas of involvement such as the liver, spleen, and paraaortic nodes (12, 14, 35) (Figure 18). Cystic masses extrinsic to the pancreas such as a renal cyst, choledochal cyst, aortic aneurysm, or fluid in the stomach are sometimes confused with a pancreatic pseudocyst, but such masses usually can be defined as separate entities clinically and by careful scanning technique (Figure 19).

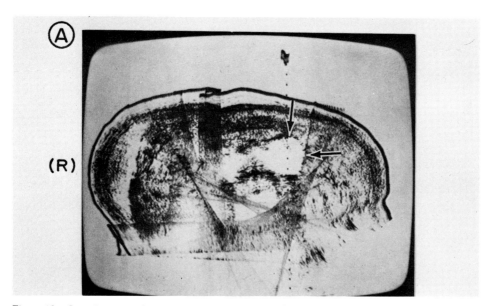

Figure 18.   Lymphoma simulating a pancreatic pseudocyst. *B* is a magnified view of *A*. Note loss of the lateral wall of the aorta due to silhouetting by the adjacent lymphoma (arrows). Arrow above *B* indicates plane of longitudinal scan *C*. The longitudinal paraaortic distribution of the mass is typical of lymphoma. (*Continued on next page.*)

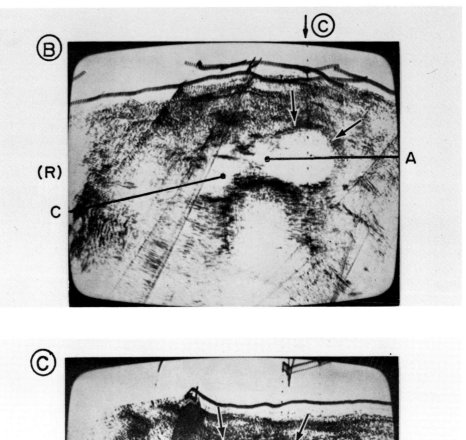

Figure 18. (Continued)

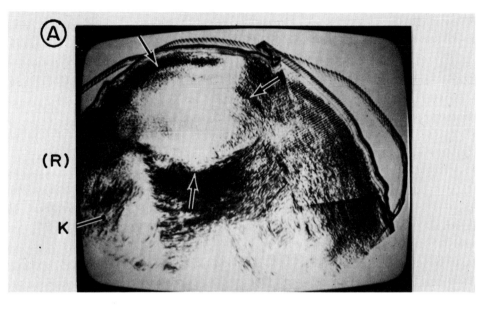

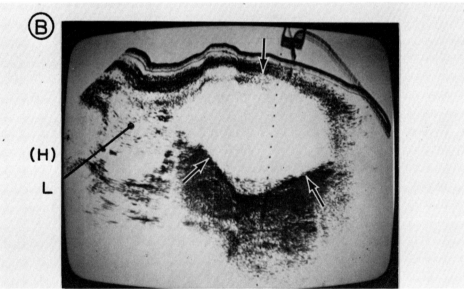

Figure 19. Large bile pseudocyst simulating a pseudocyst of the head of the pancreas. The bile pseudocyst resulted from a walled off perforation of a carcinoma of the gallbladder.

PANCREATIC CARCINOMA

Carcinoma of the pancreas presents as a focal enlargement of the pancreas (14). Any portion of the gland may be involved, however, it is most likely that a carcinoma of the head or body of the pancreas will be detected sooner than one in the tail simply because these portions of the gland are visualized more readily on ultrasound scans. Tumors as small as 3 cm in diameter have been imaged in the head of the pancreas whereas a tumor 4–5 cm in diameter might elude detection in the tail of the organ. This usually is due to air in the stomach and bowel superimposed on the tail of the pancreas. Occasionally a tumor in the tail of the pancreas may be seen only on scans over the left kidney taken while the patient is in the prone position.

Carcinomas of the pancreas may be more or less echo-producing with echoes tending to be coarser and more nonhomogeneous than the normal gland (5) (Figure 20). Characteristically the sound beam is more highly attenuated by a carcinoma resulting in poor sound transmission and a weak back wall (1) (Figure 21).

While a localized mass in the pancreas is more likely to be a carcinoma, generalized enlargement of the entire gland does not rule out carcinoma since a tumor of the head of the pancreas often can incite a secondary pancreatitis due to duct obstruction. On the other hand, pancreatitis may present as a localized involvement of the pancreatic head simulating a tumor (Figure 7). As mentioned earlier, a localized mass in the body or tail of the pancreas is most likely a carcinoma since pancreatitis seldom spares the pancreatic head (23) (Figures 22–24). Large tumors may undergo central necrosis and must be differentiated from chronic pancreatitis or pseudocyst, although this may not be possible in all cases (Figures 25 and 26).

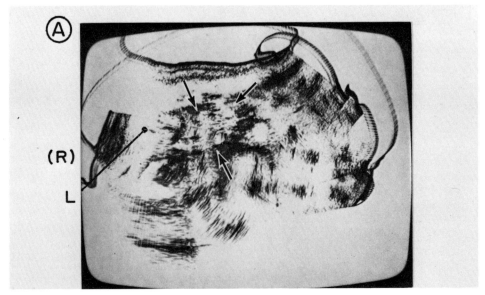

Figure 20.   Carcinoma of the head of the pancreas. Increased echogenicity of the tumor is demonstrated. *B* is a magnified view of *A*. Arrow above *B* indicates longitudinal plane of scan *C*. (*Continued on next page.*)

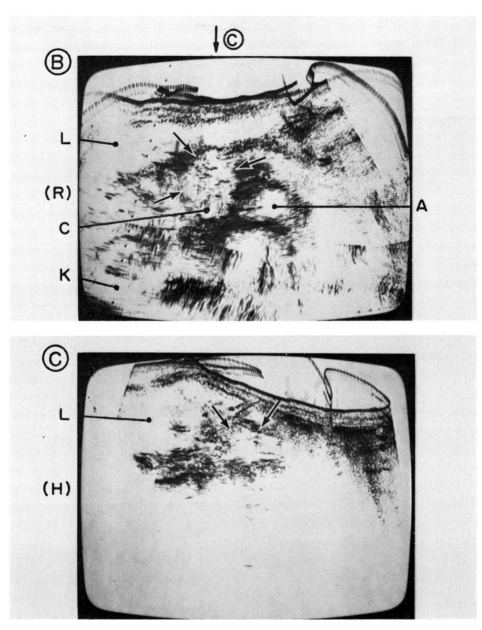

Figure 20. (Continued)

GRAY SCALE

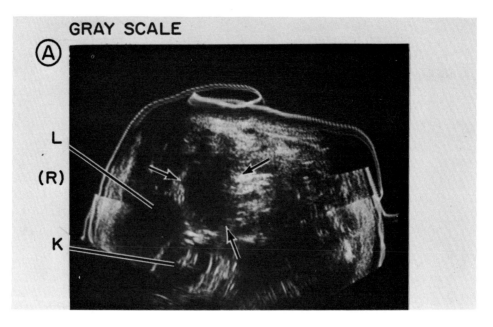

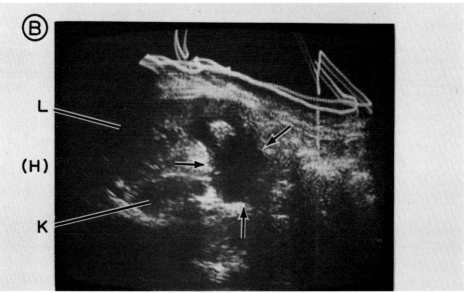

Figure 21. Carcinoma of the pancreas demonstrated in gray scale and bistable modes. Although no internal echoes are seen in the mass (arrows), the poor sound transmission beyond the mass indicates that it must be a homogeneously solid mass rather than a pseudocyst. (*Continued on next page.*)

BISTABLE

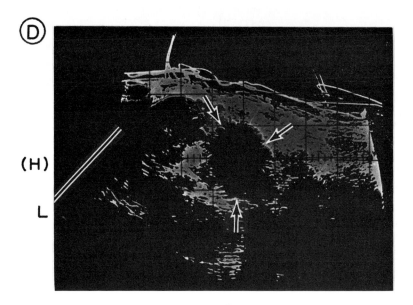

Figure 21. (Continued)

201

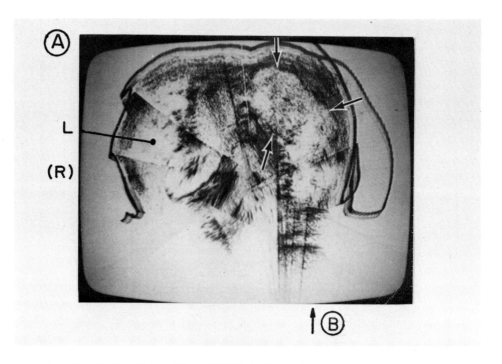

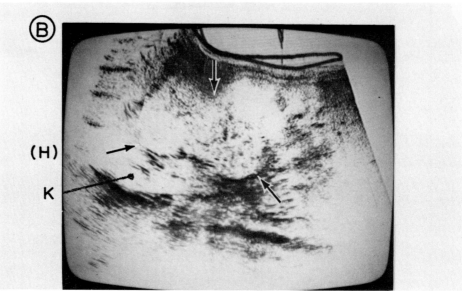

Figure 22.   Carcinoma of the tail of the pancreas (arrows). Arrow under *A* indicates longitudinal plane of *B*.

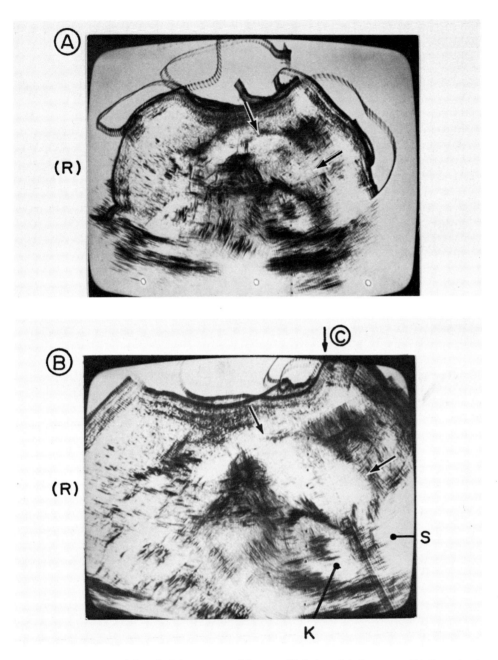

Figure 23.   Carcinoma of the tail of the pancreas. *B* is a magnified view of *A*. Arrow over *B* indicates longitudinal plane of scan *C*. (*Continued on next page.*)

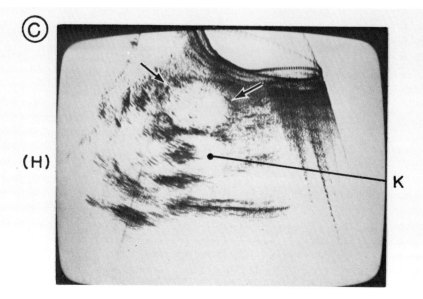

Figure 23.   (Continued)

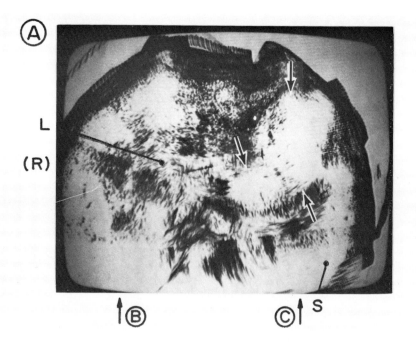

Figure 24.   Carcinoma of the tail of the pancreas with liver metastases. Arrows in *A* and *C* outline the lobu-lated pancreatic carcinoma. Arrows below *A* indicate the longitudinal planes of *B* and *C*. Patchy areas of decreased echo production in the liver in *A* and *B* represent metastases. (*Continued on next page.*)

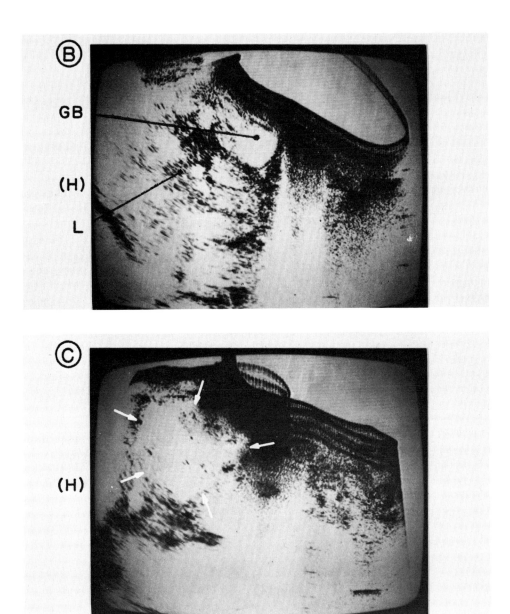

Figure 24. (Continued)

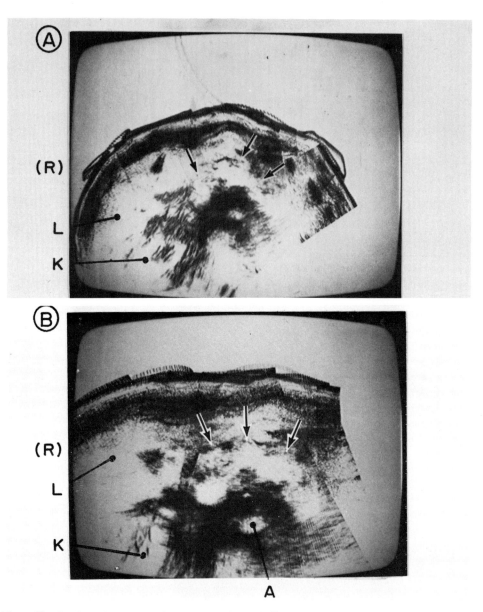

Figure 25. Cystic carcinosarcoma of the pancreas (arrows). *B* is a magnified view of *A*. Note the marked similarity of scan *B* to Figure 13B. (*Continued on next page.*)

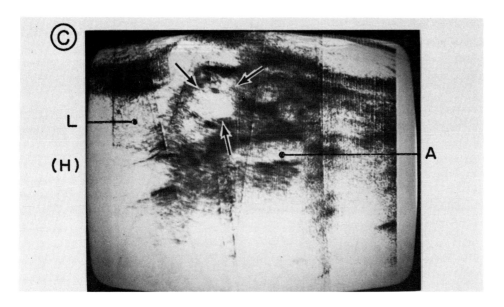

Figure 25. (Continued)

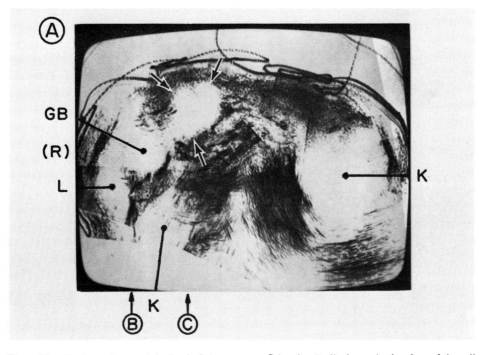

Figure 26. Cystic carcinoma of the head of the pancreas. *B* is a longitudinal scan in the plane of the gall bladder (GB), and scan *C* is in the plane of the tumor as indicated by arrows under *A*. Incidentally noted in *A* is a large benign cyst to the left kidney. (*Continued on next page.*)

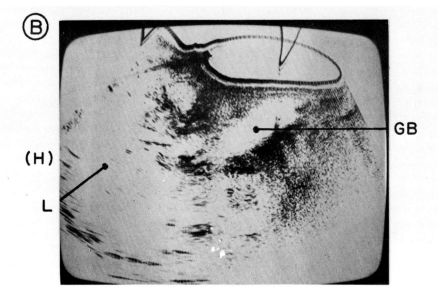

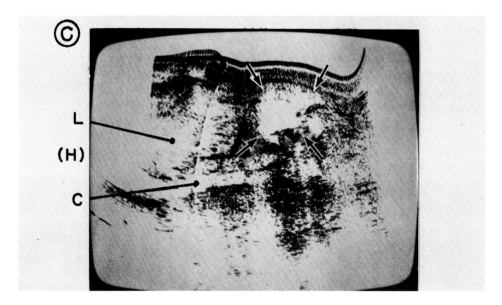

Figure 26. (Continued)

Tumors of the pancreas can be suspected even if not demonstrable in a patient with dilatation of the biliary radicles and common bile duct and a Courvoisier gallbladder. Biliary obstruction, however, is only an indirect sign since common duct stones, strictures, and chronic fibrosing pancreatitis of the pancreatic head have been shown to obstruct the biliary tract as well (17–22) (Figure 11). The patient's history and clinical course often are of great assistance in this differential diagnosis.

Metastatic tumors to the pancreas or pancreatic bed are indistinguishable from a

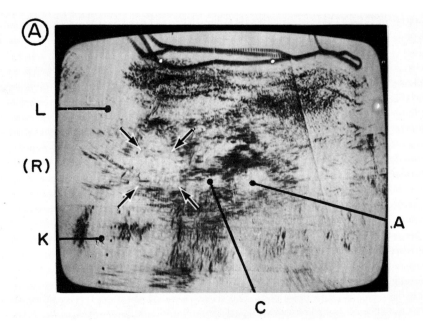

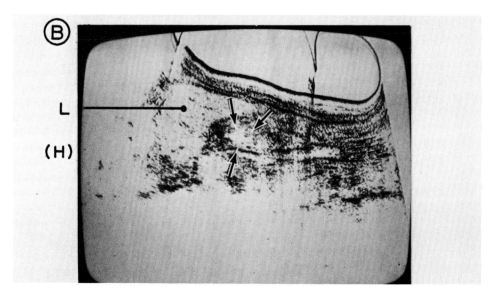

Figure 27.   Metastatic oat cell carcinoma of the lung to the head of the pancreas.

primary pancreatic carcinoma (8, 10) (Figure 27). Lymphomas with weak internal echoes can masquerade as a pancreatic carcinoma. Additional scans of the liver, spleen, and paraaortic nodes are helpful in confirming the presence of a lymphoma when these regions also are involved (Figure 28). Small islet cell tumors of the pancreas usually escape detection by ultrasound. Angiography is the diagnostic study of choice in patients suspected of having islet cell tumors.

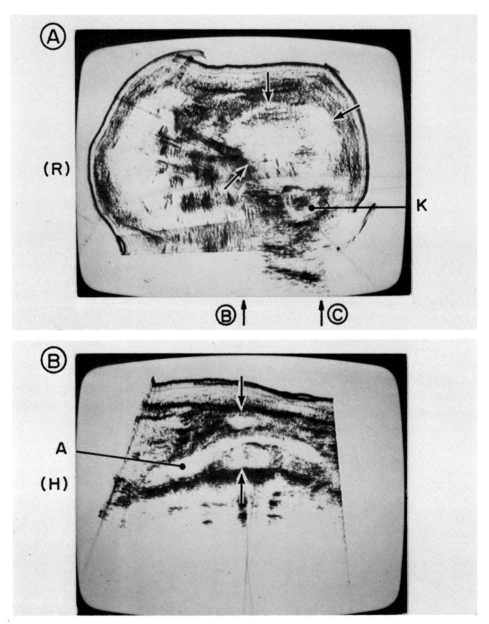

Figure 28. Lymphoma simulating a carcinoma of the tail of the pancreas. Arrows indicate the extent of the lymphoma. Arrows under transverse scan *A* indicate the longitudinal plane of scans *B* and *C*. The peri- and retroaortic location of the tumor in *B* would be unlikely for a pancreatic carcinoma. (*Continued on next page.*)

For patients having a demonstrable mass in the pancreas of uncertain etiology, be it inflammatory or malignant, there have been recent reports of an ultrasonically guided percutaneous needle aspiration biopsy method that currently is undergoing investigation. Early results suggest a high diagnostic yield and low morbidity associated with this procedure (36–38).

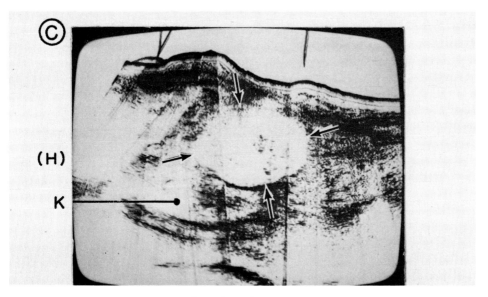

Figure 28.   (Continued)

SUMMARY

A multiplicity of diagnostic modalities are now available for imaging the pancreas. Of the noninvasive studies, ultrasound has a higher accuracy rate than barium studies and radionuclide scans. It is cheaper and more readily available than computerized axial tomography and does not require contrast enhancement. Of the invasive studies, ultrasound has a comparable accuracy to angiography except in islet cell tumors, and it probably is more accurate than endoscopic retrograde pancreatography although all the data are not yet available. Ultrasound and upper gastrointestinal series would appear to be the initial studies of choice in evaluating the pancreas.

Gray scale equipment now available affords excellent visualization of both the normal and abnormal pancreas with excessive bowel gas being the most common cause of difficulty in obtaining diagnostic images.

Pancreatitis is manifested by generalized enlargement of the pancreas, decreased echogenicity, and increased transsonicity. Carcinomas appear as localized masses with increased or decreased echogenicity and decreased transsonicity. These criteria lack specificity, however, and it is difficult at times to be certain as to whether a mass in the pancreas is inflammatory or malignant. This is probably in part due to the coexistence of both these processes in many cases.

Pseudocysts are readily detected and are relatively easy to diagnose. Care must be exercised not to confuse a pseudocyst with a lymphoma or necrotic carcinoma.

The pancreas remains a difficult organ to image and evaluate. Of the many tests available, ultrasound has become a worthwhile noninvasive method for screening and the early evaluation of pancreatic disease as well as for follow-up evaluation.

REFERENCES

1. Walls WJ, Gonzales G, Martin NL, et al: B-scan ultrasound evaluation of the pancreas. *Radiology* **114:**127, 1975.

2. Eyler WR, Clark MD, Rian RL: An evaluation of roentgen signs of pancreatic enlargement. *JAMA* **181:**967, 1962.

3. Eaton SB, Fleischli DJ, Pollard JJ: et al: Comparison of current radiologic approaches to the diagnosis of pancreatic disease. *N Engl J Med* **279:**389, 1968.

4. Landman S, Polcyn RE, Gottschalk A: Pancreatic imaging-is it worth it. *Radiology* **100:**631, 1971.

5. Doust BD: Ultrasonic examination of the pancreas. *Radiol Clin North Am* **13:**467, 1975.

6. Bookstein JJ, Reuter SR, Martel W: Angiographic evaluation of pancreatic carcinoma. *Radiology* **93:**757, 1969.

7. Rohrmann CA, Silvis SE, Vennes JA: Evaluation of the endoscopic pancreatogram. *Radiology* **113:**297, 1974.

8. Stuber JL, Templeton AW, Bishop K: Sonographic diagnosis of pancreatic lesions. *Am J Roentgenol* **116:**406, 1972.

9. Jacobson JB, Redman HC, McKay L: Diagnostic accuracy of abdominal scanning, in White D (ed): *Ultrasound in Medicine,* vol 1. New York, Plenum Press, 1975, p 183.

10. Filly RA, Freimanis AK: Echographic diagnosis of pancreatic lesions. *Radiology* **96:**575, 1970.

11. Burger J, Blauenstein UW: Current aspects of ultrasonic scanning of the pancreas. *Am J Roentgenol* **122:**406, 1974.

12. Sokoloff S, Gosink BB, Leopold GR, et al: Pitfalls in the echographic evaluation of pancreatic disease. *J Clin Ultrasound* **2:**321, 1974.

13. Kahn PC: Pancreatic Echography, in Eaton SB, Ferrucci WB (ed): *Radiology of the Pancreas and Duodenum.* Philadelphia, W.B. Saunders Company, 1973, p 276.

14. Leopold GR, Asher WM: *Fundamentals of Abdominal and Pelvic Ultrasound.* Philadelphia, W.B. Saunders Company, 1975, p 49.

15. Sample WF, Po JB, Gray RK, et al: Gray scale ultrasonography techniques in pancreatic scanning. *Applied Radiol* **4:** 63, 1975.

16. Leopold GR: Gray scale ultrasonic angiography of the upper abdomen. *Radiology* **117:**665, 1975.

17. Perlmutter GS, Goldberg BB: Ultrasound evaluation of the common bile duct. *J Clin Ultrasound* **4:**107, 1976.

18. Taylor KJW, Carpenter DA, McCready VR, et al: Gray scale ultrasonography in the differential diagnosis of obstructive jaundice, in White D (ed): *Ultrasound in Medicine,* vol 1. New York, Plenum Press, 1975, p 125.

19. Stone LB, Ferrucci JT, Warshaw AL, et al: Gray scale ultrasound diagnosis of obstructive biliary disease. *Am J Roentgenol* **125:**47, 1975.

20. Leopold GR, Sokoloff J: Ultrasonic scanning in the diagnosis of biliary disease. *Surg Clin North Am* **53:**1043, 1973.

21. Taylor KJW, Carpenter DA: The anatomy and pathology of the porta hepatis demonstrated by gray scale ultrasonography. *J Clin Ultrasound* **3:**117, 1975.

22. Taylor KJW, Carpenter DA, McCready VR: Ultrasound and scintigraphy in the differential diagnosis of obstructive jaundice. *J. Clin Ultrasound* **2:**105, 1974.

23. Leopold GR: Echographic study of the pancreas. *JAMA* **232:**287, 1975.

24. Doust BD, Malkad NF, Baum JK, et al: Ultrasonic evaluation of pancreatitis, in White D (ed): *Ultrasound in Medicine,* vol 1. New York, Plenum Press, 1975, p 141.

25. Leopold GR, Asher WM: Deleterious effects of gastrointestinal contrast material on abdominal echography. *Radiology* **98:**637, 1971.

26. Pepper HW, Keene J: Use of simethicone in abdominal echotomography, in White D, Barnes R (ed): *Ultrasound in Medicine,* vol 2. New York, Plenum Press, 1976, p 197.

27. Sarti DA, Lindstrom RR, Tabrisky J: Correlation of the ultrasonic appearance of the portal vein with abdominal angiography. *J Clin Ultrasound* **3**: 263, 1975.

28. Weill F, Eisenscher A, Aucant D, et al: Ultrasound study of venous patterns in the right hypochondrium: an anatomical approach to differential diagnosis of obstructive jaundice. *J Clin Ultrasound* **3**:23, 1975.

29. Garrett WJ, Kossoff G, Carpenter DA: Gray scale compound echography of the normal upper abdomen. *J Clin Ultrasound* **3**:199, 1975.

30. Asher WM, Nebel O, Huber K: Demonstration of the normal pancreas with gray scale ultrasound, in White D (ed): *Ultrasound in Medicine,* vol 1. New York, Plenum Press, 1975, p 194.

31. Leopold GR: Pancreatic echography: a new dimension in the diagnosis of pseudocyst. *Radiology* **104**:365, 1972.

32. Leopold GR, Berk RN, Reinke RT: Echographic-radiologic documentation of a spontaneous rupture of a pancreatic pseudocyst into the duodenum. *Radiology* **102**:699, 1972.

33. Gosink BB, Leopold GR: Abdominal echography. *Semin Roentgenol* **10**:299, 1975.

34. Kratochwil A, Rosenmayr F, Howanietz L: Diagnosis of a traumatic pancreas cyst by means of ultrasound. *Ultrasound in Med & Biol* **1**:49, 1973.

35. Bradley EL, Clements JL: Implications of diagnostic ultrasound in the surgical management of pancreatic pseudocysts. *Am J Surg* **127**:163, 1974.

36. Smith EH, Bartrum RJ: Percutaneous aspiration of abscesses with ultrasound, in White D (ed): *Ultrasound in Medicine,* vol 1. New York, Plenum Press, 1975, p 177.

37. Smith EH, Bartrum RJ, Chang YC, et al: Percutaneous aspiration biopsy of the pancreas under ultrasonic guidance. *N Engl J Med* **292**:825, 1975.

38. Holm HH, Rasmussen JK: Ultrasonically guided percutaneous puncture technique. *J Clin Ultrasound* **1**:27, 1973.

8
Reticuloendothelial System

Kenneth J. W. Taylor, M.D., Ph.D.
Associate Professor of Diagnostic Radiology
Head, Ultrasound
Yale University School of Medicine
New Haven, Connecticut

The reticuloendothelial system is a collective term for widespread tissue exhibiting phagocytosis. Cells of this system can be identified by their uptake of intravenously injected particles or dyes such as Indian ink or Trypan blue. Cells of the reticuloendothelial system, varying in number and morphology, exist in the following anatomic sites:

1. in connective tissues in which they are termed histiocytes, while in the brain they are called microglia
2. in blood, where they are represented by large mononuclear cells
3. in the spleen, liver, thymus, bone marrow, medulla of the suprarenal gland, and anterior lobe of hypophysis
4. in the lymph nodes and lymphoid aggregates throughout the body, such as the tonsils

Due to the ability of these cells to actively ingest particles, they are involved in the immediate body defense against microorganisms and also with the establishment of a specific immune response. In fetal life, the reticuloendothelial system of the spleen, liver, and bone marrow are important sites of hematopoiesis, and this function is retained postnatally in the bone marrow. However, in certain disease states, the cells of the liver and spleen may regain their hematopoietic function.

The lymphatic system comprises a network of minute capillaries that are blind-ending but are capable of absorbing lymph that has filtered out of the blood capillaries. Because of this function, obstruction to these vessels will result in the accumulation of free tissue fluid, producing edema, ascites, and so forth, depending on the anatomic site. These small lymphatic plexuses form vessels of 1–2 mm diameter that accompany the superficial veins and deep arteries. These channels are interrupted by lymph nodes. Lymph nodes are bean-shaped lymphoid masses, most of which are 2–3 mm in size, but may be as large as 2 cm in length. They act as mechanical filters for the lymph between the tissues and its return to the bloodstream, while the contained immunologically competent cells can initiate the response to microorganisms or other foreign protein.

Attempts to image this system by ultrasonography are limited largely to the display of the spleen in a normal individual, since the resolution of the method is inadequate to define the small, normal lymph nodes throughout the body. In other anatomic sites, such as the thyroid and liver, lymphoid aggregations are only apparent on microscopic examination, but these may form lymphoid masses that may be detected by ultrasound where there is abnormal cellular proliferation of these masses. Also in disease states, enlargement of the abdominal and pelvic lymph nodes may be diagnosed reliably by ultrasound.

In addition to the ability to display the primary pathologic state in such abnormalities as paraaortic lymphadenopathy and retroperitoneal lymphoid masses, ultrasonic examination frequently displays the secondary effects that are produced by the pressure of such masses on the adjacent viscera. For example, paraaortic lymphadenopathy frequently will produce varying degrees of hydronephrosis, and this may be diagnosed very reliably by simple ultrasound techniques. More rarely, upper paraaortic lymphadenopathy may produce pathologic distension of the biliary tree and these secondary effects allow one to infer the presence of abnormalities under physical conditions, such as extreme obesity or excessive air in the intestines, in which the display of the primary pathologic condition is technically difficult or impossible.

The full potential of the gray scale modifications of diagnostic ultrasound has yet to be realized in the differential diagnosis of abnormalities of the reticuloendothelial system. Using the older bistable equipment, only abnormalities of size and contour could be appreciated. However, the gray scale modifications of this technique are characterized by enhanced resolution and greatly increased signal to noise ratio, so the internal consistency or the texture of the tissue is displayed in addition to contour information. This should have important implications in the differential diagnosis of splenomegaly. With good resolution and the ability to display the tissue texture, the ultrasonologist looking at ultrasound sections through organs such as the spleen should have similar information available to him as does a pathologist looking at the cut surface of the spleen.

ABDOMINAL AND PELVIC LYMPHADENOPATHY

Lymphangiography is a most effective means for imaging the paraaortic lymph nodes, and by serial studies subsequent to opacification, the neoplastic activity in nodes may be assessed. ^{67}Gallium citrate (^{67}Ga) also is used widely to demonstrate tumor activity in nodes. The combination of ultrasound to image the size of enlarged nodes and a gallium examination to demonstrate activity within them may be an effective alternative to lymphangiography. Lymphangiography does require particular expertise which is not always available, and ultrasound examination with or without a complementary gallium study provides a meaningful alternative to lymphangiography especially under one of five conditions:

1. when operator expertise in lymphography is not available
2. where previous lymphographic examinations and/or obesity render lymphography difficult or impossible, despite operator expertise
3. in the demonstration of high para-aortic lymphadenopathy which is not opacified by lymphography
4. in patients with severe allergies to iodine in whom contrast media may produce morbidity or even mortality
5. to demonstrate nodes outside the paraaortic chain such as the mesenteric lymph nodes.

In searching for abdominal and pelvic lymphadenopathy, it is important to recall that the lymphatic channels accompany the blood vessels. Thus, it is essential for the ultrasonologist to be aware of the lymphatic drainage of each organ. For example, despite the superficial position of the testes, the lymphatic drainage accompanies the blood supply to the epigastric region and the search for lymphadenopathy from testicular tumors should be directed to the high preaortic region.

TECHNIQUE

Paraaortic lymphadenopathy should be demonstrated by both longitudinal and transverse scanning of the upper abdomen. This examination must be performed in a systematic way. The real-time ultrasound scanners that are becoming commercially available will greatly facilitate the speed with which the abdomen and pelvis can be examined. With the current generation of manually operated laminographic ultrasound scanners, a longitudinal midline scan is first performed (sagittal plane). With modern gray scale equipment, this scan can be carried out in a single linear sweep down the anterior surface of the abdomen, using paraffin oil as a coupling agent. The scanning arm is then moved one centimeter to the right and the procedure repeated. The scan can be initiated by a simple sector scan through the liver substance using previously established techniques (1) and then continued into a linear scan down the abdomen. The mechanical arm is then moved a centimeter toward the right and the procedure repeated. In this way, a series of paramedian scans are obtained to the right and left of the median plane. Lymphadenopathy is apparent as lobulated masses that are acoustically highly homogeneous, that is, relatively echo-free or producing very weak internal echoes (2).

These sagittal scans are augmented by serial transverse scanning, commencing at the xiphisternum. Although the best resolution of the upper abdominal vasculature is obtained by limited sector scans, in the demonstration of lymphadenopathy it is usually necessary to compound, to some extent, on transverse scanning. Upper paraaortic lymphadenopathy is again apparent as a lobulated highly homogeneous mass in the pre- and paraaortic position (Figure 1). The lymphadenopathy mass even surrounds the aorta (Figure 2). Mesenteric lymphadenopathy will have the same lobulated and homogeneous appearances, although it tends to be located more to the left of the midline (Figure 3). This is not apparent in routine lymphography.

In a significant number of patients, air in the gut will prevent visualization of the retroperitoneal areas. This disadvantage is particularly apparent in patients who have been hospitalized for a long period of time with consequent immobilization. Gut preparation can be carried out on these patients, initially by oral cathartics, but if necessary, enemas can be administered.

Large retroperitoneal masses tend to displace air-containing gut and render the retroperitoneal area more amenable to ultrasonic visualization. Despite all attempts at

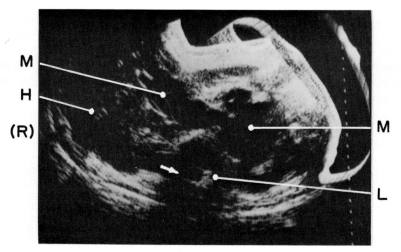

Figure 1. Transverse ultrasonogram of the level of the xiphisternum showing large, lobulated homogeneous masses (M) in the pre- and paraaortic position. These are paraaortic nodes. The liver (H) surrounds the masses. Note that the spinal canal is seen (arrow). L is the vertebral body.

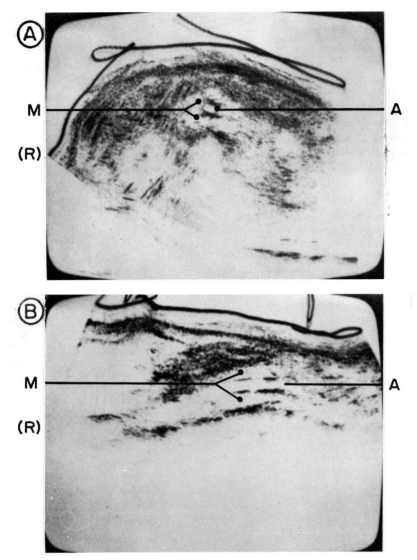

Figure 2. *A*. Transverse ultrasonogram demonstrates lymphomatous nodes (M) surrounding the abdominal aorta (A). *B*. Longitudinal ultrasonogram showing the nodal masses (M) to be located both anterior and posterior to the aorta (A).

gut preparation, there is a small number of patients, possibly 10 percent, in whom the retroperitoneal area cannot be adequately displayed. In such patients, paraaortic lymphadenopathy may be inferred if this produces a partial ureteric obstruction with consequent hydroureter and some degree of hydronephrosis (Figure 4). Both kidneys can be scanned satisfactorally by simple sector scans from the posterio-lateral aspects of the trunk, using previously established techniques (3). This technique allows a minimal degree of hydronephrosis to be reliably identified.

Upper paraaortic lymphadenopathy is shown in Figure 5, which is a longitudinal section through the abdomen 2 cm to the right of the midline and therefore shows the

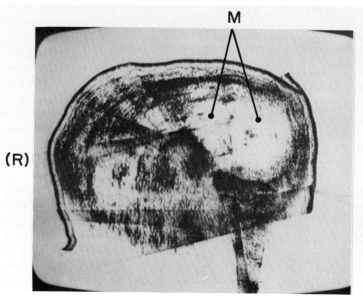

Figure 3. Transverse ultrasonogram showing lobulated, homogeneous masses to the left of the midline suggesting mesenteric rather than paraaortic nodal involvement. The lymphogram may be normal.

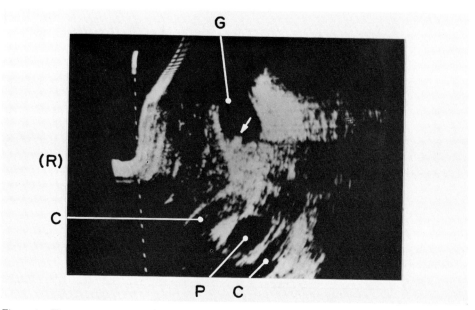

Figure 4. Transverse sector scan through the right kidney showing distension of the right renal pelvis (P) in hydronephrosis due to ureteric obstruction by paraaortic lymphadenopathy. The renal cortex (C) surrounds the dilated pelvis (P). The gallbladder (G) is seen anteriorly and contains an incidental gallstone (arrow).

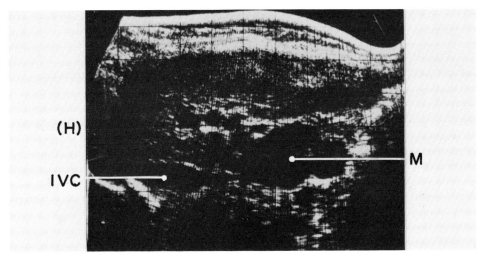

Figure 5.   B-mode ultrasonogram in paramedian plane 2 cm to the right of midline. The liver is enlarged and returns uneven echoes due to malignant involvement. There are lobulated homogeneous tumor masses (M) posterior to the liver consistent with paraaortic lymphadenopathy. These nodes compress the inferior vena cava (IVC).

lumen of the inferior vena cava which in encroached on by an accoustically homogeneous, lobulated mass. This is characteristic of upper paraaortic lymphadenopathy. This patient was a 29-year-old white female from whose leg a melanoma had been removed 2 years previously and who had presented with hepatomegaly. The ultrasound examination revealed an abnormally large liver with replacement of the normal architecture by lower echo-producing areas, and this was consistent with metastatic involvement of the liver. At subsequent postmortem examination the pathologic condition of the liver was confirmed, as well as the metastatic involvement of the upper paraaortic lymph nodes.

In such patients, the secondary changes due to such abnormal masses should be investigated. In this patient it would include the examination of both kidneys by simple sector scans to demonstrate possible signs of minimal hydronephrosis due to pressure on either of the ureters. In addition, such upper paraaortic lymphadenopathy frequently may produce distension of the biliary tree which is shown in Figure 6A. In Figure 6B lobulated masses may be seen in the region of the porta hepatis, and these frequently appear as if they are invaginated into the substance of the liver. These are very high paraaortic lymph nodes that are not demonstrated by lymphography since they lie above the cistern chyli. A section taken more laterally through the liver substance (Figure 6A), shows the gallbladder distended, and close examination of the liver reveals distended biliary cannaliculi. This is due to the enlarged lymph nodes in the region of the porta hepatis. In the experience of the author, such obstruction is not necessarily associated with biochemical changes of cholestatic jaundice in that there may be subtotal obstruction and subclinical cholestasis. This patient was treated by radiotherapy to the area of the porta hepatis and a further ultrasonic examination was carried out on completion of irradiation. The corresponding sections are shown in Figures 6C–D. These show the regression of the enlarged paraaortic lymph nodes. There is no longer any evidence of

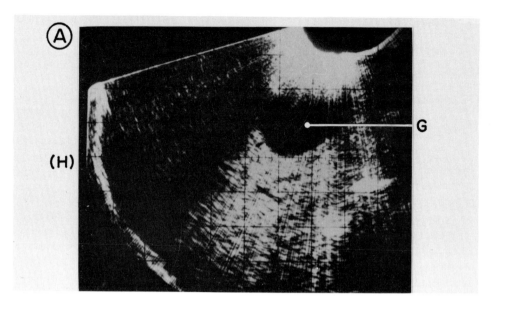

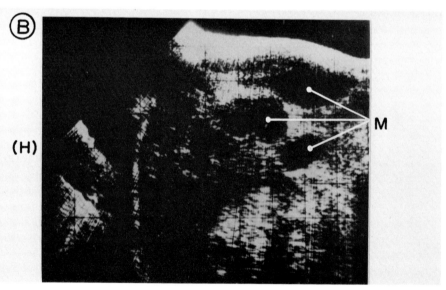

Figure 6. *A.* Paramedian ultrasonogram through liver showing distended gallbladder and posterior to this, there is evidence of dilated intrahepatic biliary canaliculi. *B.* Paramedian ultrasonogram through region of porta hepatis showing lobulated homogeneous masses consistent with enlarged lymph nodes in patient with lymphoma. It was presumed that biliary obstruction, as shown in *A* was due to these portal nodes. *C.* Region of porta hepatis following local radiotherapy showing nodal regression. *D.* Paramedian ultrasonogram correspondent to *A* after radiotherapy. Note there is no distention of the biliary tree. (*Continued on next page.*)

222

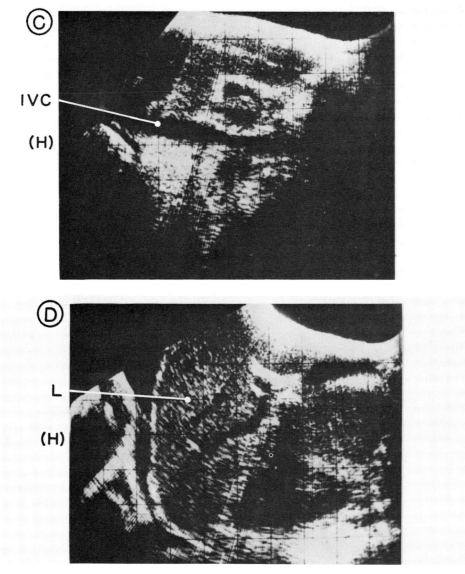

Figure 6. (Continued)

dilation of the biliary cannaliculi or of the gallbladder. The same effect of radiation therapy can be seen with lymphomatous nodes surrounding the abdominal aorta (Figure 7).

RETROPERITONEAL LYMPHOID MASSES

Like pancreatic neoplasms in a similar anatomic situation, retroperitoneal lymphoid masses may be extremely difficult to diagnose and ultrasound is the modality of choice in the initial examination for this pathologic entity. Such masses are particularly found in non-Hodgkin's lymphomas and, as with the paraaortic lymph nodes, it is important to search for secondary signs of involvement in terms of unexplained hydronephrosis or subclinical biliary obstruction. Figure 8 shows a scan of a patient who presented with a palpable epigastric mass. On ultrasonic examination at another hospital, this was considered to be cystic. Repeat examination at this center showed a mass producing low-level echoes but not as low as cystic tumors. There was also low attenuation. Careful

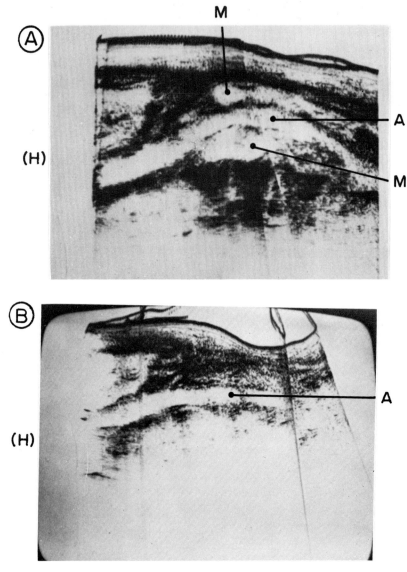

Figure 7. *A*. Longitudinal ultrasonogram demonstrates nodal masses (M) both anterior and posterior to the abdominal aorta (A). *B*. Longitudinal ultrasonogram along similar plane obtained after a course of radiation therapy shows a dramatic decrease in the masses with a return of the aorta (A) to its normal location.

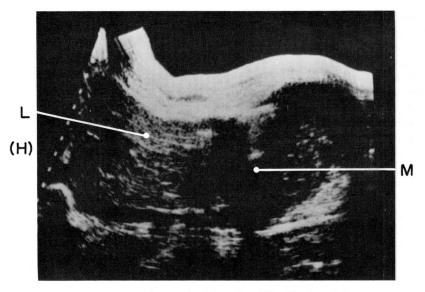

Figure 8.   Paramedian ultrasonogram 2 cm to the right of the midline showing inferior vena cava posterior to liver. Below liver (H), there is a large, very homogeneous mass (M) extending out from the prevertebral region, and this is consistent with a homogeneous tumor such as a sarcoma or lymphoma. Biopsy revealed lymphosarcoma.

examination of the adjacent liver showed signs of active invasion. Therefore, the appearances were strongly considered to be those of a retroperitoneal lymphoid mass, and this was confirmed at surgery when a lymphosarcoma was found invading the posterior wall of the stomach and the liver. Such a mass can be differentiated from paraaortic lymph nodes by the overall contour, since these lymphoid masses do not show lobulation.

SPLENIC EXAMINATION

As reported by previous authors, ultrasonic examination of the spleen can reveal its size and position even though it is not clinically palpable. If multiple serial sections are taken through the organ, the volume may be computed (4). The addition of the gray scale technique allows some differential diagnosis on the causes of splenomegaly by the tissue texture that is revealed (5).

Scanning Techniques for Splenic Examination

A normal-sized or slightly enlarged spleen is difficult to examine, and in the author's experience, it is examined most easily by scanning along the longitudinal axis of the spleen. The patient lies in the right lateral position with his left side uppermost. The patient's left arm is rested over the head and this widens the intercostal spaces on the left. The mechanical scanning arm is aligned along the eleventh intercostal space, since the long axis of the spleen lies in that plane. With the patient in this position, the spleen

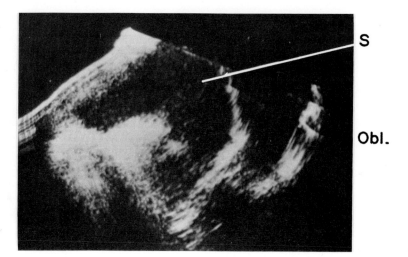

Figure 9.   Oblique ultrasonogram along eleventh intercostal space showing normal spleen (S).

will be found to be surprisingly anterior, extending from the midaxillary line to the left
subcostal margin. When the ultrasonic beam passes through normal spleen, very low-
level echoes, characteristic of lymphoid tissue, are displayed. A scan of the spleen
usually can be produced by rocking the transducer down the eleventh intercostal space
(Figure 9), and an estimation of splenic size obtained by measuring its longitudinal axis.
The limits of normality are still being assessed but a measurement of 12.0 cm is certainly abnormal; most normal spleens are less than 10.0 cm. Serial examinations of the
spleen sequentially during the treatment of a reticulosis may indicate efficacy of a treatment regime by the change in the size of the organ.

When there is a moderate degree of splenomegaly, the spleen may be conveniently
scanned transversely using a compounding technique, and if there is marked enlargement, the spleen can be displayed by the simple sector scanning technique which
produces a paramedian section (Figure 10).

DIFFERENTIAL DIAGNOSIS OF CHRONIC SPLENOMEGALY

More recently, preliminary data have become available on the significance of the various
splenic consistencies that are displayed by the gray scale technique (5). Figures 11 and
12 are axial tomograms of patients suspected of having lymphomas. Both scans were
taken at the same gain settings and it is noted that the spleen and liver in Figure 11
returns very low-level echoes compared with those seen in Figure 12. Computerized A-
scan analysis on the amplitude of the echoes from the spleens of patients with a number of
different disorders producing chronic splenomegaly was carried out, and it was found that
enlarged spleens returning very low-level echoes were often malignant. Most of those
returning high-level echoes were found to be benign and due to chronic inflammatory
states including tuberculosis, brucellosis, malaria, and sarcoidosis. However, it must be
stressed that these observations only relate to the patients when they are seen initially,
since aggressive treatment of neoplasms with chemotherapy and radiotherapy to the
spleen may considerably increase the level of echoes emanating from it.

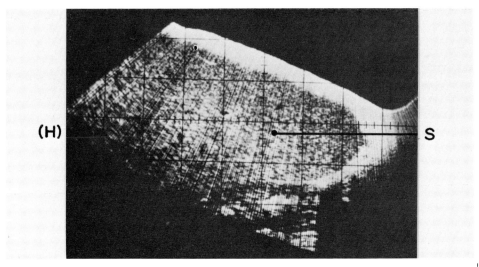

Figure 10.   Longitudinal sector scan of spleen (S) in paramedian plane in patient with brucellosis. This scanning technique can be used only in patients with moderate to marked splenomegaly in whom the spleen displaces air-containing gut.

Examination of the spleen is also useful in the assessment of portal hypertension secondary to such conditions as cirrhosis of the liver. In portal hypertension, progressive obliteration of the portal venous channels leads to a reduction of blood flow and eventually to reversal of flow in that vein. Back pressure affects the spleen, causing venous engorgement and enlargement. Oblique scans of the spleen using the technique described above, provide a linear measure of the longitudinal axis of the spleen that

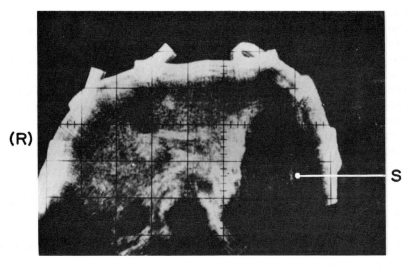

Figure 11.   Transverse ultrasound axial tomogram through upper abdomen of patient with hepatosplenomegaly. Note that the spleen (S) returns very low level echoes and hence appears black. Such appearances are found in untreated lymphomas or leukemias.

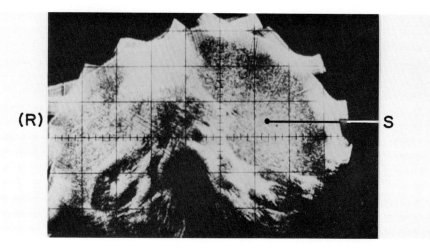

Figure 12. Transverse ultrasound axial tomogram through upper abdomen of patient with hepatosplenomegaly. Note that the liver and spleen (S) return very high level echoes and this is most characteristic of inflammatory causes for hepatosplenomegaly. This patient suffered from tuberculosis.

will confirm, and to an extent quantify, the degree of portal hypertension. In the longer term, it should be possible to differentiate the direction of the flow and measure the absolute blood flow in the portal vein using Doppler techniques.

Workmen exposed to polyvinyl chloride (PVC) monomer during its production may develop periportal fibrosis with consequent portal hypertension and splenomegaly. Preliminary data indicate that ultrasonic techniques are reliable indicators of this type of pathologic state (6).

SPLENIC CYSTS

Splenic cysts are easy to diagnose by ultrasound and appear as echo-free areas with low attenuation. Distal to the cyst, the echoes are overamplified since the compensation for tissue attenuation (TGC) is excessive for the very low attenuation by the cyst contents. Compressed splenic tissue is seen posterior to the cyst as in Figure 13.

The most common splenic cysts are echinococcal in origin although the rarer congenital epidermoid cysts also have been detected. It is usually possible to separate a splenic cyst from the left kidney; but if there is doubt as to whether the cyst arises from the kidney or spleen, an intravenous pyelogram and/or liver/spleen isotope scan is most helpful.

Cystic collections within the spleen also may result from the organization of blood in an intrasplenic hematoma. The level of returned echoes depends upon the degree of the organization of the hematoma, and such collections may be much more difficult to diagnose than simple cysts of congenital origin.

OTHER SITES OF RETICULOENDOTHELIAL PROLIFERATION

Abnormal reticuloendothelial proliferation may occur in many other sites in addition to the retroperitoneal site in various neoplastic conditions. It is important to note that lym-

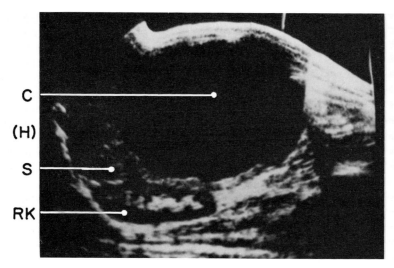

Figure 13.   Paramedian ultrasonogram through left upper quadrant mass in 11-year-old boy. A huge cystic cavity (C) is seen lying superficially with compressed spleen (S) and left kidney (LK) posteriorly.

phoid tissue in any anatomic site tends to have the same ultrasonic characteristics, which consist of low attenuation and low echo amplitude in the untreated state. Lymphomatous infiltration of the liver is common in the advanced state of the disease, and this gives rise to well-delineated areas of very low echo amplitude. (Figure 14.) Subsequent chemotherapy may alter this pattern greatly and return the levels of echoes more toward normality.

Thus, lymphomatous infiltration in other organs tends to give tumors of low attenuation and low echo amplitude. Enlargement of the thymus gland, as in a thymoma, is

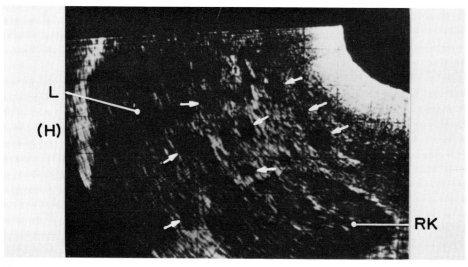

Figure 14.   Paramedian ultrasonogram through right lobe of liver (H) and right kidney (RK). Note extensive replacement of normal parenchyma by multiple small homogeneous masses (arrow). These appearances are consistent with discrete lymphomatous infiltration of the liver.

seen as a low echo-producing area anterior to the heart, while mediastinal nodes show typical lobulated low echo-producing area. Neoplastic proliferation of the lymphoid tissue in the thyroid produces accoustically highly homogeneous tumors, as do lymphomas arising in the retroorbital site.

In conclusion, the reticuloendothelial system is a diffuse anatomic entity of which only the spleen can be imaged adequately by current ultrasonic techniques in the normal person. In disease states, abnormal lymphoid masses may be visualized by ultrasound in many different sites, including the retroperitoneum and enlarged paraaortic and mesenteric regions. Such pathologic conditions may not be easily demonstrable by other diagnostic methods. Even when intestinal gas precludes visualization of the retroperitoneal area, the presence of abnormal masses sometimes may be inferred by pressure effects, such as hydronephrosis or biliary tract distension.

The recent availability of gray scale technology results in the display of the tissue texture in addition to organ contours, which should improve the ability to differentially diagnose various causes of splenomegaly.

ACKNOWLEDGMENT

We thank the editor of the *British Journal of Radiology* for permission to publish Figures 10–12.

REFERENCES

1. Taylor KJW, Hill CR: Scanning techniques in gray scale ultrasonography. *Brit J Radiol* **48**:918–920, 1975.

2. Freimanis A K, Asher W M: Development of diagnostic criteria in echographic study of abdominal lesions. *Am J Roentgenol* **108**:747–755, 1970.

3. Taylor KJW, Kraus V: Gray-scale ultrasound imaging: Assessment of acute hydronephrosis. *Brit J Urol* **47**:593–597, 1975.

4. Kardel T, Holm HH, Rasmussen SN, Mortensen T: Ultrasonic determination of liver and spleen volume. *Scand J Clin Lab Invest* **27**:123–128, 1971.

5. Taylor KJW, Milan J: Differential diagnosis of chronic splenomegaly by gray-scale ultrasonography: Clinical observations and digital A-scan analysis. *Brit J Radiol* **49**:519–525, 1976.

6. Taylor KJW, Williams DMJ, Smith PM, Duck BW: Gray scale ultrasonography for monitoring industrial exposure to hepato-toxic agents. *Lancet*, **1**:1222–1224, 1975.

9

Abscesses, Hematomas, and Other Fluid Collections

Bruce D. Doust, M.B.

Associate Professor of Radiology
Medical College of Wisconsin

Director of Ultrasound
Milwaukee County Medical Complex
Milwaukee, Wisconsin

The most striking advantage of ultrasonic studies over conventional radiographic techniques is their ability to distinguish fluid-filled structures from solid lesions. Thus, ultrasound is a particularly powerful tool in the diagnosis of abscesses, ascites, hematomas, urinomas, and lymphoceles. Even so, caution is needed in the ultrasonic diagnosis of fluid collections, particularly abscesses. A false-positive diagnosis of abscess is particularly unfortunate because it may result in inappropriate surgical exploration in a patient who is already seriously ill. Since abscesses needing surgical drainage increase in size, repeated ultrasonic examination should be used to clarify doubtful cases.

TECHNIQUE

Generally, no patient preparation is required. Administration of simethicone for 2 or 3 days prior to an ultrasound study may improve scan quality by reducing the amount of bowel gas. If there is barium sulfate in the gut, laxatives or enemas may be needed to remove it. If possible, ultrasonic studies should be scheduled prior to barium studies.

Mineral oil or aqueous gel must be used to provide sonic coupling. Mineral oil is a better lubricant and facilitates transducer motion, while aqueous gel is easier to remove, allowing dressings to be reapplied more easily and securely after the study. Dressings and colostomy belts should be loosened or removed as the first step in the examination, so as much of the abdomen as possible is exposed. Minimal cover should be left over open wounds to prevent contamination. As much of the abdomen as possible should be examined by transverse and longitudinal scans at 2 cm- or 3-cm intervals. Areas deep to incisions may be examined by an oblique approach through adjacent intact skin. A subcostal approach must be used to examine the superior part of the liver, which is inaccessible by the direct AP approach (1, 2). In the subcostal approach, the transducer is indented firmly under the right costal margin, pointed cranially, and a single slow sweep is performed while the patient holds his breath in full inspiration (Figure 1).

The posterior subphrenic areas are examined best by several longitudinal scans through the kidney and the posterior lower ribs. Patients with open abdominal wounds and colostomies cannot lie prone, so the posterior examination must be performed with the patient in the right or left lateral decubitus position. In this position the scanner arm must be angled steeply so that it moves in an almost horizontal plane. Some commercially available scanning arms are incapable of the steep angulation required to perform this examination.

A longitudinal scan with the patient sitting upright sometimes will produce clearer pictures than the same scan performed with the patient recumbent. The upright scan is facilitated by adjusting the centering controls so the trace originates in one of the upper corners of the screen. This technique is particularly useful for distinguishing between pleural and subphrenic fluid collections (3).

There are several ways of identifying the diaphragm ultrasonically. Sometimes, the diaphragm can be identified on a conventional longitudinal scan, but ribs and lung usually obscure it. If the diaphragm is seen easily, there probably is some pleural fluid. Another method uses the subcostal approach (4), in the mid-clavicular line on the right or in the posterior axillary line on the left. The transducer is swept twice—once at full inspiration and again at full expiration, so two images of the diaphragm are produced (Figure 2A). Another method, that is useful in patients who cannot cooperate, consists of an M-mode (time-motion) study of diaphragmatic motion performed with the A-mode

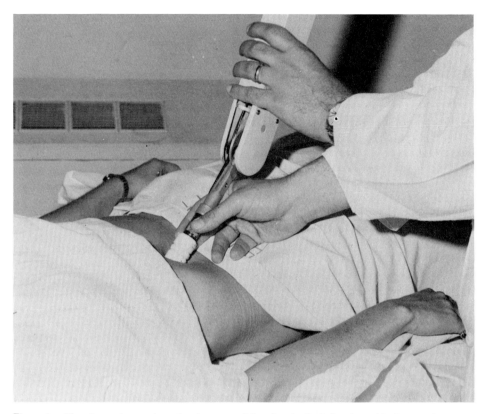

Figure 1. The ultrasonic transducer has been moved in a longitudinal direction with the transducer seen indenting the skin firmly under the right costal margin with the ultrasonic beam pointed cranially.

transducer indented under the costal margin and pointed cranially. The gain is reduced until only one echo (the diaphragm) remains, and an M-mode trace is taken of respiratory motion (Figure 2B) (5). A fourth method depends on the proximity of the diaphragm to the inferior surface of the heart. If the transducer is indented into the epigastrium, angled cranially and slightly to the left, and a slow single-sweep scan performed, a saw-tooth trace of moving cardiac structures results. The lowest level at which rhythmic motion is detected is the level of the diaphragm. This technique is useful in estimating the location of the anterior central portion of the left dome of the diaphragm (Figure 3) when the echo from the diaphragm itself is indistinct.

For a pelvic ultrasound examination, the patient's bladder should be distended. Results are unreliable when the patient's bladder is not distended. Two sets of transverse scans, one with 10-degree cranial angulation, the other with 10 to 15-degree caudal angulation, should be performed. Structures not demonstrated on one set often are seen clearly on the other, and I know of no way to predict which set will be the more revealing. The lateral parts of the pelvic cavity are best demonstrated by placing the transducer a little to one side of the midline and performing a single slow sweep sector scan by pivoting the transducer on the spot, so the sound beam sweeps the opposite pelvic wall. Oblique and longitudinal scans with tilt to the left or the right often help to demonstrate where a lesion lies in relation to the uterus and the bladder.

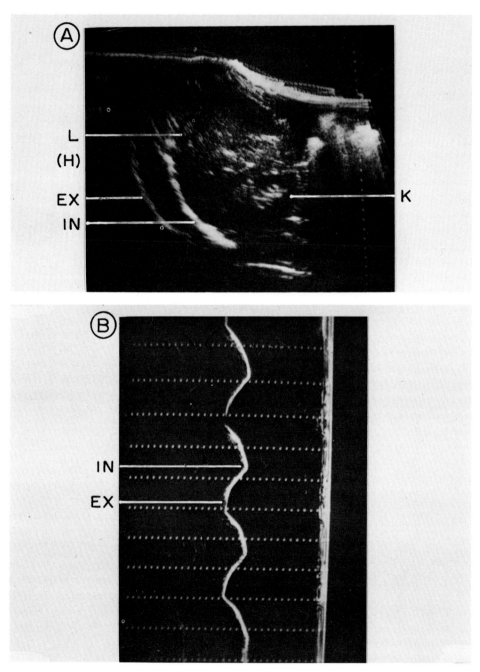

Figure 2. *A*. This longitudinal scan was taken approximately 7 cm to the right of the midline. Two sweeps of the transducer were performed: one in full inspiration, the other in full expiration. There are two images of the right dome of the diaphragm; the more cranial represents the position of the diaphragm in full expiration (K = kidney; L = liver). *B*. This M-mode scan was recorded by indenting the transducer below the right costal margin and pointing it cranially. The gain was reduced until only a single strong echo remained (the diaphragm). This M-mode trace of respiratory motion was then taken and indicates the position of the diaphragm relative to the transducer. On the left it is necessary to indent the transducer posterolaterally, as colonic and gastric gas make it impossible to get a good recording from the anterior aspect (H = head).

234

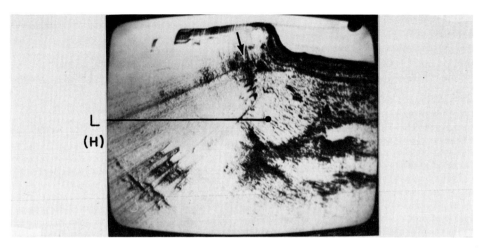

Figure 3. Identification of the diaphragm. This single-sweep sector scan was performed by indenting the transducer into the epigastrium a little to the left of the midline. (Cranial to the left, caudal to the right.) The saw-tooth configuration (arrow) of cardiac structures is due to their rhythmic to-and-fro motion. The lowest level at which this motion can be detected represents the inferior border of the heart and, therefore, the level of the diaphragm. This technique may be useful when the echo from the diaphragm itself is not clear (L = liver).

A continuous, rapid scanning technique is often valuable for surveying the entire abdomen. The transducer is moved rapidly back and forth while the screw drive of the transverse table moves the entire scanning arm slowly and continuously. Each pass of the transducer is displaced a little from the preceding one so that the transducer follows a zig-zag path. At the end of each sweep, the image is cleared from the screen and a new image forms with the succeeding sweep. Alternatively, the bistable oscilloscope can be used in the nonstorage mode. In this case, the room should be darkened. The entire abdomen can be examined quickly and thoroughly by this technique, and the best plane for demonstrating a structure can be located precisely. Unfortunately, some commercially available scanning arms do not provide continuous motion. Two-dimensional multicrystal ultrasonic instruments can be used in a similar fashion for a rapid survey.

Solid lesions may be missed easily if the gain settings are incorrect, and too high a gain also may obscure small fluid collections. The best settings vary with each patient, transducer, and scanner. The optimal settings should be determined for each study by setting the gain at a low level, scanning over a fluid-filled structure such as the gallbladder, the aorta, or the urinary bladder, and then increasing the gain until the contrast between the image of the fluid and the surrounding solid tissue is maximized. Some scanners have an output control that varies the power of the pulses that excite the transducer, and the best images usually are obtained if the highest settings are avoided. The highest settings are useful in demonstrating deeply located structures.

The transducer affects significantly the appearance of the scan. The best way to select a transducer is by trial and error, because the image quality obtained from nominally identical transducers seems to vary. The following recommendations, based on personal experience, are offered only as a guide. For anterior scans, a 2.25 MHz, 13-mm transducer focused at about 7 cm usually gives the best results. Occasionally, in emaciated patients, a 3.5 MHz, 13-mm transducer focused at 7 cm provides pictures of great clarity. A 2.25 MHz, 19-mm transducer focused at 10–12 cm is usually best for obese patients for examinations of the liver and for examinations performed through the posterior abdominal wall or the ribs.

The information obtainable from a scan depends heavily on the pattern of scanning motion. The sectored scan is best performed by an unhurried, to-and-fro brush-stroke motion that advances a little further across the abdomen with each stroke. The transducer should not be in contact with the skin at the end of a stroke, because the pause in transducer motion produces a dense line across the picture. Sectored scans can be recognized from their convoluted skin artifact (Figure 4A). They are useful for

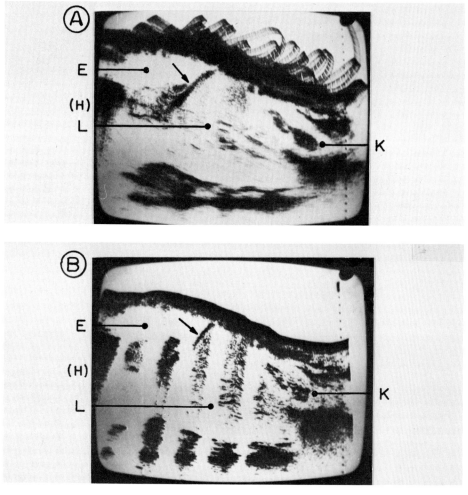

Figure 4. *A*. The sectored scan. This longitudinal scan was performed about 8 cm to the right of the vertebral column, with the patient prone. It shows the full outlines of the right kidney (K), the liver (L), the diaphram (arrow), and a large pleural effusion (E), in spite of the overlying ribs, which do not transmit sound. Note the convoluted skin artifact indicating much sectoring motion, and compare this picture with Figure 3*B*. *B*. The nonsectored scan. This scan was performed in exactly the same position as Figure 3*A*. It is a single pass scan, and care has been taken to avoid all sectoring motion. Organ outlines are incomplete, but sharper than in Figure 3*A*. Compare the image of the posterior part of the diaphragm in the two figures. Sonic shadows are very obvious and the structures casting the shadows (the ribs) can be precisely located. The same principle holds for zones of enhanced echoes deep to fluid collections.

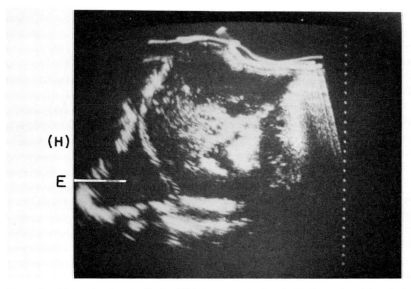

(H)

E ————————

Figure 5.   Right subpulmonic effusion. This is an anterior longitudinal scan (cranial to the left, caudal to the right) taken 8 cm to the right of the midline. There are two separate images of the diaphragm that are not quite superimposed due to respiratory movement between successive passes of the transducer. A pleural effusion (E) is seen above the diaphragm. Distinction from subphrenic abscess is easy when the diaphragm can be seen clearly.

demonstrating the complete outline of structures, for obtaining an image of an area deep to structures that do not transmit the sound (e.g., ribs), and for obtaining images of deep-seated, weakly echoing structures. However, sectored scanning decreases the sharpness of the image and obscures other diagnostically useful information. The single-sweep scan provides less complete but sharper images. The single-sweep scan may be a single sector, e.g., the subcostal longitudinal scan of the liver (Figure 5) or a single slow sweep scan that allows identification of pulsating structures, due to their saw-tooth configuration (Figure 3). A single-sweep scan performed with no retracing motion whatever is best for assessing enhanced through transmission, or sonic shadowing (Figure 4B). Even slight sectoring obscures the sonic shadow or the zone of enhanced echoes behind a small lesion. A fluid collection smaller than the diameter of the ultrasound beam may be demonstrated clearly in a single-sweep scan due to the zone of enhanced through transmission deep to it. Both sectored and nonsectored scans usually are required in the course of a study (compare Figure 4A and Figure 4B).

PROPERTIES COMMON TO MOST FLUID COLLECTIONS

Most fluid collections transmit sound well, are echo-free, and have well-defined margins. Structures greater than 2 cm in diameter that do not meet all three criteria may still be fluid collections. Renal carbuncles are exceptional and are reported to echo quite strongly. They may be indistinguishable from a hypernephroma [6]. Collections that contain much solid debris may have numerous internal echoes. Collections that are smaller than the diameter of the sound beam do not appear echo-free but can be identified by the zone of enhanced echoes deep to them.

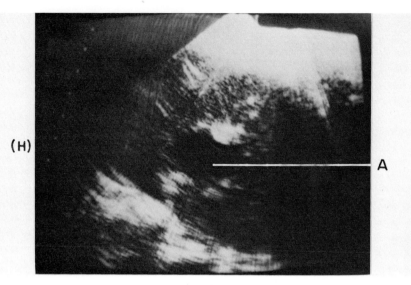

Figure 6. Small intrahepatic abscess. This longitudinal scan was taken in the anterior axillary line with the patient in the left lateral decubitus position. The abscess (A) measures less than 2 cm in its greatest diameter. It is not well marginated and is approximately circular. An abscess of these dimensions is easily overlooked. Compare with Figure 5.

Abscesses have properties that aid in distinguishing them from other fluid collections. The wall of an abscess is not as sharp as that of a cyst (Figure 6) or a fluid collection containing noninflammatory fluid such as ascites. Abscesses displace adjacent structures and are usually spherical or ellipsoidal (football-shaped), with no sharp angles.* (Right-sided subphrenic abscesses are an exception and may be crescentic because they are confined between the liver and the diaphragm.) Noninflammatory fluid such as ascites insinuates itself between organs so that the collection assumes a shape determined by the organs around it (Figure 7). Thus a collection of noninflammatory fluid often has a highly irregular outline. In summary, inflammatory fluid collections have a football-like shape of their own and indent or displace the structures around them, while noninflammatory fluid collections have more sharply defined walls and are indented and shaped by the adjacent organs. Compare Figure 12 with Figure 17.

Further clarification of the nature of a fluid collection may be obtained by fine needle puncture and aspiration of a fluid sample. Drilled and slotted transducers made specifically to guide the needle to its target are commercially available (9, 10, 11, 12).

RIGHT SUBPHRENIC ABSCESS

Right subphrenic abscesses may be purely subphrenic or may be both intrahepatic and subphrenic. The anterior right subphrenic area is best examined by the subcostal

---

* The volume of an ellipsoid is given by the formula:

$$\text{Volume} = 0.52 \times \text{length} \times \text{breadth} \times \text{depth}$$
$$\quad\text{(cc)} \qquad\qquad \text{(cm)} \qquad \text{(cm)} \qquad \text{(cm)}$$

Serial examinations allow objective assessment of the progress of an ellipsoidal fluid collection that is not drained at the time of diagnosis. Estimates of the volume of irregularly shaped fluid collections can be obtained ultrasonically, but the methods require a computer program or are laborious (7, 8).

approach. A longitudinal scan with the patient in the upright position sometimes allows clear distinction between a large intrahepatic abscess high in the right lobe of the liver, and an intrahepatic abscess with subphrenic extension (5).

A right subphrenic abscess often has a crescentic extrahepatic component, bounded by the diaphragm above, the abdominal wall laterally, and the liver below and medially. The liver capsule produces a particularly strong linear echo that indicates the boundary between the abscess and the liver, even when the liver parenchyma is unusually homogeneous.

Excessive gain setting should be avoided to minimize the confusing effects of reverberations. A gain setting that is too low makes it difficult to distinguish between the fluid collection and liver parenchyma but does not obscure the strong echo from the liver capsule. Near gain suppression should not be used to eliminate rib artifacts, because a confusing, artifactually echo-free zone results. Right subphrenic abscesses should be examined from the posterior approach, even when the anterior view suggests the liver has been fully demonstrated.

When a longitudinal (not subcostal) examination demonstrates the diaphragm with unusual clarity and ease, there is probably a pleural effusion (Figure 4). The curvature of the diaphragm insures that a clearer echo is obtained from its upper surface than from below, provided there is pleural fluid to conduct the sound. Subphrenic abscesses are commonly accompanied by pleural effusion. Distinction between subphrenic and pleural fluid depends on localizing the diaphragm (Figures 2 and 5).

INTRAHEPATIC ABSCESSES

Intrahepatic abscesses almost always are spherical and appear circular in both longitudinal and transverse scans. The margins may be ragged (Figure 6), particularly if the lesion is an amebic abscess (13). Because intrahepatic abscesses are sometimes multiple, the examination should not be concluded when the first abscess is found. Scans should

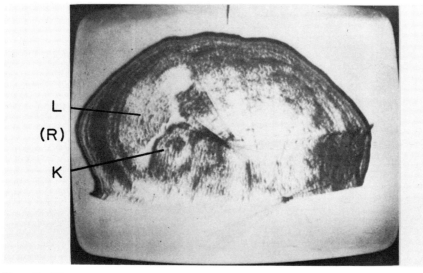

Figure 7.   The transverse ultrasonogram shows ascitic fluid collecting between the liver and kidney conforming to the shape of these organs (L = liver; K = kidney).

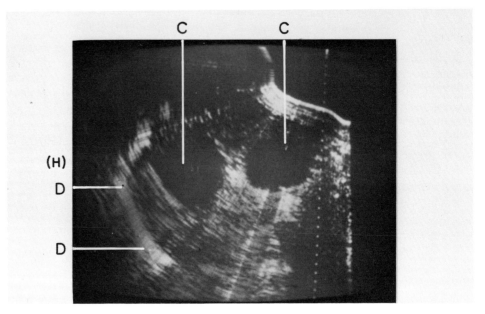

Figure 8.   Intrahepatic cysts. This is a subcostal scan of the liver. This type of scan is useful for demonstrating fine detail and for demonstrating the upper part of the right lobe of the liver and the dome of the diaphragm. Repeated sweeps blur the image. Two large cysts (C) are demonstrated. Note that their walls are very sharp in contrast to the walls of an intrahepatic abscess (compare with Figure 6).

be no more than 2 cm apart. Abscesses in the upper part of the right lobe of the liver are the hardest to detect.

During surgical exploration, it may be very difficult to identify the site of an intrahepatic abscess. Therefore, it is useful to mark the site of an abscess on the patient's skin as a guide to the surgeon, especially if there is more than one abscess.

Liver abscesses (Figure 6) occasionally must be distinguished from liver cysts (Figure 8) or a large metastasis. The patient's clinical condition usually makes the difference clear. Cysts have sharper borders than abscesses and are sometimes accompanied by polycystic kidneys. Some metastases are almost echo-free (Figure 9) but generally do not enhance echoes from structures deep to them. However, there are occasional exceptions and a solitary metastasis high in the right lobe of the liver may be particularly difficult to assess, because access to it is limited by overlying ribs and lung (1).

LEFT-SIDED SUBPHRENIC FLUID

The left-sided subphrenic region is probably the most difficult area of the abdomen to demonstrate ultrasonically, because access is restricted by the lung above, the gas-filled stomach and splenic flexure anteriorly, and the ribs laterally. Filling the stomach with water is not helpful. The best approach is through the bed of the kidney and the posterior aspect of the left lower ribs. It may be difficult to distinguish a left-sided subphrenic abscess from the spleen, which sometimes conducts sound very well and may be almost echo-free. Left subphrenic fluid collection should be diagnosed only when there is a clear difference between splenic pulp and the abscess, or when there is a clear boundary (the splenic capsule) (Figure 10) between them. Otherwise, an echo-free structure in the left subphrenic area probably represents the spleen alone (Figure 11). A radionuclide scan can be used to estimate splenic size. Comparison between the radionuclide scan and the ultrasound study determines whether the spleen is large enough to account for all the echo-free zone demonstrated in the echogram. A fluid-filled stomach could be confused with an abscess. However, a repeat examination after at least a several hour delay will usually show a decrease in size (Figure 12).

When the patient has undergone splenectomy, a left subphrenic abscess may look like the spleen, so it is important to seek a history of splenectomy prior to interpreting a study. If the left kidney is immediately below the diaphragm, the patient probably has undergone splenectomy and probably does not have a posterior left subphrenic collection.

SUBHEPATIC ABSCESS

The gallbladder may be surprisingly large in patients who have been fasting, and it must not be mistaken for a subhepatic abscess. Its pyriform shape and sharp wall usually distinguish it from an abscess. Occasionally a gallstone, which produces a strong linear echo and casts a dense sonic shadow, allows even more confident identification of the gallbladder (14, 15). Demonstration that the gallbladder is separate from the subhepatic collection (Figures 13 and 14) is the most certain way of avoiding error.

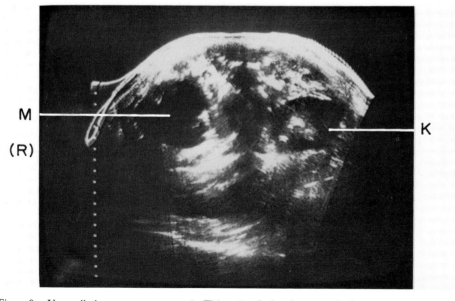

Figure 9.   Unusually homogeneous metastasis. This patient had undergone radical mastectomy for carcinoma some years previously. This transverse posterior scan taken about 8 cm above the iliac crest demonstrates a rounded, sharply defined highly homogeneous lesion (M) that potentiates the echoes from the structures deep to it. Compare the echoes deep to the metastasis with those deep to the left kidney (K). Fortunately, metastases rarely conducts sound or are as echo-free as this one.

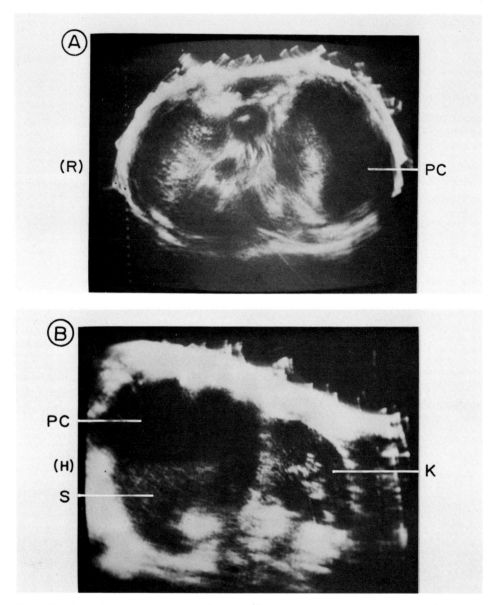

Figure 10.   Left subphrenic pancreatic pseudocyst. *A.* This transverse posterior scan was taken about 15 cm above the iliac crest. The pseudocyst (PC) resembles an enlarged spleen. *B.* This posterior longitudinal scan, taken 9 cm to the left of the midline (cranial to the left, caudal to the right) demonstrates a clear difference between the fluid within the pseudocyst (PC) and the spleen (S). If no difference can be demonstrated, it is likely that the echo-free zone represents an enlarged spleen alone.

ABSCESSES IN THE GENERAL PERITONEAL CAVITY

Diagnosis of abscesses in the general peritoneal cavity is usually straightforward. Abscesses may be multiple (Figure 15) and a thorough examination is always necessary. The question whether a fluid-filled bowel loop could be mistaken for an abscess often is raised, but this error is very rare, probably because bowel loops usually contain a little

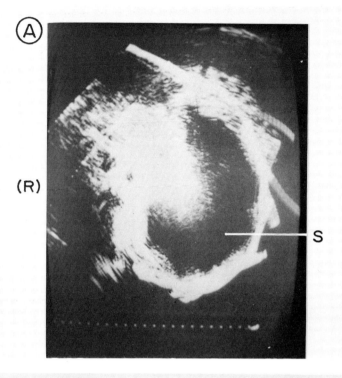

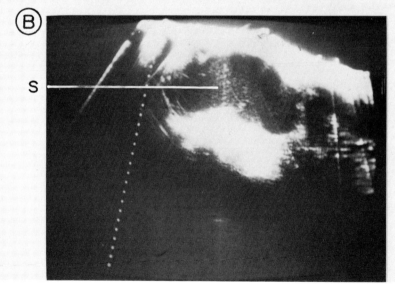

Figure 11. Enlarged and engorged spleen. The patient had suffered thrombosis of the portal venous system subsequent to blunt abdominal trauma. *A*. This transverse scan was taken with the patient in the right lateral decubitus position and the scanners set at maximum gain. The spleen (S) remains echo-free and at the time of examination was thought to represent a left-sided subphrenic abscess. Longitudinal scans supported the impression of fluidity. Note that there is no junction zone nor linear echo from the splenic capsule. *B*. This longitudinal scan taken 2 months subsequent to Figure 9A shows that the spleen now produces sufficient echoes to be recognizably solid. In this patient misdiagnosis was avoided by performing a radionuclide scan which demonstrated that the spleen was large enough to account for the entire echo-free area seen on the ultrasonic scan.

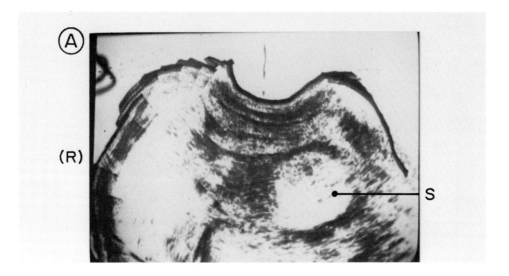

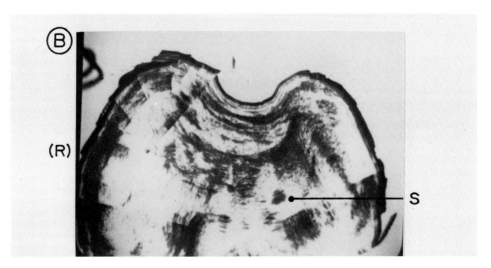

Figure 12. *A*. The transverse ultrasonogram shows a complex, predominantly cystic mass in the left quadrant of the abdomen consistent with the diagnosis of a fluid-filled stomach (S). *B*. Follow-up transverse ultrasonogram shows a definite decrease in the size of the previously detected mass due to partial emptying of the stomach (S).

gas as well as fluid and change their appearance during the study due to peristalsis. The transverse colon on longitudinal scan often has a typical "bull's-eye" appearance (Figure 16). However, dilated fluid-filled bowel proximal to an obstructing carcinoma of the cecum, and a dilated afferent loop have been reported to resemble localized fluid collections such as abscesses (16, 17). Loops of avascular, necrotic fluid-filled bowel are aperistaltic, may be indistinguishable from multiple localized extraluminal fluid collections, and may be accompanied by free intraperitoneal fluid (Figure 17).

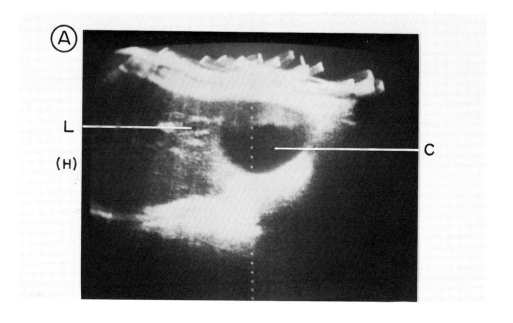

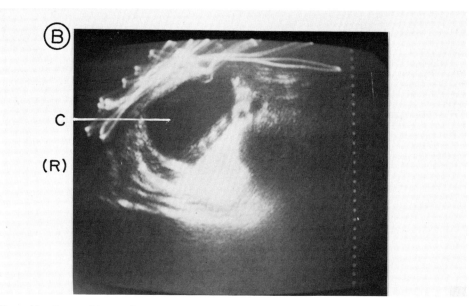

Figure 13. Large subhepatic fluid collection. *A*. Longitudinal scan, cranial to the left and caudal to the right, taken 8 cm to the right of the midline. A large, well defined fluid collection (C) is seen immediately caudal to the liver (L). *B*. Transverse scan, again showing the fluid collection a little to the right of the midline. *C*. This longitudinal scan (cranial to the left, caudal to the right) shows the gallbladder (G) separate from the fluid collection (C). Demonstration that there are 2 subhepatic fluid collections is positive proof that at least one of them is not the gallbladder. This fluid collection proved to be a large renal cyst. (*Continued on next page*.)

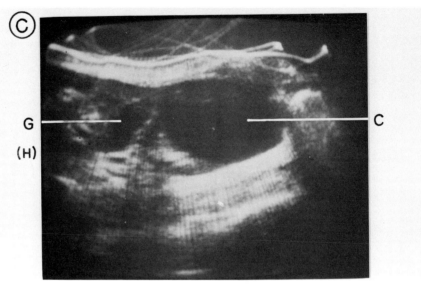

Figure 13. (Continued)

PELVIC ABSCESS

Prior to any ultrasonic study of the pelvic, the patient's bladder should be distended to push bowel loops out of the pelvis and to provide a good sound conducting medium. An anuric patient may require catheterization to fill the bladder. When the bladder is empty, results are unreliable.

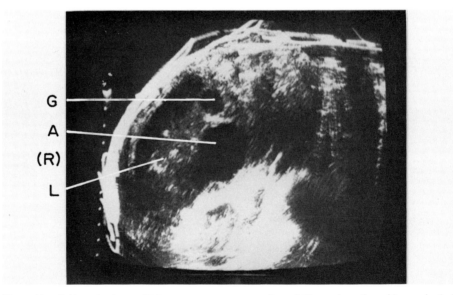

Figure 14.   Subhepatic abscess. This transverse scan was performed 18 cm above the pubic symphysis. The abscess (A) is circular and unusually well defined. It is clearly separate from the gallbaldder (G) (L = Liver).

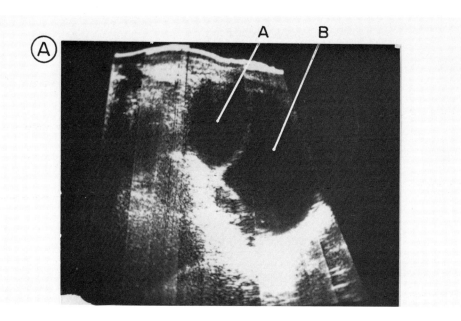

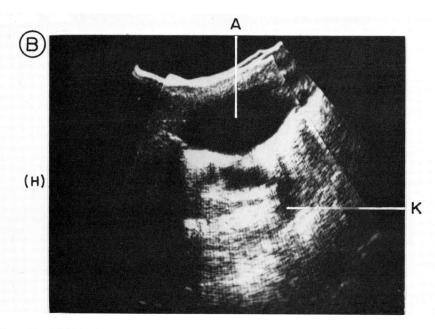

Figure 15. Multiple abscesses. *A*. This longitudinal scan taken in the midline shows an abscess (A) in direct contact with bladder (B) and immediately cranial to it. Note that the abscess indents the bladder. A collection of ascites does not indent the bladder. *B*. Same patient as Figure 12*A*. This is a longitudinal scan in the left midaxillary line. The patient is in the right lateral decubitus position. A second abscess (A) is lateral and a little anterior to the left kidney (K). Demonstration of one abscess does not preclude the presence of other abscesses.

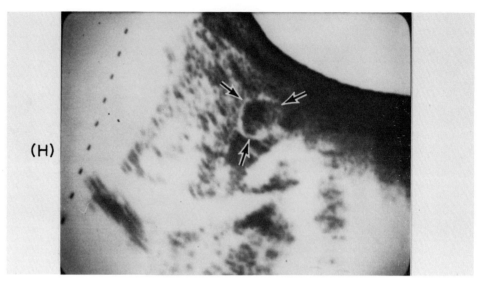

Figure 16.   Longitudinal ultrasonogram shows typical ultrasonic appearance of the transverse colon (arrows).

Pelvic abscesses have the same ultrasonic properties as abscesses elsewhere in the abdomen. They must be distinguished from an ectopic pregnancy, an ovarian cyst, and the urinary bladder. Distinction from the bladder is usually achieved by asking the patient to void. However, a large postvoid residual may cause confusion. Demonstration of two separate fluid collections is good evidence that at least one of them is not the blad-

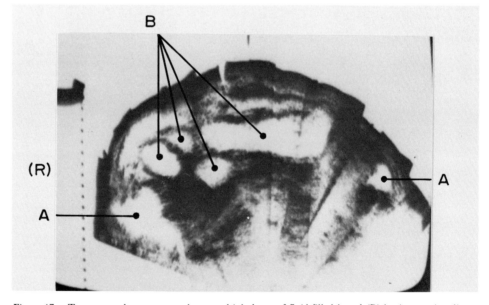

Figure 17.   Transverse ultrasonogram shows multiple loops of fluid-filled bowel (B) having varying dimensions. There is also evidence of minimal ascites (A) seen in the flanks.

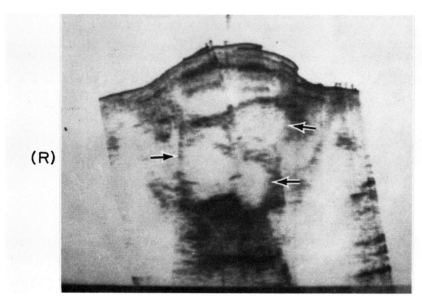

Figure 18.   Transverse ultrasonogram demonstrates multiple pelvic abscesses (arrows) producing a complex ultrasonic pattern with the walls not as sharply defined as would be expected with cysts.

der. However, if the bladder is indented by a solid mass such as an enlarged uterus, the bladder may look like two separate fluid collections. Oblique scans usually demonstrate that the two echo-free areas are really parts of the same organ.

Ectopic pregnancy is recognized ultrasonically as an adnexal mass accompanied by an enlarged uterus containing evenly echoing material (the decidual reaction). Unfortunately, false-negative diagnoses are common (25 percent) and the ultrasonic appearances may be very confusing (18). Failure to demonstrate an adnexal mass does not exclude ectopic pregnancy, since the sac may have ruptured before the examination.

Tuboovarian abscess should be suspected when the scan shows a nonpregnant uterus and a fluid-filled adnexal mass with walls that are less sharply defined than those of a cyst (Figure 18). An appendix abscess may have an identical appearance. With some abscesses layering may occur with the debris settling to the bottom producing dependent echoes. Changing position will produce a shift of the echoes related to gravitational effects.

HEMATOMAS

Usually, intraabdominal hematomas appear ultrasonically similar to abscesses but occasionally there are differences. As blood clot fragments, the number of echoes within it increases (19). Clot may form irregularly in a hematoma so that strongly echoing areas develop within the otherwise echo-free fluid. A hematoma that develops subsequent to removal of a transplanted kidney may resemble the transplanted kidney (Figure 19). Many hematomas do not show this feature and cannot be differentiated ultrasonically from other localized fluid collections.

Retroperitoneal fluid collections enhance the clarity with which the walls of the aorta and inferior vena cava can be seen (Figure 20). This property distinguishes a

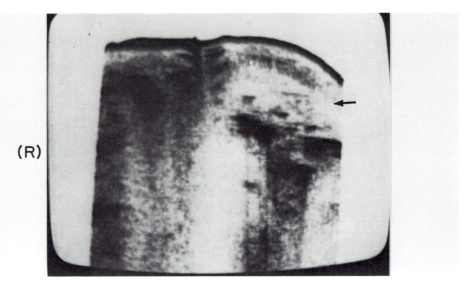

Figure 19. Organizing hematoma. A rejected kidney transplant had been removed from this patient's left iliac fossa about 1 month prior to the study. This transverse scan shows a complex structure with an outline reminiscent of a kidney, with irregular, strongly echoing structures within it (arrow). At operation, a hematoma with pieces of organizing clot within it was found.

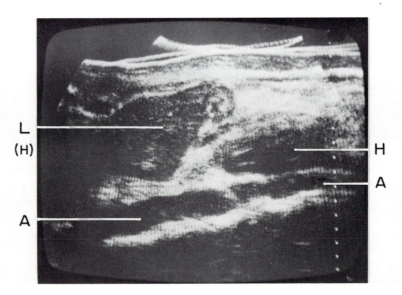

Figure 20. Retroperitoneal hematoma. A relatively echo-free hematoma (H) lies immediately anterior to the aorta (A). Note that the anterior aortic wall is not obliterated by the hematoma. At operation the patient was found to have a retroperitoneal hematoma immediately caudal to the pancreas caused by bleeding from an aneurysm on one of the pancreatico-duodenal arcades (L = liver).

250

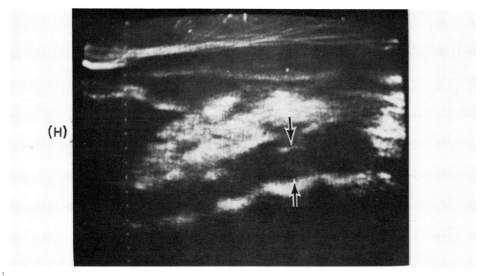

(H)

Figure 21. Enlarged retroperitoneal lymph nodes. This longitudinal scan, taken 2 cm to the left of the midline, demonstrates a large retroperitoneal mass that resembles an abdominal aortic aneurysm. Note the two faint longitudinal lines (arrows) within the mass which represent the walls of the aorta. The walls are poorly seen because of their similarity to the tissue that surrounds them. The vessel is displaced forward from the vertebral column, another sign of retroperitoneal lymphadenopathy.

retroperitoneal hematoma from a mass of retroperitoneal lymph nodes. Retroperitoneal lymph nodes often obscure the walls of the great vessels (Figure 21) and usually do not enhance the transmission (Figure 22) (20). Whenever a retroperitoneal fluid collection is found, the abdominal aorta should be examined for evidence of saccular or dissecting aneurysm.

URINOMAS AND LYMPHOCELES

Abnormal fluid collections that occur in relation to transplanted kidneys are lymphocele, urinoma, abscess, and hematoma (21). Generally the nature of the fluid cannot be predicted by ultrasonic examination, but collections with sharp, highly irregular outlines are probably not abscesses.

Soon after transplantation and during rejection, the kidney becomes swollen and (except for the calyces) it is echo-free; so that it has the properties of a fluid collection. A swollen upper or lower pole may be very hard to distinguish from fluid, particularly in sections that do not contain an image of the pelvicalyceal system. An abnormal fluid collection should be diagnosed only if the junction between the kidney parenchyma and the fluid (the renal capsule) can be demonstrated, or if the echo-free zone clearly is not related to the pelvicalyceal system or if there is an echo-free zone and the kidney has been removed. Occasionally, the psoas muscle may be nearly echo-free. Its shape and position serve to distinguish it from a fluid collection.

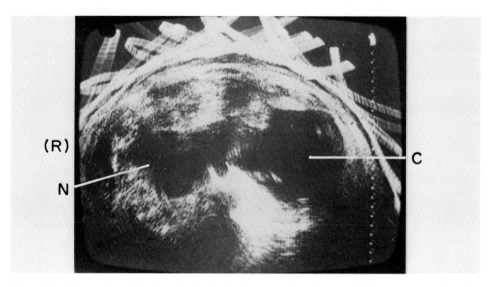

Figure 22. Retroperitoneal lymph nodes involved with metastatic malignancy. This transverse section taken 18 cm above the pubic symphysis shows two large lesions. There is a large fluid collection (C) on the left. It has very few internal echoes, has a regular margin, and strongly potentiates echoes from structures deep to it. On the right, there is a mass of enlarged lymph nodes involved by metastatic malignancy (N). The lymph node mass does not conduct sound as well as the fluid collection so that there is no potentiation of deep echoes, and detail of the retroperitoneal structures such as the aorta and vena cava is obscured. (Compare with Figure 14).

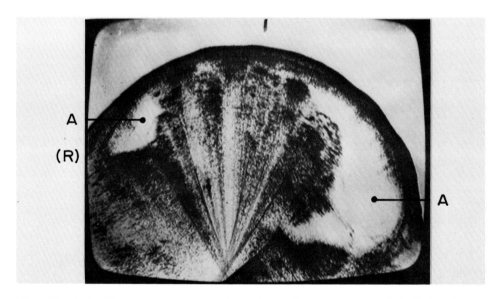

Figure 23. Ascites. Transverse ultrasonogram shows ascitic fluid (A) collecting in both the flanks and bowel loops located centrally. The greater amount of fluid has collected on the left compared to the right.

252

PANCREATIC PSEUDOCYSTS AND ABSCESSES

Colonic and gastric gas make it difficult or impossible to examine the tail of the pancreas through the anterior abdominal wall so that examinations for pseudocysts should routinely include scans performed through the bed of the left kidney as well as the usual examination through the anterior abdominal wall (Figure 9). Pancreatic pseudocysts are generally echo-free, unilocular structures with well-defined margins. However, they may contain debris, may be multiple, and may occasionally be a considerable distance from the pancreas (22, 23).

Serial estimates of the volume of a pancreatic pseudocyst give an indication of its progress. Ultrasonic monitoring of pseudocysts has recently shown that some pseudocysts resolve without surgery. They also may enlarge, migrate, remain unchanged for long periods, or rupture (22).

Provided the patient's condition allows, it is customary to defer drainage of a pseudocyst until it is stable in size and has a well-developed wall. The pseudocyst is then regarded as mature. Ultrasonic criteria of maturity have not yet been worked out, but it is likely that a pseudocyst is not mature if it has a ragged wall, contains debris, or is enlarging.

Pancreatic abscesses are very similar to pseudocysts. Pancreatic abscesses may be difficult to demonstrate ultrasonically, because the ileus of severe pancreatitis and excessive bowel gas obscure the pancreatic bed.

FREE INTRA-PERITONEAL FLUID

A massive amount of free intraperitoneal fluid has so characteristic an appearance (Figure 23) that confusion with any other condition is highly unlikely. In the supine patient with massive ascites, the bowel floats upward into the dome formed by the anterior abdominal wall, leaving the lateral parts of the abdomen filled with ascites. The fluid is echo-free, has a crescentic appearance, and separates the liver from the anterior and lateral abdominal walls.

Occasionally massive ovarian tumors appear similar to ascites both clinically and ultrasonically, but they may be distinguished because some ovarian tumors have internal septa and massive ascites does not and ascites displaces the bowel and the liver medially, whereas ovarian tumors displace the bowel and liver cranially and laterally. Therefore, in patients with a massive ovarian tumor, the central portion of the abdomen is echo-free and the liver is in direct contact with the lateral abdominal wall.

When the ascites is less extensive, it can be diagnosed by both A-mode and B-mode studies. The A-mode technique is known to be very sensitive and can detect volumes as small as 100 ml (24). The patient kneels on all fours for about 3 minutes, which allows the fluid to pool in the region of the umbilicus. The transducer is then placed in the region of the umbilicus, pointing upward, and an A-mode study recorded. Demonstration of an echo-free zone deep to the anterior abdominal wall is suggestive of ascites. If the patient then rolls onto his back and the echo-free zone disappears, the diagnosis of free intraperitoneal fluid is proven. The B-mode technique does not require as much patient cooperation, but its sensitivity compared to the A-mode technique has not been assessed (25).

The B-mode scan allows demonstration of loculated ascites and small volumes of fluid with the patient supine. Thus, ascites localized around the liver appears as an echo-free zone between the liver and the lateral abdominal wall or between the liver and the right kidney (Figure 7) or around the posterior part of the right lobe of the liver (Figure 24). Ultrasonic examination, whether A-mode or B-mode, does not distinguish between ascites and other types of free intraperitoneal fluid.

Localized collections of ascites must be distinguished from abscesses. The most useful differential points are: (a) abscesses are generally ellipsoidal and displace adjacent structures, whereas collections of ascites fill the spaces around preexisting structures and are shaped by them; (b) the wall of an abscess is less sharp than that of a collection of noninflammatory fluid; (c) loops of bowel sometimes float in collections of ascites (Figure 25) but never in an abscess; (d) loculated collections of ascites are generally more widespread and numerous than multiple abscesses. Whenever the diagnosis is in doubt, a repeat examination, to estimate change in size, is advisable.

FLUID COLLECTIONS BETWEEN ADJACENT FLAT STRUCTURES—THE LENTICULAR COLLECTION

A fluid collection (other than an abscess) that lies between two well-formed membranes takes up a biconvex lenticular shape that has a sharp, acute angle at one or both ends. This sharp angle assists in identifying the site of the collection. Abdominal wall hematomas (Figure 26), some abdominal wall abscesses (26), a hematoma or loculated ascites between the anterior abdominal wall and the liver (Figure 27) and fluid confined between the anterior abdominal wall and the greater omentum have this shape. A fluid

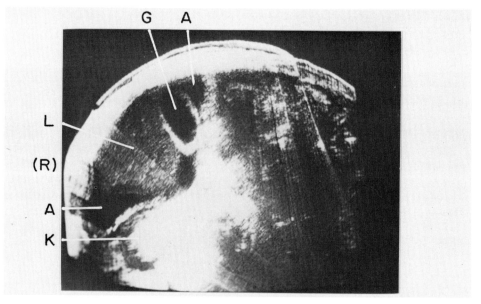

Figure 24.   Malignant ascites around the liver. Sometimes small volumes of ascites (A) separate the posterior aspect of the liver from the right kidney (K), as is seen in this transverse scan. The gallbladder (G) also is outlined by the ascites.

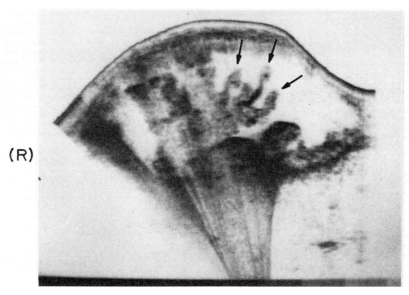

Figure 25. Noninflammatory intraperitoneal fluid. This transverse scan was taken at the level of the umbilicus. The fluid is represented by the echo-free areas on the right and left. Loops of bowel (arrows) can be seen floating in the fluid. Abscesses do not have bowel loops within them. An abscess displaces bowel.

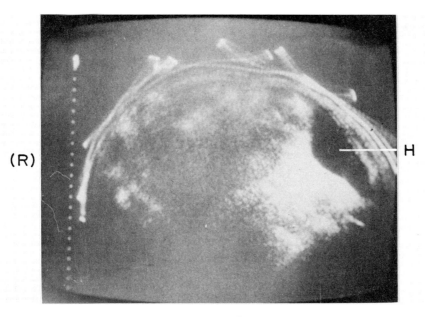

Figure 26. Hematoma of the anterior abdominal wall. The patient had fallen, striking his left side. Physical examination suggested ruptured spleen. This transverse scan taken about 20 cm above the pubic symphysis shows a biconvex (lens-shaped) fluid collection with a sharply defined inner margin, pronounced potentiation of deep echoes and a beaklike medial extremity. At operation, a hematoma of the anterior abdominal wall was demonstrated.

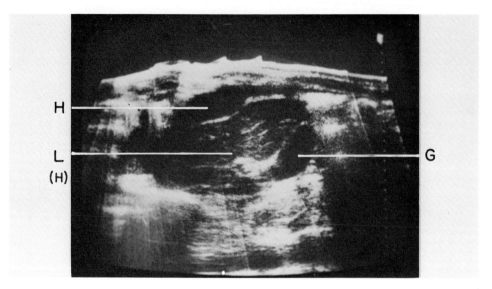

Figure 27.   Hematoma between the liver and anterior abdominal wall. This longitudinal scan, cranial to the left and caudal to the right, was taken 6 cm to the right of the midline. The hematoma (H) is bounded posteriorly by the strongly echoing, sharply defined liver capsule (G = gallbladder; L = liver).

collection that has a sharp angle but which is otherwise regular, is probably in or in contact with the abdominal wall or some other sheet-like structure.

SUPERFICIAL COLLECTIONS

Superficial abscesses and hematomas may be easily identified due to their location. Higher frequency transducers, i.e. 3.5 MgHz, may be used. Areas of pointing of the abscess, prior to its spontaneous drainage may be identified. Cerebrospinal pseudocyst collections resulting from breakage of the shunt tube from the dilated ventricle have also been diagnosed ultrasonically (Figure 28,*A* and *B*).

THE RELATIONSHIP OF ULTRASONIC EXAMINATION TO OTHER METHODS OF DETECTING INTRAABDOMINAL FLUID

Conventional radiographic techniques only demonstrate abnormal intraabdominal masses of water density if they are outlined by fat or large enough to displace normal structures. Thus, an abscess that causes little displacement of the bowel, stomach or ureter may be undetectable on plain films, barium studies and IVP. An abscess that contains gas may be visible on a plain abdominal film, but these abscesses are quite rare, and sometimes it is difficult to distinguish between gas in the abscess and bowel gas. There is little doubt, therefore, that ultrasound is greatly superior to conventional radiography in detecting abscesses. The overall accuracy of ultrasonic diagnosis of abscess is probably over 90 percent (5, 27). The only possible exception is the left subphrenic abscess, which is a difficult lesion to examine ultrasonically and which is sometimes convincingly demonstrated in left lateral decubitus films taken with barium in the stomach (28). However, no comparative series exist, and in any case, conventional radiographic techniques do not distinguish between solid lesions and fluid collections. Because barium sulfate obstructs the passage of sound (29), ultrasonic studies should preceed barium studies whenever possible. Plain radiographs are useful in detecting massive ascites and free intrapelvic fluid and are of assistance in distinguishing ascites

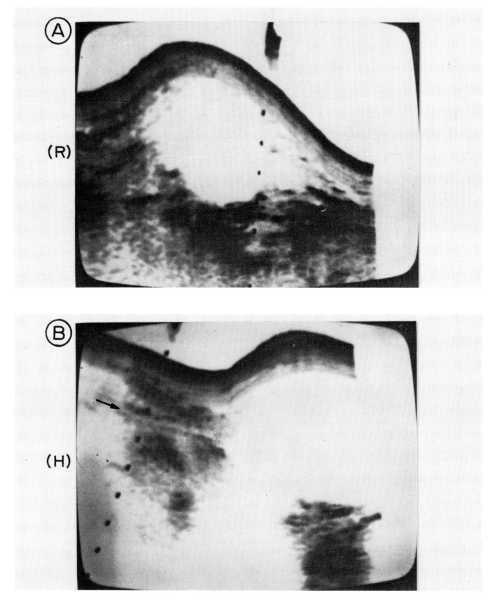

Figure 28. *A*. Cerebrospinal fluid pseudocyst. A cystic ultrasonic pattern is seen located in the superficial structures of the anterior abdominal wall, the result of a leakage of cerebrospinal fluid due to a break in the tube draining the fluid from the ventricular system into the abdomen. *B*. Oblique ultrasonogram shows the shunt tube (arrow) proximal to the point in the subcutaneous tissues where it was leaking.

from massive ovarian tumors. Small volumes are usually impossible to detect by conventional radiographic methods.

Radionuclide scans of the liver, using technetium Tc 99 m sulphur colloid, can detect intrahepatic lesions larger than 2 cm in diameter but do not indicate whether the lesion is solid or fluid. Radionuclide localization of a lesion is less precise than ultrasonic localization. Ultrasound is probably as reliable as the radionuclide scan in the diagnosis of intrahepatic fluid collections, but the radionuclide scan is more reliable in the detection of solid intrahepatic lesions such as metastases. (Not all workers agree with this statement [30].) Ultrasound is also useful in distinguishing solid from fluid-filled intrahepatic lesions detected by radionuclide liver scan.

Radionuclide liver-lung scans are used to detect right subphrenic abscesses by demonstrating separation of the right lobe of the liver from the base of the lung. Unlike the ultrasonic scan, the radionuclide liver-lung scan does not provide an image of the diaphragm and does not distinguish between subpulmonic and subphrenic fluid.

Gallium scanning has been used to detect abscesses but has several disadvantages. There is a delay of 12 to 48 hours between administration of the radionuclide and the time of scanning, gallium concentrates in inflammatory tissue, whether there is drainable fluid or not, and gallium scans do not indicate the anatomic relationship of an abscess to adjacent organs. Gallium scans are occasionally useful in determining the nature of a fluid collection that has been detected ultrasonically. Gallium is not concentrated in the region of noninflammatory fluid (unless there is an active neoplasm in the area).

When a left subphrenic echo-free zone is demonstrated ultrasonically, a radionuclide spleen scan is useful in distinguishing an enlarged spleen from a left subphrenic abscess by providing an estimate of the relative sizes of the spleen and the echo-free zone.

The ultrasonic method of estimating the volume of ascites has much the same accuracy as the dilution technique using ^{131}I-labeled human serum albumin, for volumes under 10 liters. Volumes greater than 10 liters are more accurately estimated by the isotope dilution method (24).

The role of computerized axial tomography in the diagnosis of fluid collections is not yet clear. However, it is known that computerized tomography can distinguish solid masses from fluid collections, and that less skill is required to produce a satisfactory computerized tomographic study than to produce a good ultrasonic study. Computerized tomograms have a lower resolution than ultrasonic studies, and the equipment is approximately ten times as expensive. At present, very little comparative information is available. What little literature there is compares computerized tomography to bistable ultrasound, and suggests, tentatively, that the two techniques are complementary (31).

REFERENCES

1. Leyton B, Halpern S, Leopold G, et al: Correlation of ultrasound and colloid scintiscan studies of the normal and diseased liver. *J Nucl Med* **14**:27–33, 1973.
2. Taylor KJ, Carpenter DA, McCready VR: Ultrasound and scintigraphy in the differential diagnosis of obstructure jaundice. *J Clin Ultrasound* **2**:105–115, 1974.
3. Doust BD, Baum JK, Maklad NF, et al: Ultrasonic evaluation of pleural opacities. *Radiology* **114**:135–140, 1975.
4. Haber K, Asher WM, Freimanis AK: Echographic evaluation of diaphragmatic motion in intra-abdominal disease. *Radiology* **114**:141–144, 1975.

5. Maklad NF, Doust BD, Baum JK: Ultrasonic diagnosis of post-operative intra-abdominal abscess. *Radiology* **113**:417–422, 1974.

6. Pedersen JF, Hancke S, Kristensen JK: Renal carbuncle: antiobiotic therapy govered by ultrasonically guided aspiration. *J Urol* **109**:777–778, 1973.

7. Doust BD, Baum JK, Maklad NF, et al: Determination of organ volume by means of ultrasonic B-mode scanning. *J Clin Ultrasound* **2**:127–130, 1974.

8. Kardel T, Holm HH, Rasmussen SN, et al: Ultrasonic determination of liver and spleen volumes. *Scand J Clin Lab Invest* **27**:123–128, 1971.

9. Goldberg BB, Pollack HM: Ultrasonic aspiration—biopsy transducer. *Radiology* **108**:667–671, 1973.

10. Smith EH, Bartrum RJ: Ultrasonically guided percutaneous aspiration of abscesses. *Am J Roentgenol Radium Ther Nucl Med* **122**:308–312, 1974.

11. Holm HH, Rasmussen SN, Kristensen JK: Ultrasonically guided percutaneous puncture technique. *J Clin Ultrasound* **1**:27–31, 1973.

12. Holm HH, Pedersen JF, Kristensen JK, et al: Ultrasonically guided percutaneous puncture. *Radiol Clin North Am* **13**:493–503, 1975.

13. Matthews AW, Gough KR, Davies R, et al: The use of combined ultrasonic and isotope scanning in the diagnosis of amoebic liver disease. *Gut* **14**:50–53, 1973.

14. Doust BD, Maklad NF: Ultrasonic B-mode examination of the gallbladder. *Radiology* **110**:643–647, 1974.

15. Goldberg BB, Harris K, Broocker W: Ultrasonic and radiographic cholecystography. *Radiology* **111**:405–409, 1974.

16. Hauser JB, Stanley RJ, Geisse G: The ultrasound findings in an obstructed afferent loop. *J Clin Ultrasound* **2**:287–289, 1974.

17. Holm HH, Rasmussen SN, Kristensen JK: Errors and pitfalls in ultrasonic scanning of the abdomen. *Br J Radiol* **45**:835–840, 1972.

18. Cochrane WJ: Ultrasound in gynecology. *Radiol Clin North Am* **13**:457–466, 1975.

19. Kaplan GN, Sanders RC: B-scan ultrasound in the management of patients with occult abdominal hematomas. *J Clin Ultrasound* **1**:5–13, 1973.

20. Freimanis AK, Asher WM: Development of diagnostic criteria in echographic study of abdominal lesions. *Am J Roentgenol Radium Ther Nucl Med* **108**:747–755, 1970.

21. Morley P, Barnett E, Bell PR, et al: Ultrasound in the diagnosis of fluid collections following renal transplantation. *Clin Radiol* **26**:199–207, 1975.

22. Doust BD: Ultrasonic examination of the pancreas. *Radiol Clin North Am* **13**:467–478, 1975.

23. Rosenquist CJ: Pseudocyst of the pancreas: unusual radiographic presentations. *Clin Radiol* **24**:192–194, 1973.

24. Goldberg BB, Clearfield HR, Goodman CA, et al: Ultrasonic determination of ascites. *Arch Int Med* **131**:217–220, 1973.

25. Hunig R, Kinser J: The diagnosis of ascites by ultrasonic tomography (B-scan). *Br J Radiol* **46**:325–328, 1973.

26. Weiner CI, Diaconis JN: Primary abdominal wall abscess diagnosed by ultrasound. *Arch Surg* **110**:341–342, 1975.

27. Jensen F, Pedersen JF: The value of ultrasonic scanning in the diagnosis of intra-abdominal abscesses and hematomas. *Surg Gynecol Obstet* **139**:326–328, 1974.

28. Sanders RC: Radiological and radioisotopic diagnosis of perihepatic abscess. *CRC Crit Rev Clin Radiol Nucl Med* **5**:165–211, 1974.

29. Leopold GR, Asher WM: Deleterious effects of gastrointestinal contrast material on abdominal echography. *Radiology* **98**:637–640, 1971.

30. Taylor KJ, Carpenter DA, McCready VR: Grey scale echography in the diagnosis of intrahepatic disease. *J Clin Ultrasound* **1**:284–287, 1973.

31. Alfidi RJ, Haaga J, Meaney TF, et al: Computed tomography of the thorax and abdomen; a preliminary report. *Radiology* **117**:257–264, 1975.

10
Kidney

Howard M. Pollack, M.D.
Professor of Radiology
University of Pennsylvania
Hospital and School of Medicine
Philadelphia, Pennsylvania

Barry B. Goldberg, M.D.
Professor of Radiology;
Director, Division of Diagnostic Ultrasound
Thomas Jefferson University Hospital
Philadelphia, Pennsylvania

The development of ultrasound has provided a new and important dimension in the diagnosis and treatment of renal disorders. Within the span of a relatively few years, this modality has achieved almost an indispensable status in the assessment of both medical and surgical diseases of the kidney (1). If fact, it is now not unreasonable to expect that in certain clinical situations, such as uremia of undetermined origin, ultrasound will be the diagnostic procedure first employed in the patient's evaluation. This is easily understandable in view of the ability of ultrasound to evaluate the size, shape, and internal architecture of the kidney, thus providing an immediate clue as to whether the uremia is most likely to be on a "medical or a "surgical" basis. More importantly, perhaps, ultrasound has the unique attribute of being independent of renal function for its imaging properties. This is not true of other methods of renal visualization, such as radionuclide or roentgenographic procedures. Even the newly introduced modality of computerized tomography often employs the injection of iodinated contrast material for image enhancement. Thus, in the presence of poor renal function, ultrasound appears to be the most satisfactory noninvasive method of examining the kidneys. An additional advantage of ultrasound is that it emits no radiation. It thereby becomes an important study in pregnancy, as well as in children and women in the child-bearing age. This is not to imply that ultrasound and procedures employing ionizing radiation are competitive methods of examination. Nothing could be further from the truth, since the methods are most often complementary. The point is that ultrasound enjoys properties not offered by other modalities, and whenever clinically indicated, full advantage should be taken of these attributes.

Not only can ultrasound produce excellent two-dimensional static images in shades of gray, but employing real-time techniques, it also can be used to evaluate dynamic changes, such as renal mobility. Real-time imaging also can be used to guide needles into renal masses, both cystic and solid, for either aspiration or biopsy. The aspiration-biopsy techniques will be discussed in greater detail in Chapter 12.

The future of ultrasound in renal evaluation appears quite promising. The likelihood of obtaining improved resolution is great, and with it the chances of measuring renal blood vessels, as well as detecting small stones. Experimental equipment already has been constructed for this purpose (2). Using pulsed Doppler ultrasound techniques in combination with two-dimensional imaging, it will be possible in the future to estimate renal blood flow (3). Thus, ultrasound in its present state of development and with the anticipation of new developments, will maintain and expand its place in the diagnosis of retroperitoneal diseases, especially those involving the kidney.

NORMAL ULTRASONIC ANATOMY

The kidneys are bilateral retroperitoneal structures which, in the vast majority of cases, may be found between the levels of the first and third lumbar vertebrae. There is a range of normal variation between persons, however, so that not infrequently the upper pole of a normal kidney may be found at the level of the twelfth thoracic vertebra while the lower pole of another also normal kidney may be found at the level of the fourth lumbar vertebra. The upper poles of both kidneys lie more medial than the lower poles giving the long axis an oblique course which becomes a consideration in obtaining technically satisfactory longitudinal ultrasonograms. The average renal length in adults is approximately 11–12 cm, with the left kidney being slightly longer than the right in most persons. Normally, the kidneys are mobile, and may move 1, or even 2 centimeters with respiration as well as with standing or sitting. This motion is easily detectable at sonography. In the prone position, the distance from the posterior skin surface to the posterior surface of the kidney is approximately 4 cm. It is this relatively short distance and the absence of interposed gas-filled structures that accounts for the relative ease with which excellent ultrasonic images of the kidney may regularly be obtained. The antero-posterior thickness of the kidney measures approximately 4 cm in the normal adult kidney. It is important to remember that since there is no magnification of the kidneys with ultrasound, they will appear to be smaller than their roentgenographically determined size. Of course, there are considerable variations in size, position and shape of the kidneys, all of which can be demonstrated easily by ultrasound. Examples of these variations will be shown later in this chapter.

The ultrasonic appearance of the normal kidney is quite characteristic and consists basically of two parts: a central complex of strongly reflected echoes, surrounded by a thicker, more sonolucent zone that is devoid of echoes except at high gain settings (Figure 1). The central echo complex is a composite produced by the renal collecting system (pelvis and calyces), renal vessels (arteries and veins), and renal sinus supporting tissue (fat and areolar tissue). The poor echo-producing surrounding zone represents renal parenchyma. Occasionally, the perinephric fat and the perinephric fascia (fascia of Gerota) also can be seen. The size and shape of the kidney are anatomic in depiction. On longitudinal section, the central echoes are midline and centrally distributed. In keeping with their origin from the renal hilar structures, however, the central echoes tend to be more medially located when viewed on the transverse scans. In this view, the weak echo zone of the parenchyma is distributed in a C-shaped configuration around the

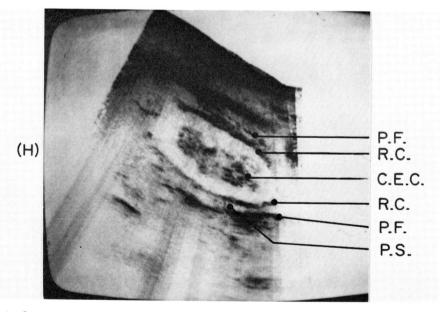

Figure 1. Longitudinal gray scale ultrasonogram of a normal kidney. Note the relatively sonolucent appearance of the renal parenchyma. The renal capsule (RC) is delineated sharply from the perinephric fat (PS). The perinephric fascia (PF) is an inconstantly recognized structure. The strong central echo complex (CEC) is from the renal pelvis and blood vessels and sinus fibroareolar tissue.

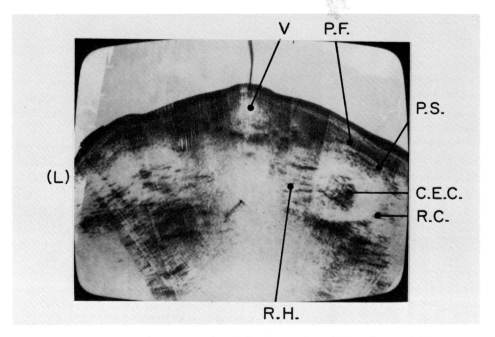

Figure 2. Transverse gray scale sonogram taken in the prone position of bilaterally normal kidneys (PF = perinephric fascia; PS = perinephric fat; CEC = central echo complex; RC = renal capsule; RH = renal hilum; V = vertebral spinous process).

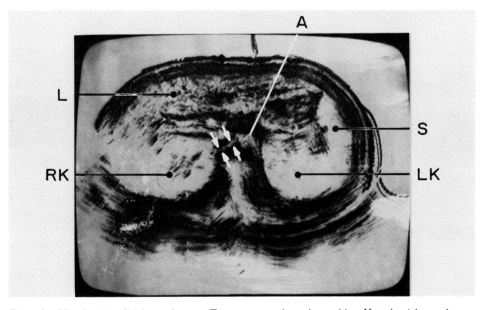

Figure 3. Visualization of right renal artery. Transverse scan in supine position. Note the right renal artery (arrows) originating from the aorta (A) (RK = right kidney; LK = left kidney; L = liver; S = spleen).

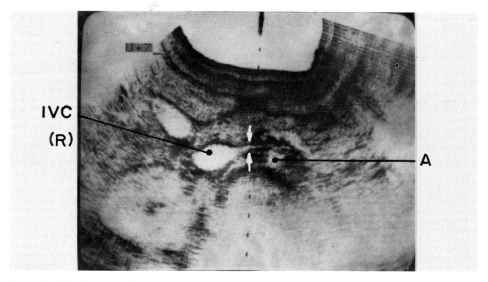

Figure 4.   Visualization of left renal vein. Transverse supine view. The left renal vein (arrows) can be seen coursing anterior to the aorta (A) and emptying into the inferior vena cava (IVC).

medial echo complex (Figure 2). Displacement, distortion, or fragmentation of the core of central echoes may be of great diagnostic significance. In similar fashion, displacement or distortion of the contour of the kidney parenchyma either by intrinsic or extrinsic masses can be easily demonstrated (see Chapter 11).

The renal artery and vein are identifiable in many patients who have been examined in the supine position. Both structures appear grossly similar, but can be differentiated from each other by means of their relationship to the aorta and vena cava respectively (Figures 3 and 4) (see Chapter 3).

TECHNIQUE

As with any diagnostic study, technique is all important and must be mastered thoroughly if credible results are to be achieved. Most mistakes in ultrasonic renal diagnosis occur not because of ignorance or misinterpretation but because of poor technique. This is turn leads to opinions being rendered on the basis of information that is, in fact, uninterpretable.

When examining the kidneys, scanning usually is performed in the prone position (Figure 5). Exceptions to this include renal transplants and other kidneys known to be anterior or pelvic in location and certain cases of right renal disease in which it may be advantageous to scan in a supine position with the sound traversing the liver before reaching the right kidney. More will be said about this later in this chapter. Either the transverse or the longitudinal scans may be performed first, the techniques being essentially the same. In general, we usually obtain initial longitudinal scans moving the transducer from the iliac crest upward toward the rib cage and beyond if necessary. With gray scale ultrasound a single linear or sector scan rather than compound sector-

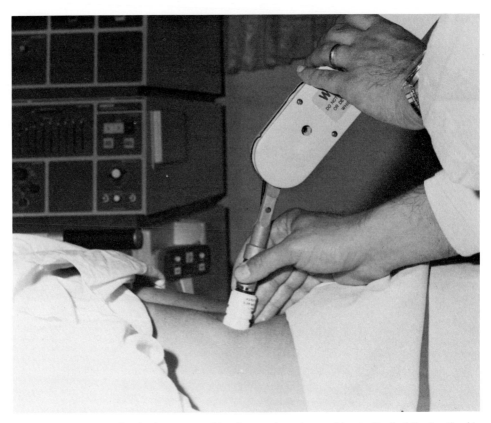

Figure 5.   With the patient in the prone position the transducer is moved longitudinally following the skin contour.

ing usually produces the best images. Once the general area of the kidney including its upper and lower extent has been localized, transverse scans are obtained. Again, these scans also should be obtained starting just at the level of the iliac crest. If the transducer is over the iliac crest, there will be no sound penetration, of course, but as soon as it is cranial to this bone, a reading will be obtained. The transverse scans are made at 1- to 2-cm intervals proceeding from the lower pole of the kidney to the upper pole and just beyond. To obtain the true longitudinal axis of the kidney, two methods may be used. One is to mark on the skin surface the maximum diameter of the kidney as shown on each transverse scan. These dots then can be connected at the completion of the transverse scanning process. The line thus made will indicate the axis of the longest diameter of the kidney (Figure 6). Longitudinal scans then can be obtained along this axis at set intervals of approximately 1–1.5 cm outlining the entire thickness of the kidney in this projection. An average of five to six sections are necessary to adequately image the kidney in this dimension (Figure 7).

The other method of determining the true long axis of the kidney is to use real-time ultrasound. With this method, it is relatively easy to obtain the true axis of the kidney by simply rotating the transducer head until the maximum diameter is obtained. Marks can be placed on the skin indicating the proper pathway for the static imaging gray scale.

While it is relatively easy to outline the lower pole of the kidney unless it extends below the iliac crest, it sometimes may be difficult to outline the upper pole. There are two major factors responsible for this: one is the interposition of aerated lung between the transducer and the kidney and the other is the presence of ribs overlying the kidney. In the presence of overlying lung, an image cannot be obtained, while ribs will produce such attenuation of the ultrasonic beam that the chances of recording echoes from beneath it are poor. Reverberations from rib edges also may produce difficulty in obtaining a satisfactory image. There are several methods of avoiding these problems. One is to obtain the scan in deep inspiration or expiration. With deep inspiration, the upper pole of the kidney may be displaced sufficiently caudad to allow a recording to be obtained (Figure 8). This does not always work, however, since the overinflated lung may accompany the kidney inferiorly and become superimposed. In such cases an expiration study may allow a recording of the upper renal pole to be obtained. Another method is to perform scanning with the patient sitting or standing (Figure 9). This usually will bring out the kidney's maximum mobility. For documentation of degrees of ptosis, comparison recordings can be made between the prone and erect positions. Another technique of visualizing the upper pole of the kidney is to angle the transducer cranially just as the lowest rib is reached. This projects the ultrasonic beam under the rib cage and tends to avoid interference from the ribs as well as from the lower edge of the lung. The lower pole of a ptotic kidney, partly obscured from ultrasonic evaluation because of the overlying iliac bone, sometimes can be elevated out of the pelvis by placing a small sand bag or pillow beneath the lower pole of the kidney.

All ultrasonic renal scanning should be performed during suspended respiration. Since the kidney is normally mobile, motion will occur during scanning unless special pains are taken to avoid it. If careful attention is not given to this point, resultant images will be blurred and small structures or masses can easily be rendered indistinguishable (Figure 10).

While the prone position is the standard one for renal sonography, it is also possible to obtain views of the kidney in the supine position. The liver provides an excellent

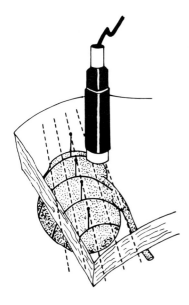

Figure 6. Diagrammatic representation of technique used to obtain the true longitudinal axis of the kidney (Black dots denote midpoints of the transverse diameters of kidney. Dotted lines denote oblique longitudinal pathways obtained from transverse scans.)

sound transmitting medium or "window" through which sound may be directed to the right kidney. Both longitudinal and transverse scans can be obtained in this manner, although the best views are longitudinal, since there is less interference from the ribs in this direction (Figure 11). Longitudinal sweeps usually are started from below the level of the umbilicus and swept upward until the costal margin is encountered by the transducer. At this point, the transducer is then angled cephalad without passing over

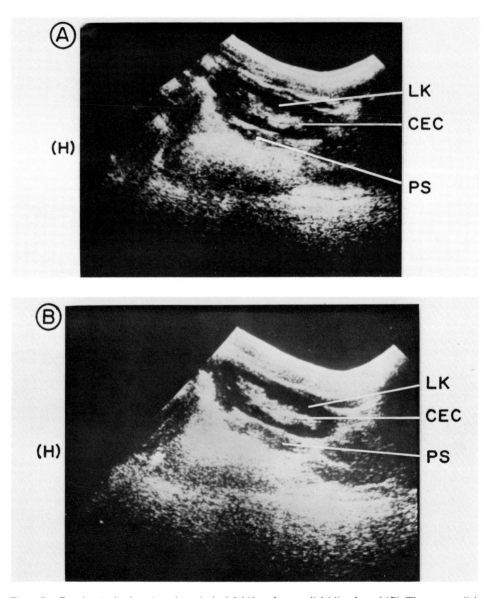

Figure 7.   Four longitudinal sections through the left kidney from medial (*A*) to lateral (*D*). The most medial sections demonstrate the central echo complex (CEC) produced by the renal pelvis and major renal vessels to the best advantage. As the scan proceeds medial to lateral, the long axis of the kidney becomes at first longer and then shorter and relatively more parenchyma is visualized in comparison to the nonparenchymal structures. (*Continued on next page.*)

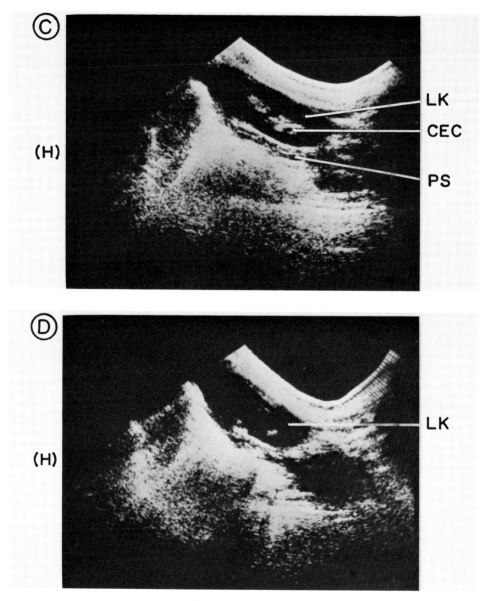

Figure 7. (Continued)

the ribs. Again, to obtain maximum resolution, the scans are obtained during suspended respiration. The scanning is usually linear in nature with very little need for sectoring. Once the upper and lower renal poles have been delineated by the longitudinal scans, transverse scanning may be begun, with care being taken to avoid interference from the anterior ribs. Satisfactory images of the left kidney usually are not obtainable in the supine position because of overlying bowel gas. Occasionally, however, an interposed parenchymal structure such as an enlarged spleen will displace the bowel and allow a sonic "window" through which the left kidney may be examined (Figure 12).

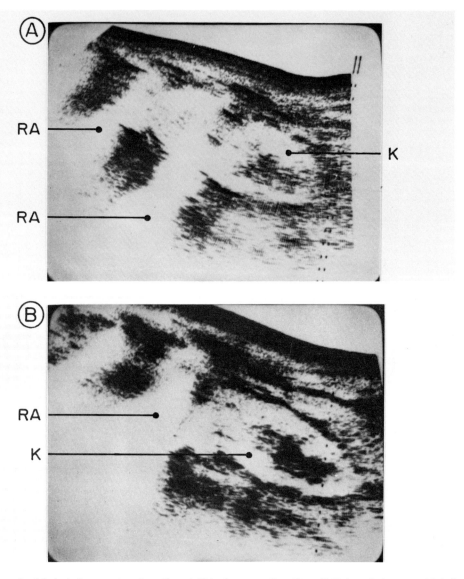

Figure 8.   Method of overcoming rib artifact. *A*. Echo-free zone rib artifacts (RA) through the upper third of the kidney produced by the twelfth rib prevent adequate imaging of the upper portion of the kidney (K). *B*. With deep inspiration, the upper pole of the kidney descends below the rib artifacts (RA). The entire kidney is now visualized.

A final approach for evaluating the kidney is the lateral or axillary view (Figure 13). In this case, the patient is in the decubitus position, with either his right or left side against the stretcher. The transducer then is moved initially in the longitudinal direction along the axillary line. Although it is not always possible to record the kidney image in this position, satisfactory information often can be obtained. If ribs are interfering, the best approach is to place the transducer in the soft tissue between the superior aspect of the iliac crest and the inferior costal margin. Sector scans can then be obtained, moving

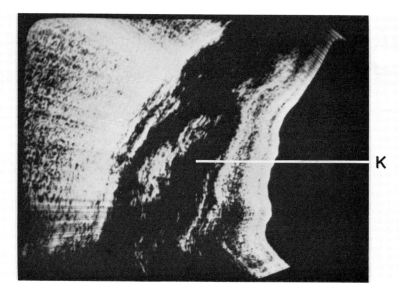

Figure 9.   Longitudinal section performed with patient upright allows complete visualization of the upper pole of the kidney (K).

the transducer a centimeter at a time until the region of the kidney is recorded. Transverse scans may be obtained if the kidney has been demonstrated in the longitudinal view. Again, suspended respiration is needed for maximum detail. Scanning should be attempted in either sustained inspiration or expiration, if initial studies do not provide adequate visualization.

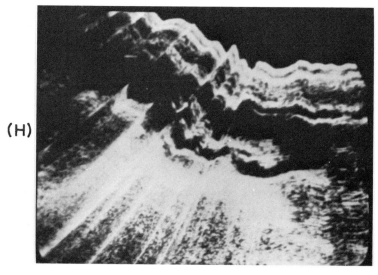

Figure 10.   The effect of excessive breathing and transducer-skin motion on appearance of kidney. Note the "rippling" effect on the kidney produced by transducer-skin motion and elongation of the kidney produced by excessive breathing.

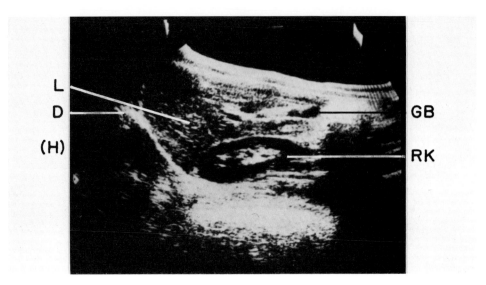

Figure 11.   Transhepatic imaging of right kidney in the supine position. Note the clear outline of the kidney (RK) through the liver (L) (GB = gallbladder; D = diaphragm).

If visualization of the main renal vessels is desired, scans are obtained in the supine position. The abdominal aorta is first localized in a longitudinal direction, and the level of the origin of the superior mesenteric artery (SMA) is demonstrated. The renal arteries usually originate just distal to this point. A mark is made on the skin at the level of the SMA-aortic junction during longitudinal scanning, and the patient then is repositioned for transverse scanning. Recordings are obtained starting at the level of the SMA and moving in a generally caudad direction 3mm at a time. The transducer sweep

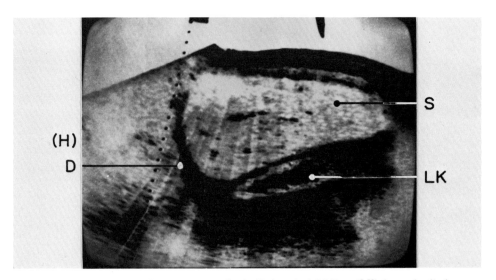

Figure 12.   Supine longitudinal ultrasonogram clearly displays the left kidney (LK) due to the displacement of bowel by an enlarged spleen (S).

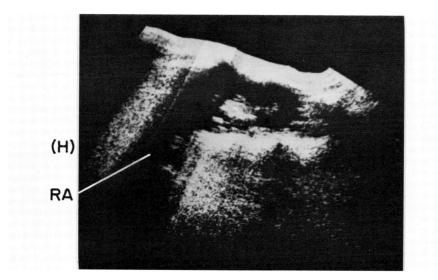

(H)

RA

Figure 13. Longitudinal axillary view of the left kidney. Note echo-free zone due to absorption and reflection of the ultrasonic beam by a rib (RA).

should be short over these areas without sectoring and with all scans obtained during suspended respiration. In thin patients, it is possible to obtain images of the kidney in this position too, but obesity or the presence of bowel gas usually preclude this. Demonstration of the renal arteries also allows their depth beneath the skin surface to be measured. In the future, by using combined gray scale B-scan or real-time gray scan in association with pulsed Doppler ultrasound, it is likely that not only the luminal diameter of these vessels can be obtained but that the flowrate of blood within them also may be calculated. In many cases, the renal veins also can be visualized. The left renal vein often will be seen as it passes transversely between the abdominal aorta and superior mesenteric artery before entering the vena cava. The right renal vein enters directly into the vena cava.

Experience has suggested that, in general, the better hydrated the patient, the easier it is to depict that patient's kidneys ultrasonically. The reason for this is not clear but may be related to the kidney's increased fluid content during diuresis. The difference in the appearance of the hydrated and nonhydrated kidney is not vast, however, and even in the presence of severe dehydration adequate renal sonography should be attainable. If the renal images are not entirely satisfactory, repeat examination with hydration should be considered. It should be noted that the use of iodinated water-soluble contrast agents does not interfere with adequate visualization of the kidneys.

RENAL MASSES

One of the earliest and perhaps still most frequently employed urologic uses of ultrasound is in the differential diagnosis of renal masses. Because of the relative frequency of asymptomatic masses, most of which are serous cysts, the development of a safe, reliable, and inexpensive method of investigating renal masses based on ultrasound as the keystone study, has been a boon to patients, physicians, and third-party medical

TABLE 1.   DISTRIBUTION OF TYPES OF
RENAL MASSES IN 336 ADULT
PATIENTS

	Number	Percent
Cysts	231	69
Pseudotumors	40	12
Tumors	26	7
Abscesses	10	3
Hydronephrosis	9	3
Polycystic disease	9	3
Hematomas	8	2
Perirenal pseudocysts	3	1

intermediaries alike (4). In addition to simple serous cysts, there are many other masses that can involve the kidney including neoplasms, abscesses, hematomas, multilocular cysts, granulomas, and others (Table 1). The differentiation of these masses is based to a great extent on their sonographic patterns of which three main types are recognized: the cystic pattern which is obtained from fluid-filled masses such as cysts, the solid pattern which is obtained from parenchymatous lesions such as neoplasms, and the complex pattern which is seen with masses having both fluid and solid components. There is further refinement of classification within these categories as will be discussed in the following paragraphs.

Cystic Masses

The typically cystic renal mass will be seen as a sharply defined echo-free zone having strong far-wall echoes (Figure 14). Since sound passing through a uniform fluid is not reflected, but sound encountering a fluid-solid interface is strongly reflected, both the echo-free zone and the strong far-wall echoes are required to make a diagnosis of a cystic mass. Failure to adhere to this admonition will result in mistakes in diagnosis. Since the distal wall of the cyst is seen as a smooth surface, the display of echoes from this area will appear as a smooth line. Closer to the transducer, the proximal wall also presents a strong interface, but because of reverberation echoes, frequently lacks the smooth, even contour of the far cyst wall. With increasing sensitivity the more likely are reverberation echoes to be recorded. Reverberation echoes or "false" echoes are present with solid masses as well as with cystic ones, but they are not normally recognized with the former because they are obscured by the true echoes. When there is a problem differentiating false from true echoes, scans should be obtained in two planes and compared. Echoes truly originating from within a mass will not change with changes in the patient's position, and they will be stronger and more persistent than reverberation echoes (Figure 15). An additional important finding in cystic masses is that the through sound transmission is great, but with solid masses, the opposite is true (Figure 16). If there is any question about the strength of the through transmission, comparison can be made with the filled urinary bladder. In fact, any mass can be compared with the equivalent-sized bladder. With masses smaller than the bladder this viscus can be compressed until its diameter which lies in the path of the ultrasonic beam becomes roughly equal to that of the mass in question.

The minimum sized lesion that can be imaged reliably by ultrasound depends on both the frequency employed and the depth of the mass. Because of beam divergence, the deeper the mass, the larger it must be to allow satisfactory resolution. When a standard 2.25 mHz transducer is used, superficial masses 1 cm in diameter can be assessed accurately, while with deeper masses, at the approximate depth of the kidney, a

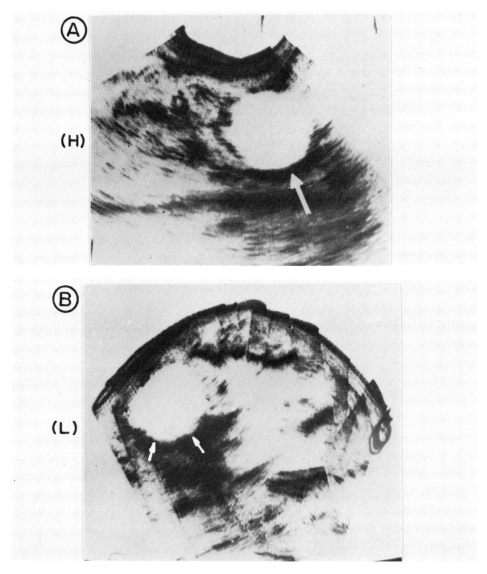

Figure 14. Typical renal cyst. *A*. Longitudinal image of the left kidney taken in the prone position. The large renal cyst at the lower pole of the kidney is transsonic. There are no echoes within it and there is accentuation of sound transmission through the mass with especially strong echoes at the immediate far wall (arrows). *B*. Same lesion imaged transversely in the prone position.

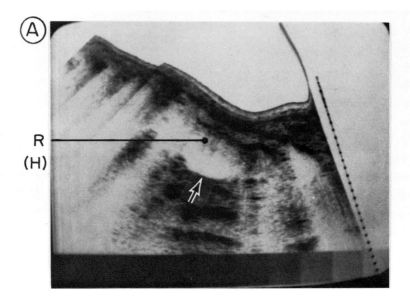

R
(H)

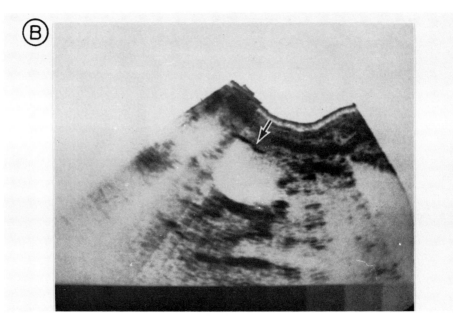

Figure 15. Sound reverberation mimicking internal echoes. *A.* Longitudinal image of a kidney containing a cyst (arrow) taken in the prone position. A number of reverberation echoes (R) are seen concentrated near the proximal wall. *B.* Patient in same position but with the transducer angled slightly. Sharply outlined anterior wall echoes are seen (arrow with no evidence of the reverberation echoes. The changing appearance of the echoes with change in position of patient or the transducer is characteristic of reverberations.

276

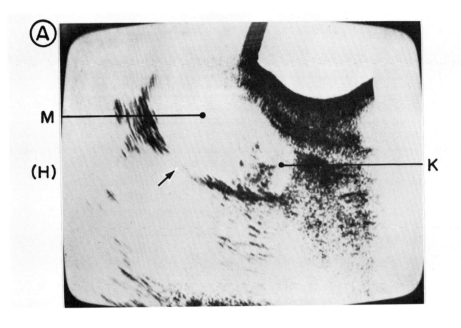

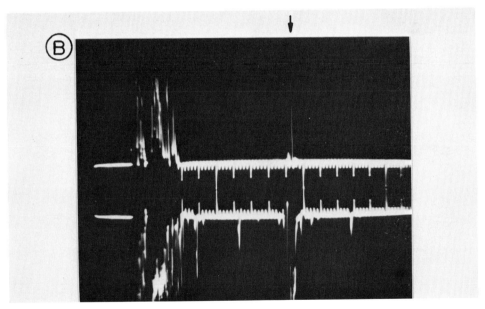

Figure 16. *A.* Longitudinal scan taken in the prone position shows a tumor of the upper pole of the right kidney. Although no echoes are demonstrated within the mass (M), there is attenuation of the ultrasonic beam transmission through the lesion (arrow) (K = lower pole). *B.* A-mode examination demonstrates more vividly the absorption of sound through the mass with occasional echoes seen at high gain (arrow denotes distal-wall echo). *C.* Longitudinal scan taken in the prone position shows a renal cyst (M) of the upper pole of the left kidney. Again note the absence of echoes within the upper pole mass, but in this case there is accentuation of sound transmission. Numerous strong echoes are seen just beyond the far wall (arrow) (K = normal lower pole). *D.* A-mode examination demonstrates an echo-free zone corresponding to the mass with no appreciable loss of sound transmission (arrow denotes distal-wall echoes). (*Continued on next page.*)

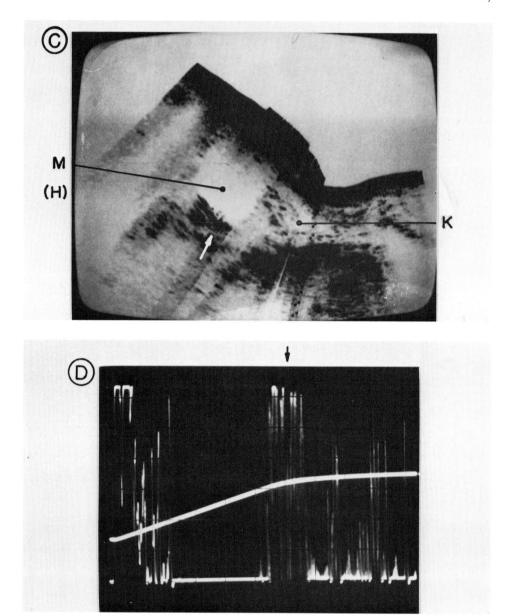

Figure 16.   (Continued)

diameter of approximately 2 cm is required to allow accurate evaluation (Figure 17). By
using higher frequency transducers, masses much smaller than 1 cm in diameter can be
differentiated, but the depth of penetration, of course, falls off as the frequency increases.
The ability to differentiate a deeply placed mass is related to the width of the ultrasonic
beam at the level of the mass and, therefore, to beam divergence. Since the lateral resolution is inversely proportional to the beam width, there will be poor resolution of those
structures smaller than the diameter of the beam itself. In such cases, echoes produced

from the structures immediately adjacent to the mass will appear to originate from within the mass, thus imparting a complex quality to cystic masses (Figure 18). In the future, with the use of electronic focusing and variable frequencies, it will be possible to differentiate much smaller masses.

It must be emphasized that cystic patterns can be reproduced not only by liquids but by any tissues or substance that acoustically behaves like a liquid (5). For example, uniform gelatinlike clots, abscesses consisting only of leukocytes without debris and, of course, unclotted blood all will show cystic patterns. In addition, there are a few solid lesions that occasionally produce a pattern which so closely simulates a cystic one, that only the most scrupulous and meticulous technique can be depended upon to differentiate them. This is described in more detail in the section on solid masses. Masses in the upper pole of the kidney can be particularly troublesome in this regard, because of potential interference in transmission of the ultrasonic beam by the overlying lung and ribs. We have found it of benefit in the study of renal masses to confirm all gray scale images with a simple A-mode recording from the mass. With A-mode the pattern produced is only that contributed by passage of the sound beam through the mass (Figure 16).

In our hands, the accuracy with which a renal cyst can be identified by ultrasound including combined gray scale and A-mode imaging is approximately 98 percent. That is, approximately 2 percent of all renal cysts will be misrepresented as tumors or overlooked completely. This figure should be distinguished from the reliability rate of a demonstrable cystic pattern which has approximately a 95 percent confidence level. That is, for each 100 renal cyst patterns obtained, only 5 will be attributable to noncysts. The reasons some cysts are incorrectly diagnosed or missed are: (a) the diameter is less than 2 cm, (b) the wall is calcified, (c) technical pitfalls (i.e., breathing, gain setting too low), (d) faulty interpretation. The most frequent noncystic lesions that may be misinterpreted as renal cysts are listed in Table 2.

Comparisons of gray scale and bistable B-scanning indicate that the accuracy of renal cyst detection has been increased only slightly by the advent of the gray scale modality, although smaller lesions are probably more clearly depicted. A great improvement,

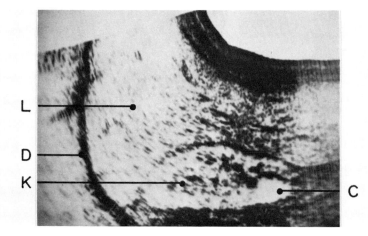

Figure 17.   Longitudinal ultrasonogram taken in the supine position reveals a small renal cyst (C), measuring 2 cm, located in the lower pole of the right kidney (K) (L = liver; D = diaphragm).

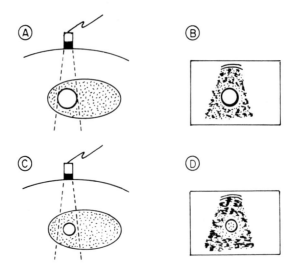

Figure 18. *A.* Lateral width of the ultrasonic beam is equal to the diameter of cyst. Image produced (*B*) gives true representation of the sonic properties of the lesion. No internal echoes are seen. *C.* Since the diameter of the cystic mass is smaller than that of the beam, echoes produced from structures surrounding the mass appear to originate from within the mass (*D*) giving a false appearance of a complex mass.

however, has been noted in the ability to evaluate more critically certain complex lesions, such as Wilms' tumors, which will be discussed later in this chapter.

Complex Masses

Complex masses may be considered to be essentially cystic masses which differ, however, in that they contain echo-generating internal reflecting interfaces. These echoes, unlike reverberations, are persistent and constant in location. Since complex masses are composed mainly of material that transmits sound well, their far-wall echoes will be strong, although less so than cysts of the same size. They will, however, be discernibly stronger than the far-wall echoes emanating from solid masses. This can be confirmed in most cases by comparing the far-wall echoes of the complex mass in question with the distal wall-echoes of the opposite, normal kidney (Figure 19). Normal kidneys transmit sound

TABLE 2.   LESIONS POTENTIALLY MISDIAGNOSED AS
RENAL CYSTS BY ULTRASOUND

Intrarenal vascular malformations (i.e., AVMs, aneurysms)
Hematomas
Abscesses
Urine collections (i.e., localized hydronephrosis, urinoma)
Cysts containing small mural tumors*
Necrotic, hemorrhagic tumors*
Lymphoma*

* rare cause.

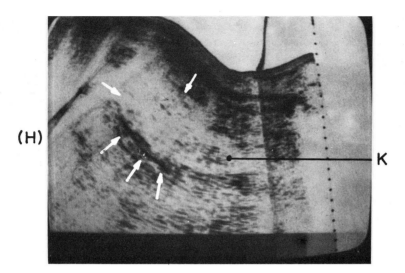

Figure 19. Longitudinal ultrasonogram taken in the prone position of an upper pole complex mass (upper arrows) containing multiple internal echoes with excellent sound transmission through the mass shown by accentuation of the far-wall echoes (lower arrows) (K = normal lower pole of kidney). Diagnosis: necrotic carcinoma.

less well than complex masses. The most common renal lesions associated with complex patterns are listed in Table 3.

The most important mass yielding a complex pattern is a renal neoplasm. Although these lesions usually produce solid patterns, there are certain morphologic variants that are seen primarily as fluid-filled structures. Thus, those renal cell carcinomas that are partly cystic, as well as those associated with a great deal of hemorrhage (Figure 20), take on fluidlike characteristics which, acoustically, may overshadow their basically solid nature. The same is true for neoplasms that have lost much of their blood supply and have become necrotic as a result (Figure 21). The necrotic debris within the tumor becomes jellylike, and acts as a homogeneous transmitting medium. If the internal echoes, sometimes sparse, are not recognized, the propensity for misdiagnosis is great. It is primarily this fact, in addition to the occasional small tumor which may occur in a renal cyst, that has led to the recommendation that cystic masses be aspirated whenever possible to insure that they are not, in fact, complex masses masquarading as cysts (6).

Cysts may produce complex patterns when they are multilocular (Figure 22) or when they are multiple and placed very close together, as in polycystic disease. Here, they

TABLE 3. RENAL LESIONS PRODUCING COMPLEX
SONOGRAPHIC PATTERNS

Neoplasms (i.e., cystic, hemorrhagic, or necrotic only)
Cysts (Infected, multilocular, bloody, or multiple)
Abscesses
Hematomas or Hemorrhagic infarcts
Hydronephrosis

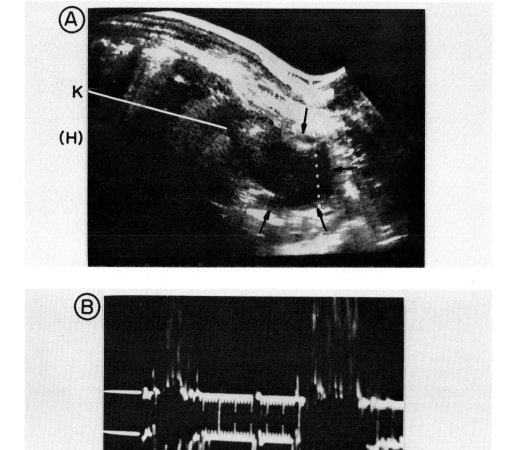

Figure 20. Complex renal mass. *A*. Longitudinal B-scan ultrasonogram taken in the prone position of a complex renal mass (arrows) with only a few internal echoes (K = upper pole). *B*. A-mode ultrasonogram also demonstrates only a few internal echoes (arrow). Diagnosis: extensively hemorrhagic renal cell carcinoma.

may be seen as an overall complex mass, although each clear space actually represents an individual cyst (Figure 23). If the cysts are larger than 2 cm in diameter, as in the adult form of polycystic disease, they will be identifiable as individual lesions (Figure 24). If, on the other hand, they are smaller than this, as in infantile polycystic disease, they will not be individually recognizable (Figure 25). Cysts that contain either debris or a clot also will be complex (Figure 26). Hematomas (Figure 27) and abscesses may be either complex or cystic depending on the physical state of their internal milieu. Often the walls of these lesions are not as smooth as the walls of uncomplicated renal cysts would be expected to be. Hemorrhagic infarcts, as are seen in renal vein thrombosis, for example, also produce a cystic pattern; internal echoes may occur from the edges of dilated calyceal rims and fornices, converting the pattern to a complex one. Parapelvic and central renal cysts may be confusing at times, since their central location places them into apposition to the larger renal vessels and the renal pelvis. As a result, extraneous echoes from these normal structures may give a complex quality to the ultrasonogram (Figure 28).

Ultrasound has been of great value in differentiating parapelvic and central renal cysts from an entity frequently confused with them—sinus lipomatosis (7). The latter is a condition characterized by the heavy deposition of fat in the renal sinus, often seen in the nephrosclerotic or aging kidney. Although the roentgenographic picture in the two conditions is somewhat similar, they can be distinguished ultrasonically, since a cystic or complex pattern will be seen with parapelvic and central cysts, while there is no sonographic evidence of fluid in sinus lipomatosis (Figure 29).

As discussed in the previous section, false complex patterns may occur with cysts smaller than the width of the ultrasonic beam. Such artifacts are hardly disastrous, however, since, if anything, they may cause cystic lesions to appear complex and, therefore, raise the clinician's index of suspicion, rather than falsely lower it.

Solid Masses

There are two main features that characterize solid masses, and these may occur singly or together. First, these masses have the capacity to generate internal echoes that increase in number and intensity as the equipment sensitivity is increased (Figure 30). Second, the sound absorption through the mass is much greater than that seen with cystic and complex masses, resulting in much weaker distal-wall echoes (Figure 31). When identifiable, the back wall is less smooth than in cystic lesions. When compared to the opposite kidney, the sound transmission will be no greater; in fact, if the mass is larger than the kidney, the transmission through it will be less than through the normal

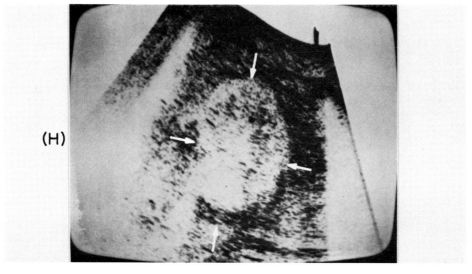

(H)

Figure 21. ·Necrotic tumor. Longitudinal ultrasonogram taken in the prove position demonstrates a complex mass (arrows) consistent with a diagnosis of necrotic renal tumor.

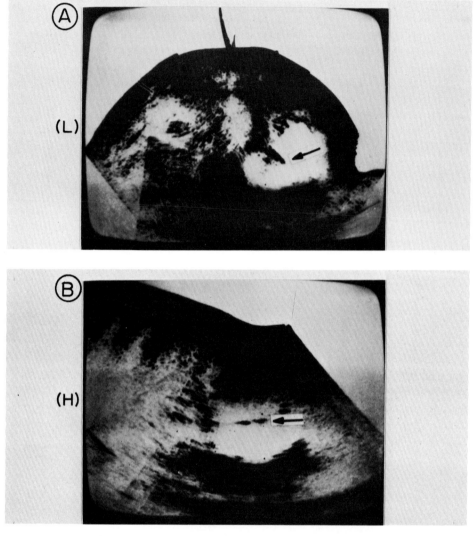

Figure 22.   Septated renal cyst. *A*. Transverse ultrasonogram taken in the prone position of a right-sided renal cyst shows a linear echogenic structure (arrow) representing a septum within the cyst, producing a bilocular configuration. *B*. Longitudinal ultrasonogram of the same lesion. Septum (arrow) is visualized as echo-producing structure.

kidney unless internal necrosis has occurred. In the same way, the urinary bladder may be used as a standard of comparison for the back wall of cystic lesions. Thus, if there is confusion in judging the nature of the far wall of any renal mass, comparison with these two readily available normal structures always will provide a reliable background for comparison.

Not all masses in this category are uniformly solid; many have areas of hemorrhage or necrosis and some have cystic components. It is possible to distinguish both the liquid and solid tissues, and the overall diagnosis of a predominantly solid mass containing mixed elements can be made. Echoes need not originate uniformly from the entire mass, since there may be homogeneous areas containing very few reflecting interfaces. The most important quality of solid masses is the absorption of sound within the mass and the resultant decrease in through transmission. Thus, the strength of the back wall becomes the key point in differentiating these masses from complex and cystic ones.

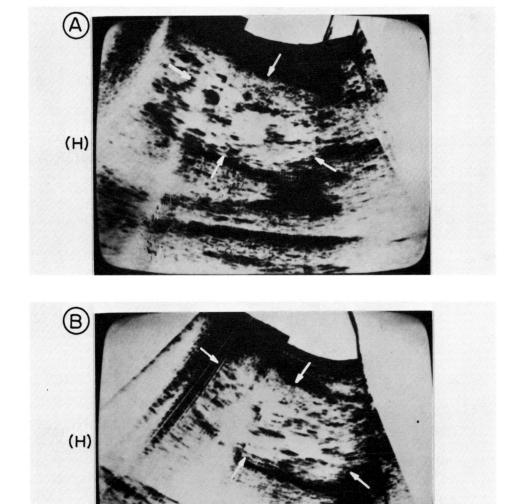

Figure 23.   Bilateral polycystic disease—adult variety. *A*. Longitudinal view taken in the prone position of an enlarged right kidney (arrows) with the normal parenchymal appearance replaced by multiple nondescript echoes. A few of the larger cystic areas are well defined. *B*. Longitudinal ultrasonogram of enlarged left kidney (arrows) shows a similar pattern. *C*. Transverse ultrasonogram of same patient's large kidneys (arrows).

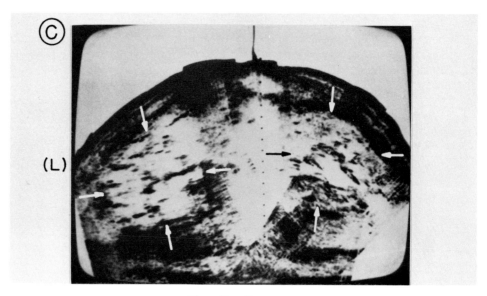

Figure 23.   (Continued)

Although the typical solid pattern will include multiple internal echoes, one must not depend on these to make such a diagnosis, for to do so, is to invite disaster.

The reason for the variation in echo-generating properties between solid masses is not understood clearly, but several factors are thought to play roles. One factor is the size of the mass. The larger the mass, the more sound absorption, thus lessening the chances that the weaker echoes will reach the transducer for recording. Another is related to the blood supply of the mass. In general, those solid masses having very sparse vascularity, and usually of uniform cell type, will produce few echoes since the interfaces between blood vessels and surrounding tissue are one of the major causes of echo production within masses (Figure 32). This atypical solid mass pattern should not be confused with

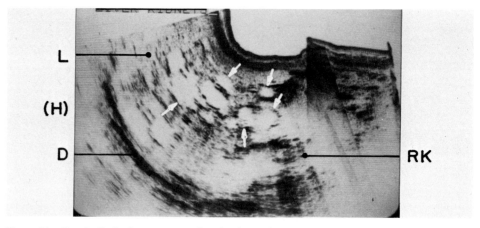

Figure 24.   Longitudinal ultrasonogram taken in the supine position of a polycystic kidney and liver demonstrates several clearly defined cysts (arrows) (D = diaphragm; L = liver; RK = right kidney).

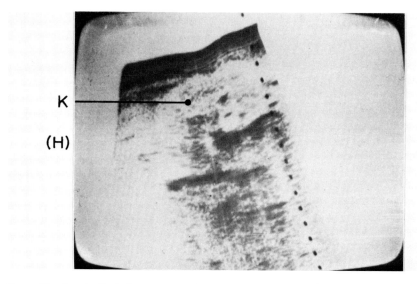

Figure 25. Longitudinal ultrasonogram taken in the prone position of a case of infantile polycystic disease. In this condition, the cysts are extremely small and impossible to visualize individually. There is disruption of the normal kidney architecture (K).

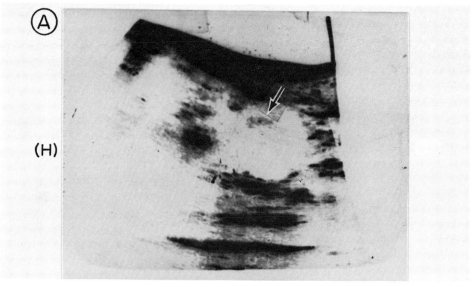

Figure 26. *A*. Longitudinal ultrasonogram of a lower pole necrotic renal cyst shows a few well-defined internal echoes (arrow) making this a complex rather than a cystic lesion. *B*. A-mode ultrasonogram with similar internal echoes (arrows). (*Continued on next page.*)

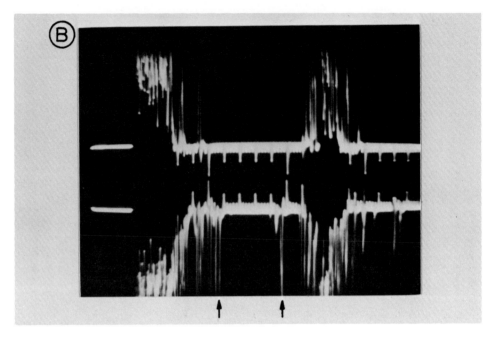

Figure 26.   (Continued)

cystic or complex masses that have a strong back-wall echo pattern. Conversely, vascular masses will contain many echoes (Figure 33). Poor vascularity should not be confused with necrosis, which as has been pointed out, results in a complex pattern. Hypovascularity occurs frequently in neoplasms of certain cell types. For example, papillary cystadenocarcinomas (a variant of renal cell carcinoma), lymphomas, sar-

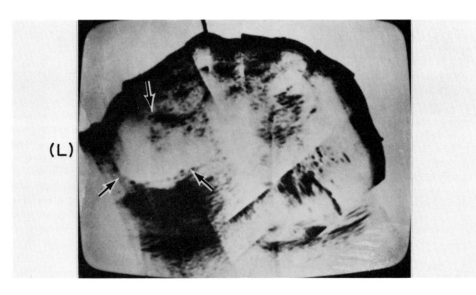

Figure 27.   Transverse ultrasonogram taken in the prone position of a left-sided renal hematoma (arrows) producing a complex pattern.

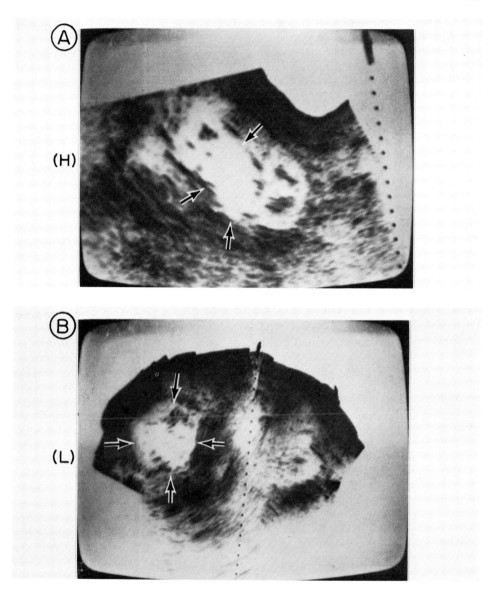

Figure 28. Complex renal mass. Parapelvic cyst. *A.* Longitudinal image taken in the prone position demonstrates a predominantly cystic pattern arising from a parapelvic renal mass (arrows). *B.* Transverse image shows the mass (arrows) to have internal echoes attributable to the multiple extensions of the cyst through the renal hilar structures and into the periinfundibular areas.

comas, and most metastatic tumors to the kidney are usually hypovascular. Although there is not an absolute correlation between lack of echoes and sparse vascularity, the association is frequent enough to allow fairly reliable predictions to be made. Still another factor related to the cause of anechoic masses is tissue homogeneity. If a mass is composed of fairly uniform tissue type, the differences in specific acoustic impedance between its internal structures will be slight, and echo production in turn will be

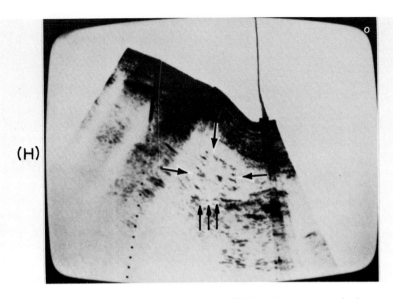

Figure 29. Sinus lipomatosis. Longitudinal prone image of kidney shows the central echo complex (arrows) to be somewhat dispersed but without the presence of strong distal-wall echoes (triple arrow). The splaying of the central structures is due to the deposition of large quantities of sinus fat. A parapelvic cyst also could produce breaking up of the central complex but would be associated with a definite cystic pattern.

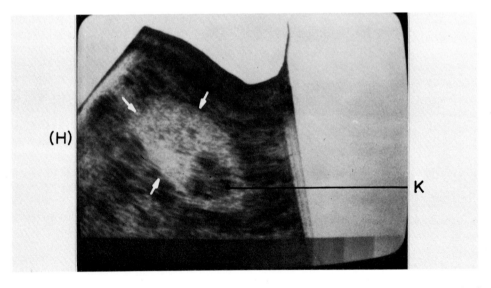

Figure 30. Longitudinal ultrasonogram taken in the prone position shows a large mass in the upper pole of the kidney (arrows) containing innumerable internal echoes with no difference in sound transmission compared to the normal lower pole (K). This is the typical appearance of a solid renal tumor.

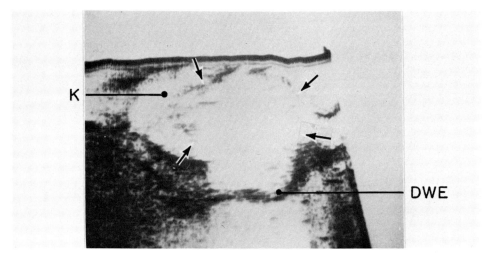

Figure 31. Longitudinal prone ultrasonogram taken in the prone position of a lower pole renal cell carcinoma (arrows) demonstrates weak distal-wall echoes (DWE) compared to the rest of the kidney, due to its absorption by the tumor. At this sensitivity setting there are few internal echoes.

diminished in number and intensity. Lymphomas, in particular, have been noted to exhibit this characteristic.

Rarely, a solid pattern will be obtained from a renal mass other than a tumor. In our experience this has only happened in the presence of mural calcification, usually in the wall of a cyst, but occasionally in the wall of a hematoma or abscess. The marked reflec-

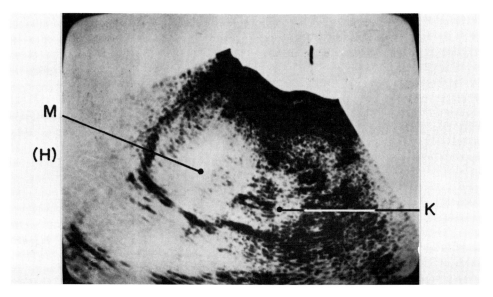

Figure 32. Longitudinal ultrasonogram reveals a renal mass (M) having an atypical solid pattern with sparse internal echoes and weak distal-wall echoes. This was a poorly vascularized renal cell carcinoma (K = lower pole of kidney).

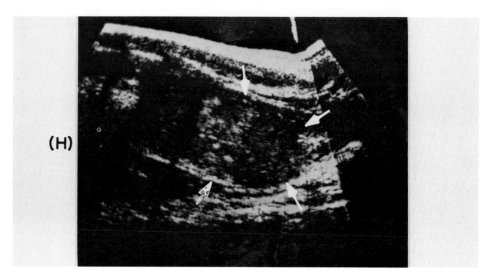

Figure 33. Longitudinal ultrasonogram taken in the prone position of a large renal cell carcinoma with innumerable internal echoes (arrows). These echoes were attributable to its abundant blood vessels.

tion of sound produced by the calcium prevents the through transmission of enough sound to define the far wall. It is important, therefore, to correlate the ultrasonic findings with those seen on the roentgenograms at all times, lest obvious oversights such as failure to detect calcification, occur. In the same vein, it cannot be overemphasized that ultrasound cannot be depended on to diagnose solid tumors that are completely intrarenal, and do not bulge the renal contour. The presence or absence of a renal mass should be ascertained clearly at the time of urography, before the sonographic examination is performed. An intrarenal tumor may be difficult or impossible to distinguish sonographically from normal renal parenchyma. If, at urography the presence or absence of a bona fide renal mass cannot be ascertained, then radionuclide scanning should be performed to differentiate between a pseudotumor and a pathological mass (8). Figure 34 is an in vitro sonogram of an excised kidney that harbored a carcinoma in the lower pole and a benign serous cyst in the upper pole. In this one kidney can be seen the typical ultrasonic findings in both solid and cystic masses.

Renal masses in infants and children also may be assessed reliably by ultrasound (9). As in adults, three basic types of patterns are encountered. A cystic pattern in a neonate suggests multicystic kidney (Figure 35) or hydronephrosis (10). Such a pattern is not seen with solid lesions. The sonogram of a Wilms' tumor (Figure 36) or leiomyomatous hamartoma is either solid or complex. This is true also of neuroblastoma, but the latter usually can be differentiated from an intrinsic renal mass by adequate urography (see Chapter 11).

In children, when the presence of disease in one kidney presages the possible development of disease in the other, such as in the case of a Wilms' tumor, ultrasound can be used for follow-up evaluation of the remaining kidney for as long as desired. In a long-term setting this approach has obvious advantages when compared to roentgenographic techniques, but more data regarding the comparative sensitivity of the two methods in detecting early abnormalities are required before ultrasound can be recommended confidently as a substitute for urography in such situations. Similarly children at risk for the

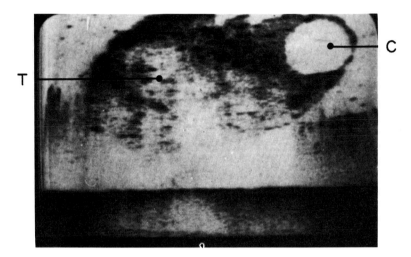

Figure 34. Comparison of sonographic properties of renal cysts and tumors. Renal specimen containing cyst in the upper pole (C) and tumor in the lower pole (T). Both lesions are approximately the same size. However, the sound transmission through the cyst is excellent, whereas the sound transmission through the tumor is largely attenuated and has produced a shadowing effect. There are in addition many echoes seen within the tumor, but none within the cyst.

development of renal tumors, such as those with aniridia, hemihypertrophy, or the Beckwith-Wiedeman syndrome can be kept under surveillance for the appearance of a renal mass. Adults, too, with familial histories such as polycystic disease and tuberous sclerosis may be examined periodically by ultrasound to detect the appearance of renal masses. In fact, such renal monitoring can be extended to encompass innumerable

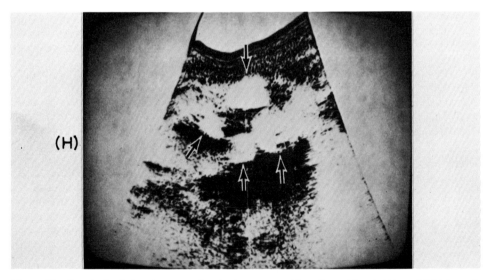

Figure 35. Longitudinal ultrasonogram taken in the prone position of a multicystic kidney. Multiple cystic masses are seen (arrows) in the absence of a definite renniform shape.

clinical situations in which periodic reassessment is mandated. In this category are such diverse entities as patients with renal trauma who are being observed for the development of an expanding hematoma, patients with hydronephrosis, patients undergoing nonsurgical management of renal tumors (i.e., radiation therapy), and patients with renal and perirenal urine collections to name only a few.

ASSESSMENT OF RENAL ANATOMY

Ultrasonic renal imaging may be of immense value when renal insufficiency precludes adequate depiction of the kidneys by traditional means of study such as excretory urography. Thus, in a uremic patient, about whom little else is known, an ultrasound examination may provide the necessary information to allow a therapeutic plan to be formulated, or a presumptive diagnosis to be made (11). For example, with sonography, the following facts may be ascertained: the number of kidneys present, their location, their size, their shape, and the status of the renal pelvis. With these data, it is possible to accurately assess the likelihood of certain entities such as chronic end-stage renal disease, which produces bilaterally small kidneys with nondilated renal pelves. It also can be used to rule out obstructive uropathy, polycystic disease and various anomalies that produce distinctive sonographic patterns. Similar information is helpful when only one kidney is abnormal such as in the case of a nonvisualizing kidney on urography (12, 13). It is sometimes difficult to be certain whether such a kidney is actually present. Ultrasound represents a quick, relatively effortless, and accurate way to find out.

Number of Kidneys

Unilateral renal agenesis occurs in approximately 1 in 1000 persons (14). Frequently such individuals as well as an occasional patient who has had a nephrectomy, are unaware that they have only one kidney. Even patients having this knowledge are sometimes too ill to impart it to their physician. Ultrasonic examination readily provides this information, although ordinarily urography would have detected it first. However, in severely uremic or traumatized patients urography may not prove definitive, and it is here that ultrasound achieves its maximum value, possibly obviating the need for retrograde pyelography or angiography. Obviously, the knowledge that patients in either of the above categories have only one kidney is of critical importance in their management. If a kidney cannot be imaged in the usual flank location, a search should be made for it in the pelvis. If not found here, the kidney must be either absent or so small as to be undetectable (Figure 37). The knowledge that a second kidney is present is equally important. We have seen several cases of newborns with hydronephrotic kidneys who were thought by urography to have only one kidney but were shown by sonography to have small contralateral kidneys (Figure 38).

Locations of Kidneys

Although ectopically located kidneys usually are noted at urography, an occasional case will be overlooked because of impaired function or perhaps because of obscuration by the underlying skeleton. Fortunately, it is possible to image pelvic kidneys by ultrasound

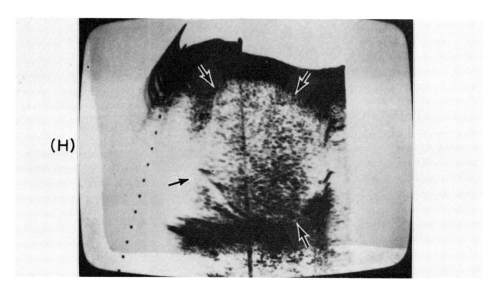

Figure 36. Longitudinal ultrasonogram taken in the prone position of a complex predominately solid renal mass (arrows) consistent with Wilms' tumor. The good sound transmission is the result of areas of internal hemorrhage and necrosis.

in most instances, although obviously this must be done in the supine position and preferably with a filled urinary bladder (Figure 39). Ectopic kidneys may be located at any point between the upper abdomen and the pelvis and the search for them must be very purposeful and complete. The diagnosis is suspected when it is discovered that both kidneys are not present in their normal location. The long axis of the pelvic kidney is frequently at an unconventional angle, making it difficult to obtain detailed visualization of the central echo complex. Real-time ultrasound is often helpful in rapidly obtaining the long axis. The detection of a pelvic kidney is especially important in female patients who are scheduled to undergo exploratory laparotomy for a "pelvic mass." Ectopic kidneys often exhibit associated pathology especially ureteropelvic junction obstruction and calculi, and these complications also may be recognized. The location of kidneys that have been displaced from their normal locations by masses or other abnormalities also may be ascertained by ultrasound as well as by roentgenography. This will be discussed further in Chapter 11.

Renal Size

The size of the kidneys is one of the most important determinants of prognosis in patients with renal failure. Generally speaking, those patients with small kidneys have a poor outlook, usually suffering from so-called "medical" renal disease which is the contracted end-stage kidney of chronic glomerulonephritis, chronic pyelonephritis, nephrosclerosis, and so forth, or rarely from congenital hypoplasia (Figure 40). Surgery plays little if any role in the management of such patients. Patients with normal-sized or even enlarged kidneys usually have a better prognosis. Acute pyelonephritis, renal

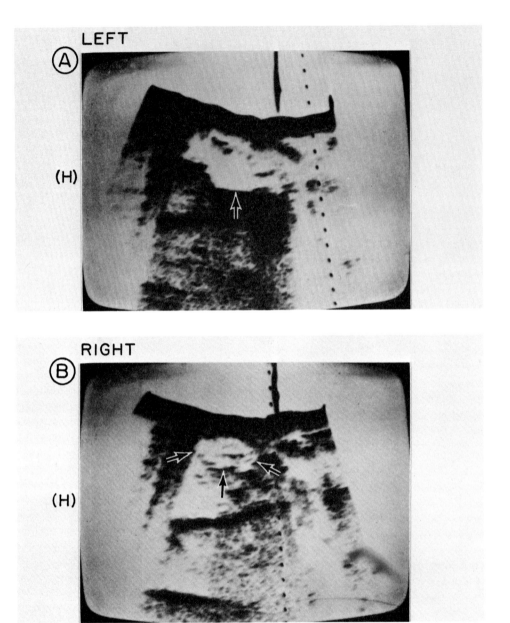

Figure 37.   Value of sonography in detecting the presence of unsuspected renal tissue. *A.* Longitudinal image taken in the prone position of left kidney in a newborn demonstrates a fluid-filled central mass (arrow) consistent with a diagnosis of hydronephrosis. *B.* A longitudinal image of the right flank demonstrates the presence of a small nonhydronephrotic kidney (arrows), which later was proved to contain moderate functional capability.

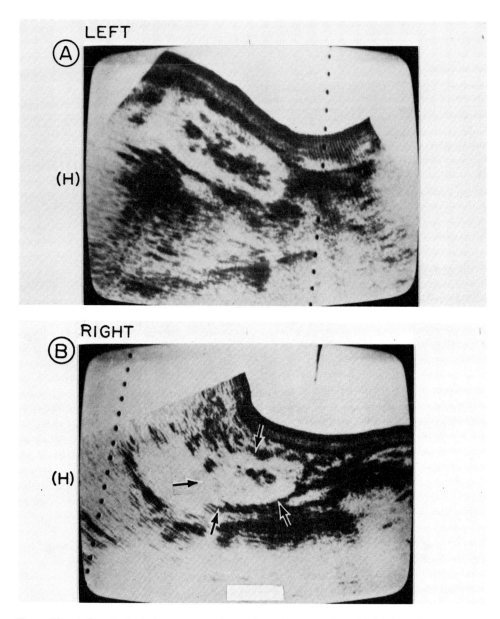

Figure 38. *A.* Longitudinal ultrasonogram of a newborn shows an enlarged left kidney. *B.* Longitudinal ultrasonogram of the opposite side reveals a hypoplastic right kidney. (arrows).

cortical necrosis, and renal tubular necrosis fall in this category, although the former is a rare cause of renal failure. Those who can be helped surgically by stone removal or relief of obstruction usually are found in this category. Renal vein thrombosis (Figure 41), xanthogranulomatous pyelonephritis, and leukemic infiltration usually cause renal enlargement, although the most common causes are duplicated kidneys and compensatory hypertrophy.

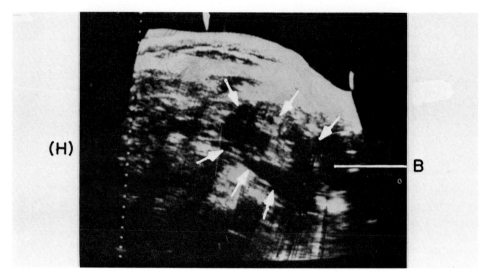

Figure 39. Longitudinal image taken in the supine position shows a pelvic kidney (arrows). The presence of a distended urinary bladder (B) is usually helpful in visualizing the most caudal portions of an ectopic kidney.

Renal Shape

Abnormalities in the shape of kidneys occur primarily as a result of congenital anomalies. Polycystic and multicystic disease, which have been discussed previously, are examples of disturbances in morphology that can be evaluated nicely by ultrasound. To these can be added fusion abnormalities such as horeshoe kidney which also can be depicted sonographically. The isthmus usually can be identified as it crosses anterior to the aorta and vena cava by scanning in the supine position transversely (Figure 42).

Renal Pelvis and Collecting System

Hydronephrosis is the most important entity in this category. Fortunately, ultrasound has proved to be of great value in the detection of this problem, for often the hydro-nephrotic kidney is severely damaged and does not excrete urographic contrast agents well (15). Several sonographic patterns are indicative of hydronephrosis (16). An early sign is an echo-free area in the region of the renal pelvis, surrounded by well-defined echoes from the wall of the renal pelvis—the so-called ballooning of the central echo complex (Figure 43). At times, dilated infundibula and calyces also may be identified. Later, the central echoes no longer can be identified, while strong echoes can be detected from compressed renal tissue surrounding the dilated pelvis (Figure 44). Finally, with advanced hydro-nephrosis, renal tissue no longer can be identified, the diseased area giving the appearance of a cyst because of the fluid-filled sac that has developed (Figure 45). In cases of bilateral hydronephrosis, the urinary bladder always should be examined to rule out infravesical obstruction as a cause for the renal changes.

Hydronephrosis is an important and often unrecognized cause of renal failure. Since it is potentially one of the more remediable causes, it is important that its presence not be overlooked. Since hydronephrosis is relatively easy to detect by ultrasound, it would seem reasonable to state, that unless obstruction has been ruled out unequivocally by some other means, ultrasonic evaluation of the kidneys should be performed on all patients in renal failure. It is appropriate to note, as well, that ultrasound also may be employed to guide the procedure of percutaneous needle pyclostomy (17).

Hydronephrosis occurs frequently during pregnancy, and is thought to be a contributing cause of the urinary tract infections that are so frequent in pregnant women. In

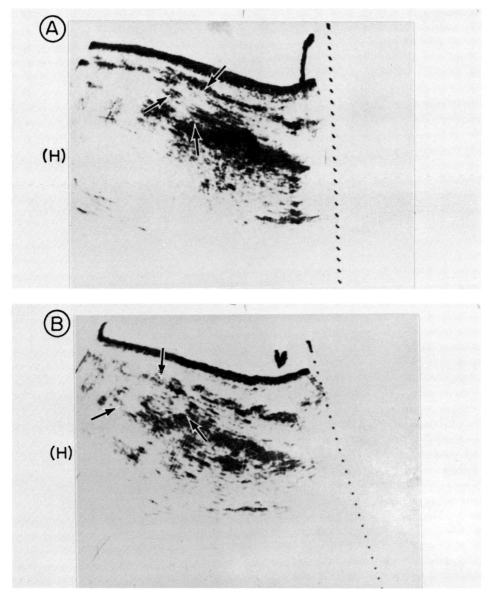

Figure 40. *A*. Longitudinal image taken in the prone position of the right kidney reveals a very small reniformlike structure (arrows). *B*. A similar ultrasonic finding is present on the opposite side (arrows). In this newborn these findings are consistent with a diagnosis of congenital bilateral hypoplasia.

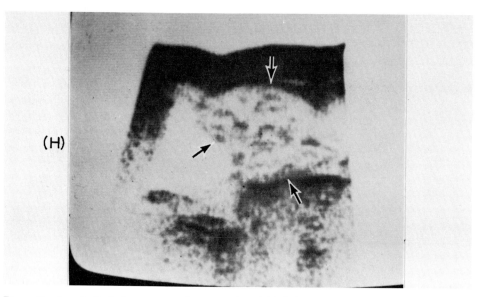

Figure 41.   Longitudinal ultrasonogram shows an enlarged left kidney in a newborn with a nonvisualizing kidney on IVP. The normal parenchymal outline is replaced by numerous ill-defined amorphous echoes. This is a nonspecific pattern, but it is compatible with an engorged and congested kidney.

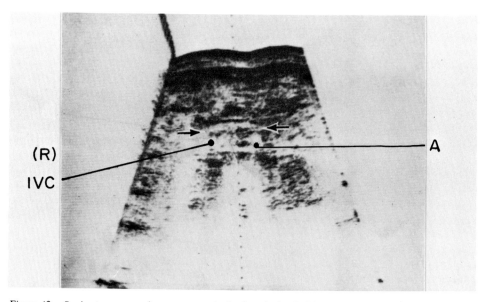

Figure 42.   Supine transverse ultrasonogram obtained at the level of L-5 shows the renal isthmus (arrows) just anterior to the aorta (A) and inferior vena cava (IVC).

those women who are symptomatic, ultrasound can be used to assess as well as continually monitor the degree of hydronephrosis and thereby decrease the need to use ionizing radiation in their investigation.

Gray scale ultrasonography has allowed satisfactory recording of renal calculi that heretofore were detectable poorly or not at all by conventional bistable imaging. Hallmarks of nephrolithiasis are the presence of acoustic shadowing, resulting from the

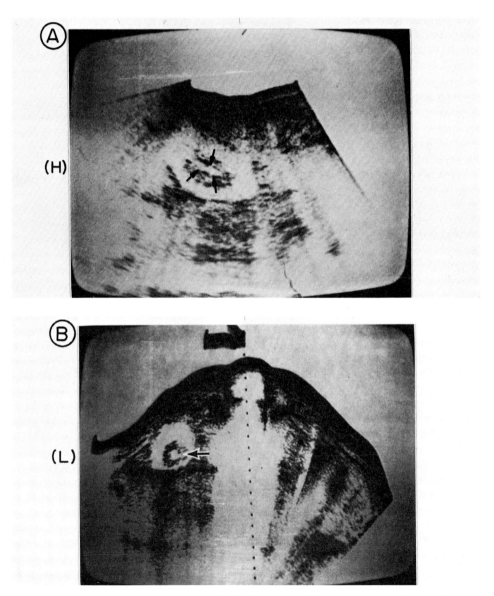

Figure 43. *A*. Longitudinal ultrasonogram taken in the prone position demonstrates a slight ballooning of the central echo complex (arrows). *B*. A similar appearance of central ballooning (arrow) can be seen in the transverse section.

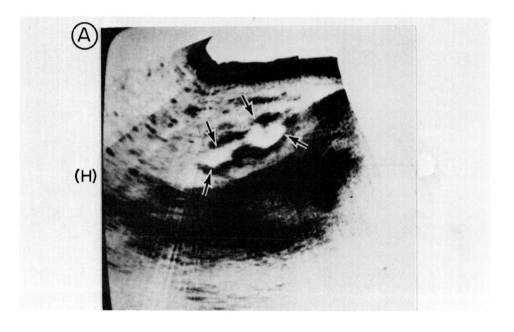

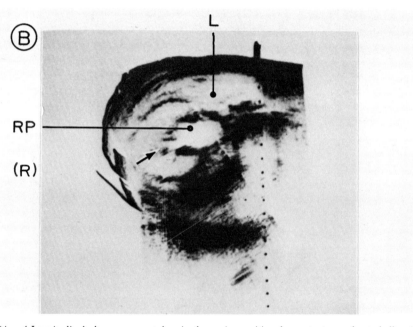

Figure 44. *A.* Longitudinal ultrasonogram taken in the supine position demonstrates moderate ballooning of the central echo complex (arrows). This is consistent with moderate hydronephrosis. *B.* Transverse ultrasonogram shows a similar pattern of a dilated renal pelvis (RP). Note dilated infundibulum and calyx (arrow).

302

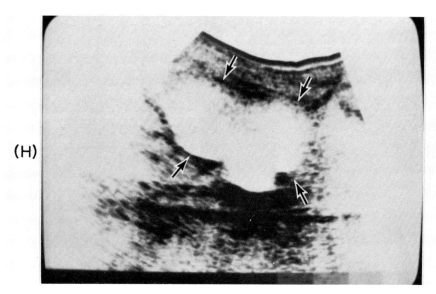

Figure 45. Longitudinal image taken in the prone position of the right kidney demonstrates a large nondescript fluid-filled structure (arrows). There is no evidence of normal renal architecture. The kidney was markedly hydronephrotic, and the renal cortex was represented by a thin shell.

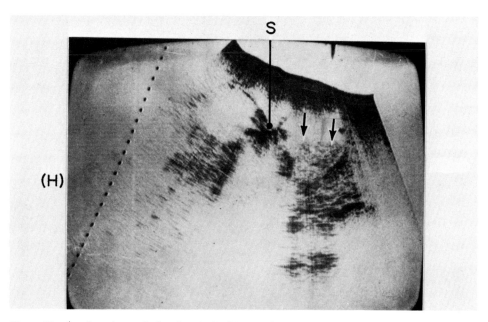

Figure 46. Renal staghorn calculus. Longitudinal image taken in the prone position reveals multiple fluid-filled cystlike structures representing large hydrocalyces. A densely echo-producing stellate structure (S) in the center of the kidney is associated with marked sound absorption and pronounced shadowing effect. This represents a staghorn calculus (S). Note the leveling off of echo-producing tissue in the lower half of the kidney representing debris (arrows) that has settled to the bottom of the hydronephrotic sac.

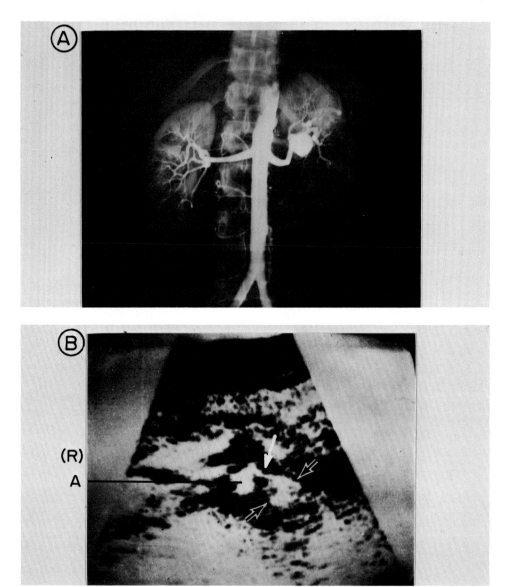

Figure 47. *A*. Arteriogram demonstrates an aneurysm of the left renal artery. *B*. Transverse ultrasonogram taken in the supine position shows the renal artery aneurysm (black arrows) arising from the left renal artery (white arrow) (A = abdominal aorta).

stone's reflecting and absorbing most of the ultrasonic beam (Figure 46). Generally speaking, stones produce stronger reflecting echoes and allow less sound transmission than soft tissue masses of the same size. This property has been utilized successfully for intraoperative localization and removal of occult renal calculi (18). Attempts to differentiate the chemical components of renal calculi on the basis of their ultrasonic behavior appear promising, but as yet have produced no clinically useful results (19).

RENAL BLOOD VESSELS

Before the development of gray scale ultrasonography detailed imaging of the main renal artery and vein was not possible. Now, however, employing the gray scale modality, a great deal of clinically important information about these structures can be obtained easily. Renal artery aneurysms, for example, can be recorded (Figure 47), as can thrombi in the renal veins. In the presence of a renal neoplasm, the demonstration of a thrombus in the renal vein bespeaks intravascular extension of the tumor and has great prognostic significance (Figure 48). The demonstration of aneurysms in patients with, as well as without, hypertension can greatly influence their management. Certainly future developments in ultrasound will make it possible to examine the renal vasculature in detail, a capability heretofore obtainable only with invasive techniques.

THE TRANSPLANTED KIDNEY

The transplanted kidney is, of course, prone to many complications covering a wide spectrum of immunologic, inflammatory, and vascular disorders as well as problems developing as a result of mechanical derangements. Ultrasound is extremely important in the evaluation of the patient with a transplant since most these complications lend themselves readily to sonographic assessment.

Scans are obtained in the supine position, and may be carried out as early as the second or third postoperative day, if necessary, without risk of infecting the surgical inci-

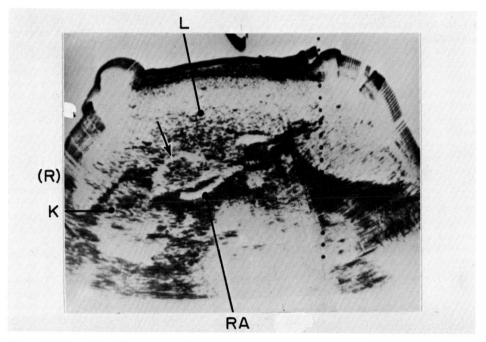

Figure 48. Transverse ultrasonogram taken in the supine position demonstrates an enlarged renal vein that contains echogenic tissue (arrow) representing tumor thrombus in the vein from a renal cell carcinoma (K). The renal artery (RA) also is visualized. (L = liver).

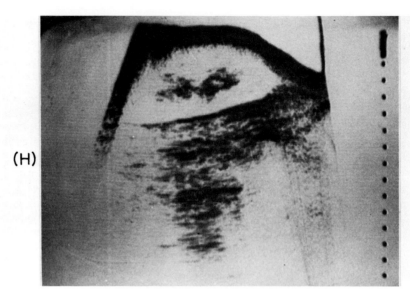

Figure 49. Longitudinal ultrasonogram of a normal transplanted kidney obtained on the tenth postoperative day. Aside from its location, the kidney has a normal sonographic appearance.

sion. If possible, and mainly for the patient's comfort, direct application of the transducer to the skin incision should be avoided, but this is not critical. The scanning axis should be parallel and at right angles to the longitudinal axis of the kidney, which is often at a 45-degree angle with the patient's long axis. The true axis of the kidney can be determined easily by real-time scanning, or if this is not available, by making two approximately transverse sections at different levels and marking the midpoint of the kidney on the skin at each level. The long axis of the kidney may be constructed by con-

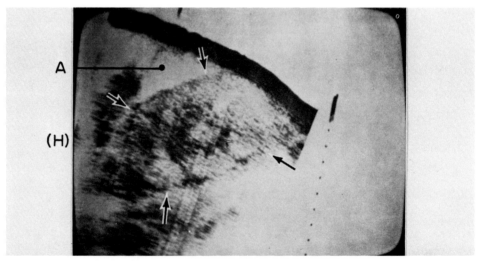

Figure 50. Longitudinal supine ultrasonograms obtained 2 weeks after surgery demonstrate the kidney to be enlarged (arrows) with innumerable echoes originating from the parenchyma. Note the presence of ascites (A).

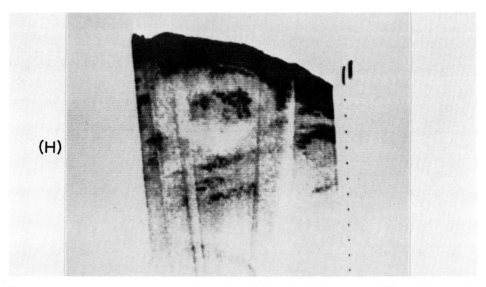

Figure 51. Longitudinal ultrasonogram of transplanted kidney in which severe renal failure had occurred 1 week after surgery. Although the kidney is enlarged slightly, the internal echoes seen with graft rejection are not present here. Findings are compatible with acute tubular necrosis.

necting these two points. The iliac areas and the entire pelvis should be included in the ultrasonic field, and the bladder should be full.

Because postoperative changes in renal size may hold the key to the differential diagnosis of the unique complications inherent in this population group, it is recommended that all patients with transplants be scanned routinely. A baseline study at approximately seven days will suffice in the patient without complications, while scans as often and whenever needed should be done on the others.

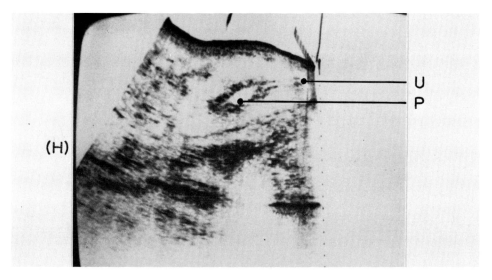

Figure 52. Longitudinal ultrasonogram taken in the supine position of a renal transplant demonstrates a minimally dilated renal pelvis (P). Note that the ureter also is visualized (U).

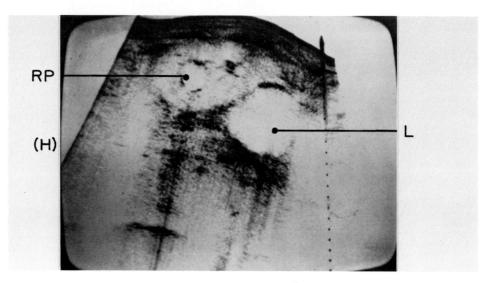

Figure 53. Longitudinal oblique ultrasonogram reveals an extrarenal inferiorly located cystic mass (L) consistent with a diagnosis of lymphocele that is producing hydronephrosis (RP = dilated renal pelvis).

Normally, the transplanted kidney increases slightly in volume, with changes detectable as early as the second week. A slight but progressive increase over the next month is not unusual. The kidney outline is smooth, and the parenchyma is relatively anechoic (Figure 49). No pararenal masses are detectable and the calyceal echoes are compact, although the renal pelvis may show a slight fullness. Kidneys undergoing real or threatened rejection demonstrate a more acute increase in volume (20), and in advanced cases we have observed disruption of the normal pattern with scattered echoes recorded from the renal parenchyma due to areas of hemorrhage and necrosis (Figure 50). If the rejection is reversible the renal size diminishes, and this can be followed easily ultrasonically. Acute tubular necrosis also may cause renal enlargement, but usually is not accompanied by the extensive internal echoes seen in advanced graft rejection (Figure 51). Ultrasound can detect hydronephrosis easily in the transplanted kidney (21) (Figure 52) as well as pararenal and pelvic fluid collections, neither of which are rare and which, when they occur, may be due to lymphocele, urinoma, abscess, or hematoma, singly or in combination (Figure 53). While it is not possible to differentiate these fluid collections consistently with accuracy, based on sonography alone, there is a tendency for abscesses to produce more complex masses with less sharp borders than the others (22). Needle aspiration of the collection using ultrasonic guidance usually will shed more light on the correct diagnosis.

REFERENCES

1. Vallance J, et al: Gray scale ultrasonic imaging of the kidney. *Brit J Radiol* **49**:635, July 1976.

2. Marich KW, Zatz LM, Green PS, Suarez, JR, Macovski A: Real-time imaging with a new ultrasonic camera. Part 1: In vitro experimental studies on transmission imaging of biological structures. *J Clin Ultrasound* **3**:5, March 1975.

3. Mozersky DJ, Hokanson DE, Baker DW, Sumner DS, Strandness DE: Ultrasonic arteriography. *Arch Surg* **103**:663, December 1971.

4. Pollack HM, Goldberg BB, Morales JO, Bogash M: A systematized approach to the differential diagnosis of renal masses. *Radiol* **113**:653, December 1974.

5. Green WM, King DL, Casarella WJ: A reappraisal of sonolucent renal masses. *Radiol* **121**:163, October 1975.

6. Pollack HM, Goldberg BB, Morales JO, Bogash M: Differentiation of renal masses: a systematized approach, in *Radiologic and Other Biophysical Methods in Tumor Diagnosis.* Chicago, Yearbook Medical Publishers, Inc, 1975, p 235.

7. Becker J, Schneider M, Staiano, S, et al: Renal pelvic lipomatosis: A sonographic evaluation. *J Clin Ultrasound* **2**:299, December 1974.

8. Pollack HM, Edell S, Morales JO: Radionuclide imaging in renal pseudotumors. *Radiol* **111**:639, June 1974.

9. Goldberg BB, Pollack HM, Capitanio M, Kirkpatrick JA: Ultrasonography: an aid in the diagnosis of masses in pediatric patients. *Pediatrics* **56**:421–428, September 1975.

10. Bearman SB, Hene PL, Sanders RC: Multicystic kidney: a sonographic pattern. *Radiol* **118**:685, March 1976.

11. Sanders RC, Jeck DL: B-scan ultrasound in the evaluation of renal failure. *Radiol* **119**:199, April 1976.

12. Marangola JP, Bryan PJ, Azimi F: Ultrasonic evaluation of the unilateral nonvisualized kidney. *Am J Roentgen* **126**:853, April 1976.

13. Sanders RC: Place of diagnostic ultrasound in examination of kidneys not seen on excretory urography. *J. Urol* **114**:813, December 1975.

14. Longo VJ, Thompson CJ: Congenital solitary kidney. *J Urol* **68**:63, 1952.

15. Taylor KJW, Kraus V: Gray scale ultrasound imaging: assessment of acute hydronephrosis. *Brit J Urol* **47**:593, December 1975.

16. Sanders RC: Renal ultrasound. *Radiological Clinics NA* **13,** 417, December 1975.

17. Pedersen JF, Cowan DF, Kristensen JK et al: Ultrasonically-guided percutaneous nephrostomy. *Radiol* **119**:429, May 1976.

18. Andaloro VA, Schor M, Marangola J: Intraoperative localization of a renal calculus using ultrasound. *J Urol* **116**:92, July 1976.

19. Cunningham JJ, Cunningham MA: Characterization of renal stone models with gray scale echography. *Urology* **7**: 315, March 1976.

20. Bartrum RJ, Smith EH, D'Orsi CJ, Tilney NL, Dantono J: Evaluation of renal transplants with ultrasound. *Radiol* **118**:405, February 1976.

21. Rosenfeld AT, Taylor KJW: Obstructive uropathy in the transplanted kidney: evaluation by gray scale sonography. *J Urol* **116**:July 1976.

22. Koehler PR, Kanemoto HH, Maxwell JG: Ultrasonic "B" scanning in the diagnosis of complications in renal transplant patients. *Radiol* **119**:661, June 1976.

11
Retroperitoneum

Howard M. Pollack, M.D.
Professor of Radiology
University of Pennsylvania
Hospital and School of Medicine
Philadelphia, Pennsylvania

Barry B. Goldberg, M.D.
Professor of Radiology
Director, Division of Diagnostic Ultrasound
Thomas Jefferson University Hospital
Philadelphia, Pennsylvania

Unquestionably, the retroperitoneum is the blind spot of abdominal diagnosis. The retroperitoneal space contains many structures and can give rise to many problems that defy identification. The recognition of disease in this area is rendered difficult by the fact that most roentgenographic studies that reflect disease therein (for example, barium enemas and excretory urograms) provide evidence of an indirect nature, such as displacement or compression of a contiguously involved structure. For this reason, primary retroperitoneal tumors, abscesses, and fluid collections frequently still defy conventional radiographic efforts at detection. Physicians concerned with such diseases have long sought a reliable method of evaluation. One answer, in the form of ultrasound, now seems at hand. In the previous chapter, it was shown that ultrasound is of great value in the assessment of renal disease. In this chapter, it will be shown that ultrasound is no less valuable in illuminating the nature and extent of retroperitoneal diseases. Although a relatively new modality, ultrasonography now occupies a primary position in the evaluation of such disorders and should be employed routinely whenever retroperitoneal disorders, especially masses, are under consideration.

With the exception of retroperitoneal fibrosis, most disease processes in this anatomic area are masses. They may occur anywhere in this relatively large space, and in general, they produce displacement of adjacent structures, especially the kidneys. Ultrasound cannot only detect these masses but can show their relationship to other retroperitoneal structures in the majority of cases. The ureters are not seen normally, but if significantly dilated, portions of the proximal as well as the distal ureters may be recorded. The urinary bladder, of course, provides a standard of reference to confirm the cystic or solid nature of a mass. Evaluation of the size of the bladder, as well as the presence of internal abnormalities such as tumors and stones, also can be carried out. The prostate and adjacent structures may be visualized by any of several different approaches. The techniques utilized will be discussed in general in the following paragraphs and specifically in the appropriate sections of this chapter.

TECHNIQUE

The techniques employed for evaluating the retroperitoneal area are identical to those discussed in the previous chapter. The evaluation of retroperitoneal structures is first attempted in the prone position and then, if necessary, supine and axillary imaging may be added. Essentially the area of interest is located with reference to the kidney. Preliminary information usually is available through physical examination or on urography demonstrating either a palpable mass or renal displacement. Thus the kidneys initially are localized and the mass is defined with reference to the ipsilateral kidney. For suprarenal masses, as with upper pole renal masses, several methods may be required to produce satisfactory imaging. These include sustained inspiration in an attempt to displace the mass downward or, if this results in interference by the lung, sustained expiration during each scan. Scanning with the patient erect also may be used if these two techniques fail to displace the mass sufficiently caudad. For the right side, the supine position may be helpful for transhepatic scanning, using the same techniques described in the earlier chapters, with initial longitudinal scans followed by transverse scans during suspended respiration.

When evaluating medially located masses or dilated ureters, the longitudinal scans are continued medial to the kidney. For lateral masses, the opposite is true. Masses located inferior to the kidney may be difficult to evaluate in the prone position, since the iliac crest will prevent the penetration of the ultrasonic beam. If the mass is large, and projects into the abdomen, it may displace the bowel sufficiently to allow for satisfactory imaging in the supine position. In this case, the techniques followed are similar to those used elsewhere in the abdomen. First, the area of interest is localized; then scans are obtained at uniform distances in both longitudinal and transverse directions. One must exercise care to avoid the overlying bowel, not only because of the deleterious effect of gas on the ultrasonic beam but because of similar effects that may be produced by barium. Such interference is not a problem, of course, when examining in the prone position.

The presence of normal structures capable of simulating masses always must be kept in mind. The spleen, for example, at times may show a large retroperitoneal surface and, if care is not taken, this may be confused with a left suprarenal mass (Figure 1). The characteristic shape and complex ultrasonic pattern, however, usually allow the spleen to be identified readily. On the right, a large caudate lobe of the liver may produce the same effect. If necessary, correlation with roentgenograms or radionuclide scans may be employed to assist in the anatomic localization of an unusually shaped liver or spleen.

Examination of the urinary bladder is, of course, performed in the supine position. Initial midline longitudinal scans are obtained extending from the pubis toward the umbilicus and beyond if necessary. Scans then are obtained at intervals of 1 or 2 centimeters on each side of the midline until the entire pelvic region has been examined. Next, transverse scans are obtained at set intervals, again starting at the level of the pubis and continuing upward to the umbilicus and beyond if needed. As with most gray scale techniques, there is little need for compound sectoring and linear or simple sector sweeps provide excellent results. A single sweep per scan is desirable rather than a retracing of areas already examined as the latter will tend to produce falsely positioned

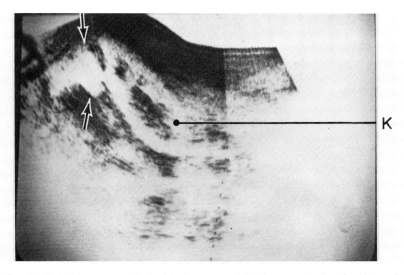

Figure 1.   Longitudinal ultrasonogram obtained in the prone position demonstrates the spleen (arrows) simulating suprarenal mass at the superior anterior border of the kidney (K). The sonographic appearance of the spleen is that of a complex mass due to its high blood content.

echoes if there is any movement of structures within the body or change in position of the transducer. Bowel gas is usually not a problem in urinary bladder evaluation, since this organ is anteriorly located and will displace bowel as it distends. It is helpful if the sweeps, which start at the pubis in both longitudinal and transverse planes, are angled caudally into the pelvis so that the deep pelvic structures, such as the bladder trigone and structures adjacent to the pouch of Douglas, may be evaluated adequately. It is easy to do this when performing longitudinal sweeps by merely angling the transducer under the pubic bone. With transverse scans, the transducer arm must be angled. Abnormalities of the urachus or cystic areas in the pelvis can be evaluated throughly using the same technique as that applied for the bladder. Similarly, the female pelvic organs and the prostate can be examined if the transducer is angulated steeply toward the pelvic floor in both the longitudinal and transverse scans. In general, it is a good rule to perform pelvic ultrasonography with a full urinary bladder. Not only does this provide information about the relationship of the bladder to contiguous pelvic masses but serial examinations with controlled decreases in bladder volume through a catheter allow an estimate of the presence or absence of bladder wall fixation, which may accompany certain neoplastic and inflammatory processes. In addition, the sound conducting properties of fluid allow the water- or urine-filled bladder to act as an excellent transmitting medium for ultrasonic evaluation of structures posterior or caudal to the bladder, such as cul de sac collections, deep pelvic cysts, and even the prostate gland itself (Figure 2). Of course, the filled urinary bladder also serves as a standard against which to compare other masses for their sonographic properties.

The ultrasonic examination of the prostate may be conducted either externally or internally. The external approaches to the prostate include the suprapubic method described above and a perineal approach in which the transducer traverses the area

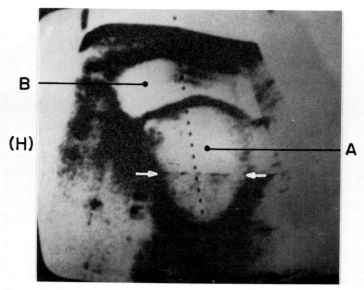

Figure 2.   Longitudinal ultrasonogram demonstrates a complex pelvic mass (A) elevating the floor of the urinary bladder (B), with a clearly defined echo pattern (arrows) denoting the level of the settled debris in this abscess. (Courtesy of Dr. L. Rosenbaum, Department of Radiology, Delaware Memorial Hospital, Wilmington, Delaware.)

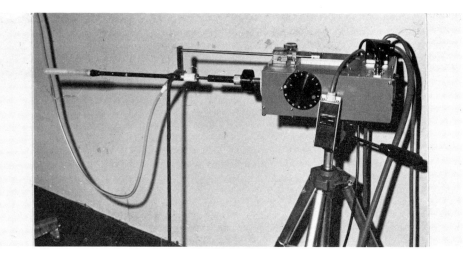

Figure 3. Ultrasonic endoscanner equipment used to obtain transrectal prostatic image. Transducer tip, which is inserted into the rectum, is located to the far left.

between the anus and scrotum. Although the latter avenue provides only a small window through which to gain sonographic access to the prostate, it is usually sufficient to record this structure. At times, a combined approach using both suprapubic and perineal access, may be employed. Here, a transducer is moved downward from the umbilicus to the pubis, angling deeply under the symphysis for an anterior recording before moving the transducer (without erasing the scan) to the perineum where the transducer is swept from scrotum to anus, obtaining a second recording. Transverse scans in the perineal area can be obtained, but they are more awkward and usually will not add additional information. Of course, the perineal scan can be obtained both in the midline and to either side as needed. The internal method of prostatic imaging uses specially constructed equipment known as an endoscanner in which a transducer is affixed to the end of an arm slightly smaller than a standard sized sigmoidoscope. The transducer and arm apparatus can be covered by a protective plastic bag and then inserted into the rectum (Figure 3). Once appropriately positioned, the plastic bag is inflated with water to displace rectal gas and feces. The transducer is then free to rotate through 360 degrees without discomfort to the patient. Scans produced during these rotations produce images of the prostate, bladder, or seminal vesicles, depending on the depth of insertion of the transducer. The unit can be repositioned at set increments, usually at 0.5-cm intervals, to obtain serial transverse images of the entire prostate or of the bladder base and seminal vesicles as well as adjacent pelvic organs or masses. This modality has been adapted successfully to gray scale techniques by the addition of a scan converter. With this modification, not only can the size of the prostate by evaluated but also its internal sonographic nature. The technique also shows promise for the evaluation of other pelvic structures, including the female internal genitalia. Endovaginal scanning also may be carried out with this type of scanning apparatus.

The scrotal contents can be examined ultrasonically either by a direct contact technique, moving the transducer over the surface of the scrotum in the area to be examined or by immersing the scrotum in a water bath in which the transducer can move freely or mechanically around the area. Gray scale images have been produced successfully by both techniques. Since the testis is a superficial structure, high frequency transducers (5–10 MHz) similar to those employed for the breast and thyroid can be used for its evaluation with resultant increased resolution.

ADRENAL GLAND

Since the normal adult adrenal gland rarely measures more than 3 cm in its maximum diameter, special scanning techniques usually are required to record ultrasonic images of this structure. Sample has reported an 80–90 percent success rate in obtaining satisfactory images of normal adrenal glands employing a technique based on a specific alignment of the left kidney with the aorta and the right kidney with either the aorta or inferior vena cava (1). Alignment of the adrenal with these reference structures is obtained while scanning the patient transversely in the lateral decubitus position. Diagnostic images then are obtained by scanning the patient longitudinally, in the same position, based on the alignment observed on the transverse scans (Figure 4). Scanning through the liver for the right adrenal often allows satisfactory recording of this gland, while scans carried out in the prone position are also valuable if the adrenals are significantly enlarged (2). Imaging in the erect position may be helpful when lung and rib interference render the prone position unsatisfactory. Changes in the normal triangular or lunate configuration of the adrenal, for example, a rounded appearance, may indicate the presence of an adrenal mass. A pathologic process also is suggested strongly if the gland measures more than 3 cm in diameter, or if its echogenicity, which ordinarily is greater than the nearby kidney, liver, or spleen is lost.

Adrenal lesions seen in clinical practice consist primarily of tumors and cysts although large adrenal hematomas sometimes are encountered especially in infants (3). In our

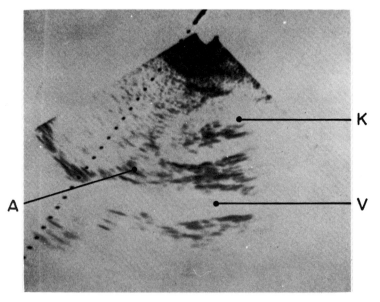

Figure 4. Longitudinal section obtained with axillary approach shows a normal adrenal gland (A) (K = Kidney; V = Vena cava). (Courtesy of W. F. Sample, M.D. Department of Radiology, U.C.L.A.)

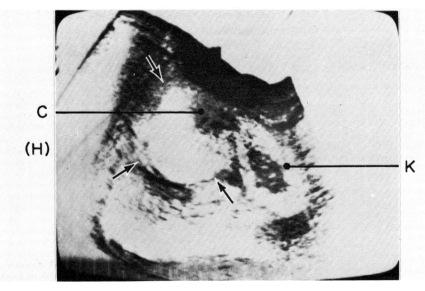

Figure 5. Longitudinal section obtained in the prone position shows a large complex predominantly cystic mass (arrows) located above the right kidney (K). Along its dorsal aspect is an echogenic mass of tissue that later was found to be composed of adherent clot with calcification (C). This was a benign hemorrhagic adrenal cyst.

experience, adrenal cysts represent the single largest group of suprarenal masses. Their ultrasonic pattern in most cases is that of a typical cystic mass, but exceptions may be encountered when the cyst wall is calcified or when the cyst lumen contains clots or other large particulate matter (Figure 5). Here, a complex pattern will be produced. Adrenal hematomas also may show more than one type of pattern producing either a cystic or a complex picture depending on the degree of liquefaction of the hematomas (3).

Adrenal tumors may be either benign or malignant. Cortical adenomas, ganglioneuromas, and pheochromocytomas comprise most of the benign lesions and usually lend themselves well to ultrasonic imaging. Solid patterns are the rule in these cases (4) (Figure 6), although pheochromocytomas exhibit suprisingly good sound transmission in many instances. Perhaps this is attributable to their uniform cell structure or to the frequent areas of hemorrhage encountered with this lesion that results in a complex ultrasonic pattern. At any rate, it is often possible to demonstrate a well-defined capsule surrounding both pheochromocytomas and cortical adenomas (Figure 7). In patients with pheochromocytoma, careful attention should be given to the contralateral suprarenal area, since in 10–15 percent of cases bilateral tumors will be found. The most common malignant lesions affecting the adult adrenal gland are metastatic tumors. The sonographic appearance may be either solid (Figure 8) or complex depending on the presence or absence of internal hemorrhage in the gland. Of the two, the complex pattern is seen more often. Adrenal cortical carcinoma, which is much less common, may be seen as a solid or complex mass. In children, adrenal neuroblastoma is a relatively common malignant tumor and frequently grows to a large size before becoming clinically detectable. Ultrasonic visualization of this tumor presents few difficulties, and the pattern is that of a solid lesion. Occasionally, as with retroperitoneal tumors elsewhere,

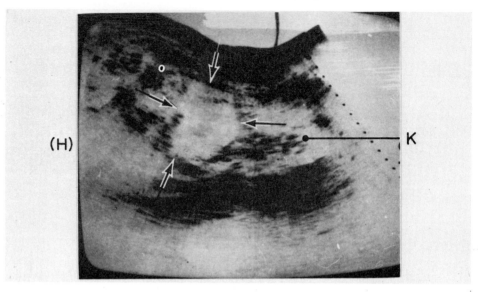

Figure 6. Longitudinal section obtained in the prone position reveals a large mass (arrows) in the left suprarenal area, overlapping in part the upper pole of the kidney (K). Although the mass contains few if any internal echoes, the sound transmission through it is the same or slightly less than that through the normal kidney parenchyma caudal to the mass. Therefore, it is not a fluid-filled structure. This was a neurilemmoma of the adrenal gland.

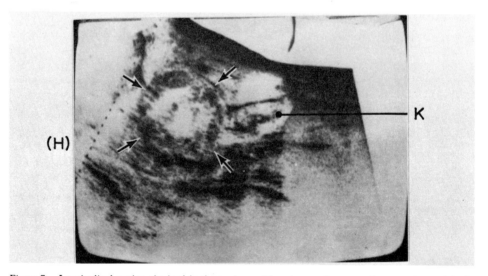

Figure 7. Longitudinal section obtained in the supine position shows a large complex mass (arrows) in the right suprarenal area. A central sonolucent area is attributable to hemorrhage within the tumor. The mass is seen to be well defined. This was a pheochromocytoma. (Courtesy of Department of Radiology Allentown-Sacred Heart Hospital, Allentown, Pennsylvania.)

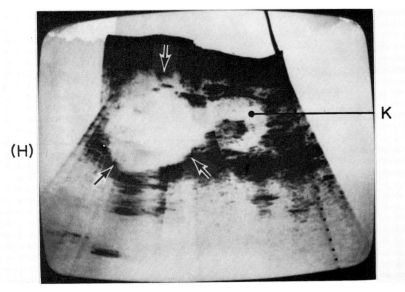

Figure 8. Longitudinal section taken in the prone position reveals a large solid mass occupying the left suprarenal area (arrows). Although few or no internal echoes are present, the sound transmission is less than that seen through the kidney, indicating that it is not cystic but rather a solid mass with relatively few internal reflecting interfaces. This was a metastatic adrenal tumor.

ultrasonic assessment will allow differentiation between a primary adrenal mass and a renal tumor that appears to involve the adrenal. This is possible, of course, only when ultrasonic evaluation reveals one of the two structures to be anatomically intact.

PERI- AND PARANEPHRIC COLLECTIONS

The retroperitoneal space in the renal area is divided into two anatomic subdivisions. The space immediately surrounding the kidney is known as the perinephric space and has as its peripheral boundary the renal fascia (fascia of Gerota). Surrounding the renal fascia is another compartment known as the paranephric space, which in effect, includes the remainder of the retroperitoneal space. The perinephric space is closed superiorly but open inferiorly and allows fluid collections to spread downward. Fluid accumulations in these areas consist of hematomas, abscesses, and urinomas (5). Generally speaking, precise localization of fluid collections to either of the anatomic subcompartments of the retroperitoneum cannot be accomplished by ultrasound, but localization adequate to guide the surgeon in planning a proper operative approach is provided easily.

While it is difficult or impossible to distinguish one type of fluid from another with certainty, uninfected urinomas usually show a typical cystic pattern on sonography (Figure 9). Hematomas may do likewise, but this is dependent on their degree of liquification (Figure 10). The presence of infection tends to convert the pattern to a complex one as seen, for example, with perinephric abscesses; but cystic patterns, too, may be seen with abscesses (Figure 11).

The prone position is usually the most informative in retroperitoneal fluid collections,

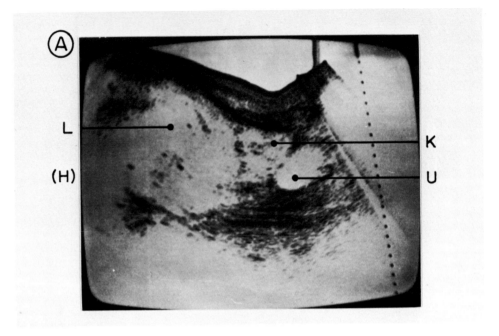

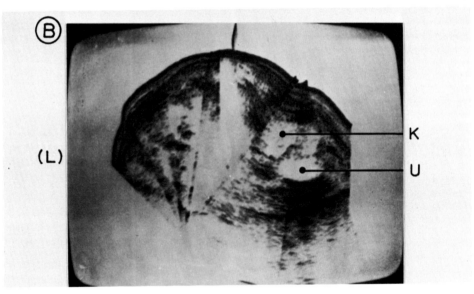

Figure 9 *A.* Longitudinal ultrasonogram obtained in the prone position 1 week following partial nephrectomy. A fluid-filled mass (U) is seen just caudad to the remaining half of the kidney (K). This is consistent with a diagnosis of urinoma (L = liver). *B.* Transverse section shows the urinoma (U) to lie just anterior to the nonresected portion of the kidney (K). Note its typical cystic ultrasonic pattern.

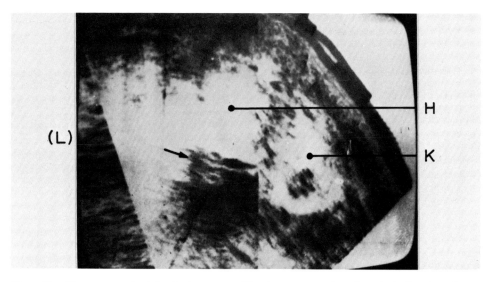

Figure 10.   Transverse section taken in the prone position demonstrates a large irregularly shaped sonolucent mass (H) seen just medial to the kidney (K) and dorsal to the renal artery (arrow). This was a retroperitoneal hematoma, which developed following needle-biopsy of the kidney. The kidney actually is displaced somewhat laterally and the renal artery is stretched.

and scanning should be initiated in this position. In some cases, particularly with pelvic collections, the supine position will prove to be very helpful. It has been mentioned that one of the main benefits of ultrasonic evaluation of retroperitoneal fluid collections is the ability to aid the surgeon in determining the optimum operative approach for these sometimes elusive masses. It should be pointed out, however, that sometimes needle aspiration rather than open surgical drainage is the treatment of choice, and in these instances, ultrasound also can be used to provide guidance for inserting the needle. This is covered in more detail in Chapter 12. Ultrasound also may be used to determine the adequacy of drainage, as well as to provide a ready means of evaluating for satisfactory resolution of the collection or perhaps its recurrence. Of particular importance in this regard is the use of ultrasound to examine for hematoma formation following renal trauma, including needle biopsy of the kidney (Figure 12). It also has been very helpful in excluding abscesses in those patients who, following renal or ureteral surgery, develop unexplained fever (Figure 13).

THE RETROPERITONEAL SPACE

The retroperitoneal space contains abundant soft tissues that are not organized into well-defined organs. The space contains, for example, much loose fibroareolar tissue, fat, neurogenic elements, lymphatics, and other structures mainly of mesenchymal origin. The great vessels and their branches and the major abdominal lymph node aggregates also are found here, but since specific chapters in this book have been allotted to them, they will not be discussed further. Masses occur in the retroperitoneum that are not derived from any organ and appear to originate directly from the mesenchymal soft

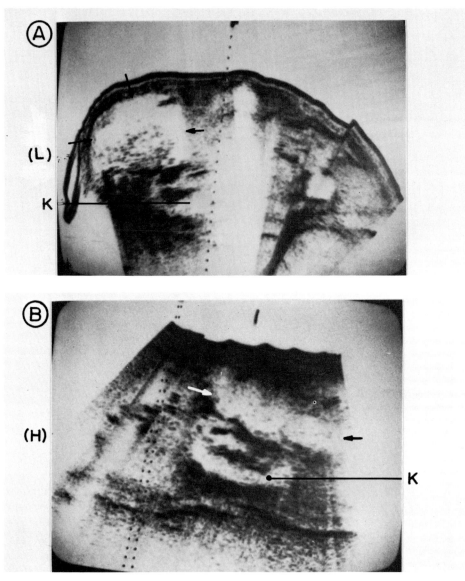

Figure 11. *A.* Transverse scan obtained in the prone position delineates a large complex mass (arrows) occupying the retroperitoneal area extending posterior to the left kidney (K) proven to be an abscess. *B.* Longitudinal ultrasonogram again demonstrates the retroperitoneal abscess (arrows) posterior to the kidney (K). (Courtesy of Dr. L. Wurtele, Holy Redeemer Hospital, Meadowbrook, Pa.)

tissues. These are not to be confused with masses arising from organs that are partially or completely retroperitoneal such as the pancreas, kidneys, and adrenals or with masses primarily or secondarily involving bone and spinal cord. Primary retroperitoneal masses may be neoplastic or nonneoplastic, and either cystic, complex, or solid. The majority of such lesions are neoplasms, however, and of these most are malignant (6). The major nonneoplastic lesion is the retroperitoneal cyst, which, in conjunction with the benign neurogenic and smooth muscle tumors, constitutes the vast majority of benign masses.

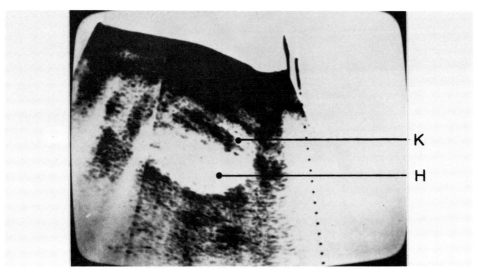

Figure 12.   Longitudinal ultrasonogram taken in the prone position shows a complex mass (H) just anterior to the kidney (K). It is predominantly of a cystic nature, but several internal echoes are seen. The mass was a retroperitoneal hematoma.

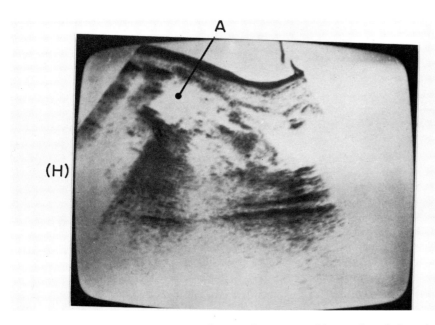

Figure 13.   Longitudinal ultrasonogram taken in the prone position, performed 1 week following nephrectomy because of persistent fever, reveals a complex predominantly fluid-filled mass occupying the renal fossa (A). This retroperitoneal abscess was drained surgically.

Excluding primary and secondary lymph node tumors, liposarcoma, leimyosarcoma, and hemangiopericytoma comprise the bulk of the malignant tumors.

The sonographic patterns of these masses depend on their physical makeup. Retroperitoneal cysts, like cysts elsewhere, will demonstrate a cystic ultrasonic pattern. Solid tumors, too, behave like their counterparts in other areas and will produce either solid (Figure 14) or complex ultrasonic patterns, depending on the presence or absence of hemorrhage, necrosis, or cystic degeneration within the tumor. With ultrasound, it is often possible to differentiate a pararenal retroperitoneal tumor from a primary renal tumor even when this distinction is not possible by urography. The sonographic images may delineate clearly a separation between the two structures although they may appear to be indistinguishable roentgenographically (Figure 15). Some retroperitoneal tumors, however, actually may invade the kidney making it all but impossible to determine their true origin. Because these lesions so often affect the ureters—usually by extrinsic compression but occasionally by invasion—hydronephrosis frequently accompanies retroperitoneal masses of all types (Figure 16).

Retroperitoneal fibrosis is a disease of unknown origin characterized by the presence of thick sheets of fibrous tissue in the retroperitoneal space. Although not well appreciated, it is possible in some cases to demonstrate such thick fibrous deposits by ultrasound (7). Scans carried out in the supine position usually are more informative than those in the prone position. The fibrous tissue may be demonstrated as a mass lying anterior and lateral to the great vessels. The surgical approach to patients requiring intervention for this disease—usually because of obstructive uropathy—may be facilitated by preoperative ultrasonic demonstration of the extent of the disease.

Hypertrophy of the psoas muscle is a physiologic phenomenon seen in some muscularly well-developed individuals and, while ordinarily of no importance, can be associated with deviation of the ureters. Visualization of an unusually thick ileo-psoas muscle mass by ultrasound allows confirmation of this diagnosis that only may be suspected by urography (8).

THE URETER

At present, ultrasonic imaging of the ureters enjoys only limited usefulness because of the relatively small diameter of the ureter. If the ureter is significantly dilated, however, it may be detected ultrasonically and imaged in surprisingly good detail. In the syndrome of anterior abdominal wall agenesis for example, (prune-belly syndrome) in which the ureters are characteristically widely dilated, a clear depiction of the degree of ureterectasis frequently may be obtained (Figure 17). This is particularly helpful when renal function is inadequate to produce satisfactory opacification by urography and may be quite useful in following the changes in ureteral caliber after treatment has been instituted.

If the ureter can be rendered echo-producing, as for example, by inserting a ureteral catheter, then its position can be recorded ultrasonically. This technique can be employed in cases of suspected retrocaval ureter (Figure 18). Enlarged lymph nodes may produce obstruction of the ureter causing hydronephrosis or ureterectasis (Figure 19). Another example of ultrasonic visualization of the ureter occurs in cases of ureterocele, which sometimes may be imaged through the fluid-filled urinary bladder, giving a "cyst within a cyst" appearance.

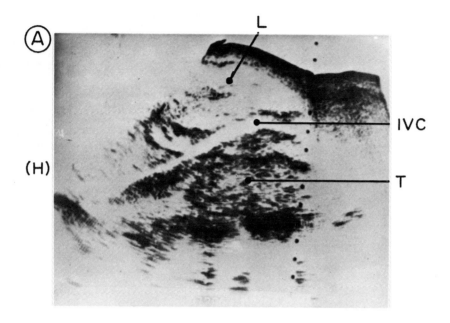

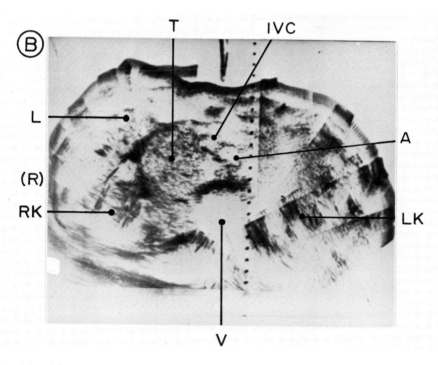

Figure 14. *A.* Longitudinal ultrasonogram obtained in the prone position to the right of the midline reveals a large echo-producing solid retroperitoneal mass (T). The inferior vena cava (IVC) is displaced anteriorly (L = Liver). *B.* The transverse image shows the large tumor (T) to be displacing the right kidney (RK) laterally. Histologically, it proved to be a retroperitoneal choriocarcinoma (V = Vertebra; LK = Left kidney; A = Aorta). (Both figures Courtesy of Dr. R. Binder, Oakland, California.)

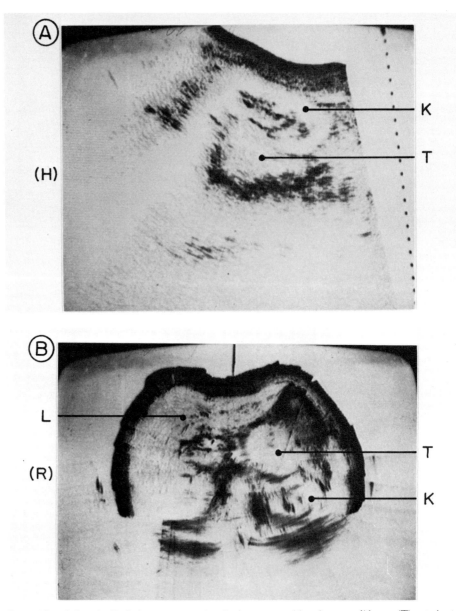

Figure 15.   *A*. Longitudinal ultrasonogram taken in the prone position shows a solid mass (T) anterior to the kidney (K) that proved to be an ectopic pheochromocytoma. *B*. Transverse image obtained in the supine position reveals that the mass (T) is separate from the kidney (K) (L = liver).

URINARY BLADDER

As a fluid-filled structure close to the anterior abdominal wall, the bladder enjoys the distinction of being one of the easiest of all organs to examine ultrasonically. Because of its typical ultrasonic appearance (Figure 20), it frequently is used as a standard against which other masses are compared. Sonographic study of the bladder has proved of particular value in the following situations.

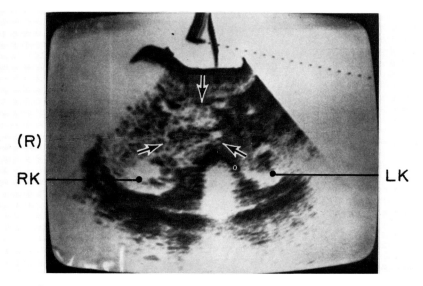

Figure 16. Supine Transverse ultrasonogram taken in the supine position delineates a large solid mass (arrows) anterior and medial to the right kidney (RK). Kidney contains central echo-free area due to hydronephrosis. Mass proved to be a retroperitoneal rhabdomyosarcoma in an 8-year-old child.

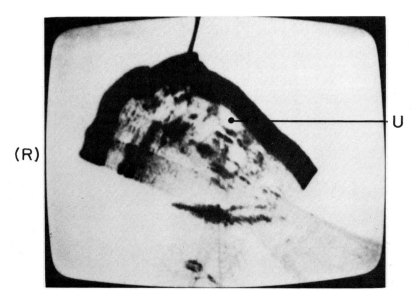

Figure 17. Supine axillary ultrasonogram shows a large fluid-filled structure (U) just beneath the abdominal wall skin representing a tortuous dilated ureter. Although the abdominal wall appears thick on this image, the thickness is artifactually produced by the prominent transducer-skin wall reflections.

327

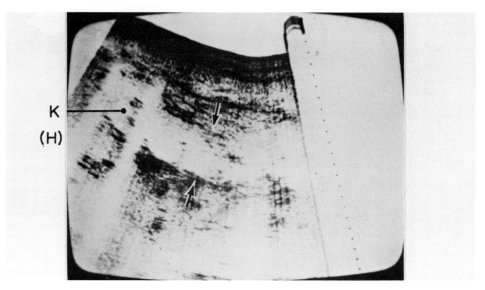

Figure 18. Longitudinal ultrasonogram obtained in the prone position demonstrates a markedly dilated proximal ureter (arrows) due to its retrocaval course (K = Kidney).

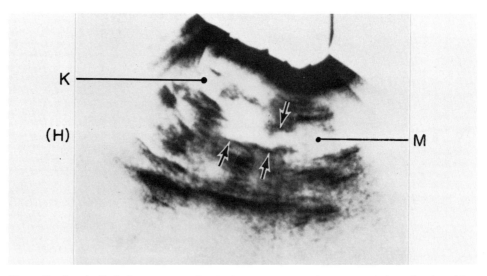

Figure 19. Longitudinal ultrasonogram taken in the prone position demonstrates hydronephrosis and hydroureter secondary to a retroperitoneal carcinoma. Ureteral entrapment has occurred, and the dilated ureter and renal pelvis are easily recognized (arrows). (K = Kidney; M = Mass) (Courtesy of Department of Radiology, Allentown-Sacred Heart Hospital, Allentown, Pennsylvania.)

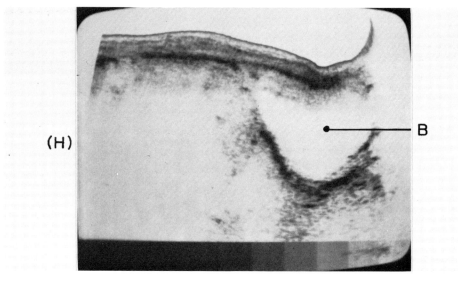

(H)   B

Figure 20. Longitudinal ultrasonogram obtained in the supine position reveals a normal urinary bladder that is typically round to triangular in shape (B). It transmits sound unusually well, as evidenced by accentuation of the far-wall echoes. It contains no internal echoes except for reverberations located near the anterior bladder wall.

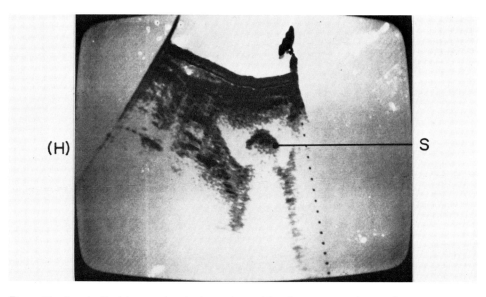

(H)   S

Figure 21. Longitudinal image taken in the supine position demonstrates a large, echo-producing defect within the urinary bladder, representing a stone (S). The marked absorption of sound by this stone is indicated by the echo-free zone (shadowing effect) beyond it.

Intraluminal Masses

Echoes can be recorded from intraluminal tumors, stones (Figure 21), and blood clots (Figure 22) as well as from the less common entities, foreign bodies (Figure 23) and ureteroceles. The characteristic echo-free pattern of the urinary bladder, with accentuated back-wall echoes is interrupted by echoes originating from the intraluminal mass, and in the case of stones, there is a corresponding marked diminution in transmitted sound through the mass ("shadowing effect"). Bladder tumors may be seen to be arising from the bladder wall while blood clot will be free within the lumen and will often change its pattern with a change in position of the patient. A tumor sometimes may be seen to extend from the bladder to the perivesical tissues. Bladder diverticula, including those arising from the urachus (Figure 24), may be seen as fluid-filled structures immediately adjacent to the bladder (Figure 25).

Staging of Bladder Tumors

Ultrasound has been used to determine the extent of invasion of bladder neoplasms into and beyond the bladder wall (Figure 26). Correlation with other methods of staging including operative assessment have been proved to be good, and an accuracy of 80 percent has been reported (9). When planning radiation therapy of bladder tumors, ultrasonic visualization of the tumor and its relationship to other pelvic structures also can be of great value. Transverse scanning with a full bladder is usually the best approach for evaluating bladder tumors, since extension of a bladder tumor may be recognized by the presence of amorphous masses of echo-producing solid tissue spreading peripherally from the bladder toward the pelvic wall (Figure 27). Unilateral fixation of the bladder wall may result in an uneven or atypical shape of the distended bladder.

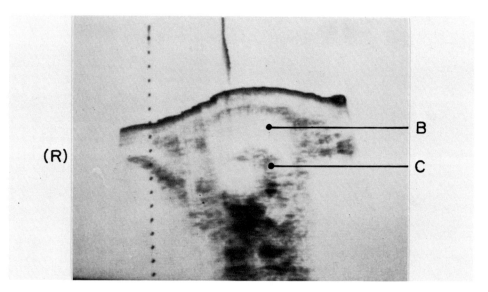

Figure 22. Transverse ultrasonogram obtained in the supine position shows the urinary bladder (B) to contain an echogenic defect representing a blood clot (C). No significant shadowing effect is produced. Blood clots usually change their location with positional changes of the patient which is not the case with bladder tumors.

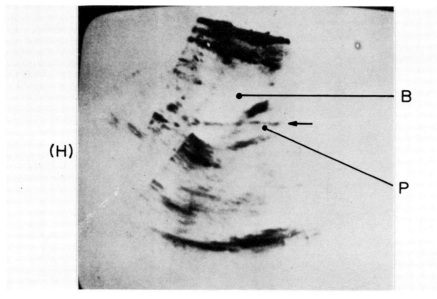

Figure 23.   Longitudinal ultrasonogram taken in the supine position demonstrates a foreign body in the urinary bladder (B) producing a linear echogenic pattern (arrow). This later was found to represent a glass cocktail stirrer. A portion of the stirrer is seen to be passing through the prostatic urethra (P). (Courtesy of Dr. Fudell, Department of Radiology, Parkview Hospital, Philadelphia, Pennsylvania.)

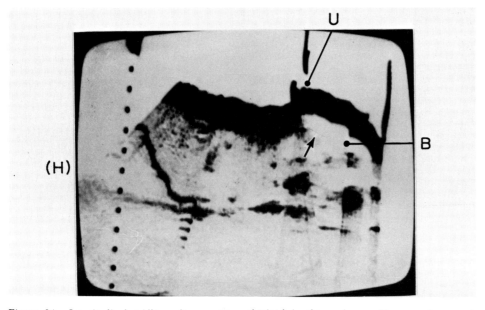

Figure 24.   Longitudinal midline ultrasonogram obtained in the supine position reveals a cystic diverticularlike projection (arrow) extending from the anterior surface of the urinary bladder (B) toward the abdominal wall. This represened a urachal cyst that drained intermittently through the umbilicus (U).

331

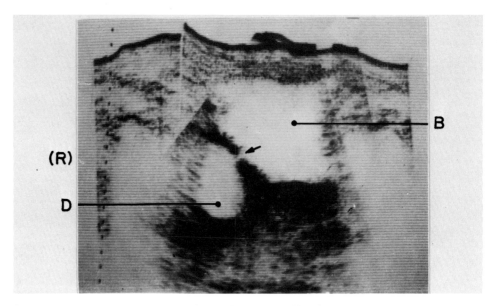

Figure 25. Transverse ultrasonogram taken in the supine position demonstrates diverticulum (D) arising from wall of bladder (B). Neck of diverticulum (arrow) is clearly visualized.

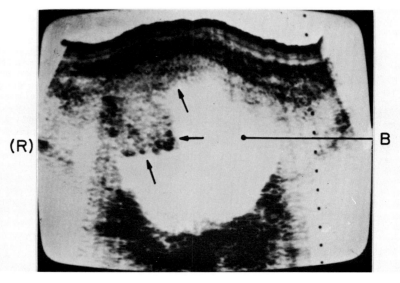

Figure 26. Transverse image taken in the supine position reveals a solid echo-producing mass (arrows) arising from the right superior wall of the bladder (B). The bladder tumor does not extend beyond the bladder wall.

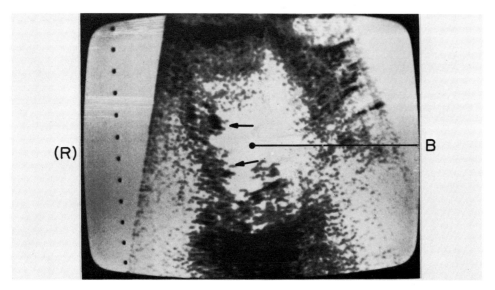

Figure 27.   Transverse image obtained in the supine position shows the wall of the urinary bladder (B) to be irregular (arrows) because of the presence of an infiltrating bladder tumor. The walls of the bladder cannot be identified. There is blending of the echoes into the perivesical soft tissues and loss of any normal boundaries. This finding usually is associated with tumor invasion into the perivesical areas.

Measurement of Residual Urine

While not strictly speaking a unique property restricted to gray scale imaging, the bladder may be assessed for its emptying capabilities by recording its dimensions in both transverse and longitudinal planes immediately following voiding (10). Empirical formulas have been devised that provide estimates of residual urine which correlate exceedingly well with actual measured values. This is a valuable technique in those patients in whom it is desired to avoid catheterization or in whom catheterization cannot easily be performed (11).

Suprapubic Aspiration of the Bladder

This has proved to be a useful method and will be discussed in detail in the Chapter 12.

PROSTATE AND SEMINAL VESICLES

Ultrasonography of the prostate has been used to differentiate between benign and malignant enlargement of the gland and in the estimation of prostatic size. Utilizing the transrectal approach, the diagnostic accuracy of the method has been reported to be approximately 80 percent in differentiating carcinoma of the prostate from benign hyperplasia (12). This compares favorably with the results of other methods, including needle biopsy.

The most reliable ultrasonic indicator of prostatic malignancy is the shape of the capsule (12). In the benign gland, the capsule may be visualized as a smooth continuous structure circumscribing the prostate (Figures 28A and B). In carcinoma, however, the capsule is usually irregular and discontinuous, as a result of its infiltration by malignant elements (Figure 28C). Other features of prostatic malignancy include asymmetry and

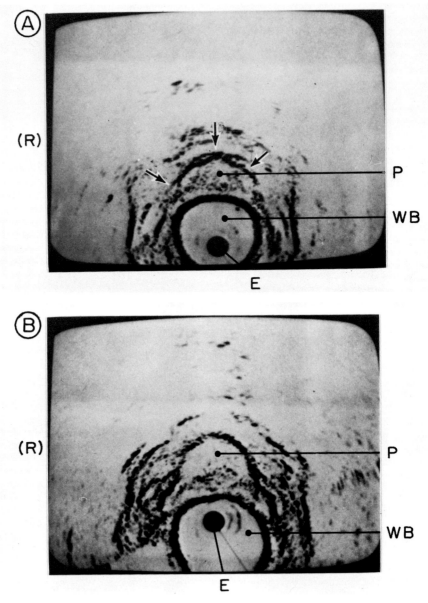

Figure 28.   Transrectal endoscans of the prostate depicting the endoscanner surface (E), the water-filled protective bag (WB), and the prostate (P). A. Normal prostate. The arrows denote the intact prostatic capsule. B. Benign prostatic hyperplasia. C. Prostatic carcinoma. The black arrow shows disruption of the capsule. (Courtesy of the Department of Urology, Bowman Gray University, Winston-Salem, North Carolina.) (Continued on next page.)

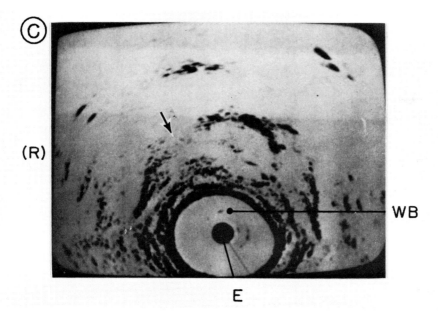

Figure 28. (Continued)

irregular clusters of internal echoes. The mere presence of internal echoes is not of itself, however, sufficient to allow a diagnosis of carcinoma to be made since neither the normal nor the benign hyperplastic prostate is echo-free. Careful attention to the appearance of the capsule, therefore, is mandatory, as well as to the distribution of the internal echoes.

Prostatic size can be estimated by either external or transrectal scanning and a correlation of 95 percent with the measured volume of the prostate has been reported (13) (Figure 29). Using external scanning, the transverse section showing the largest prostatic diameter is selected and this measurement is used to calculate its volume, using the formula for a sphere (13). With the transrectal method, transverse dimensions also are employed, with the volume calculated on the basis of the sum of the areas. Since the specific gravity of prostatic tissue is approximately 1.0, the volume will be approximately equal to the prostatic weight.

Cysts of the seminal vesicles, prostate, and Müllerian duct anlagen have been described and may be visible as cystic areas visualized through the transonic bladder (14).

SCROTAL CONTENTS

Ultrasonic scanning of the scrotum is of value in the differentiation of intrascrotal swelling (15). Although the most common scrotal swelling, hydrocele, is usually quite easy to diagnose clinically, some thick-walled hydroceles as well as pyoceles and hematoceles may simulate tumors. Additionally, in infants and children, it is sometimes difficult to differentiate hydroceles from hernias. Ultrasonography of the scrotal contents can be used to make these distinctions, since the fluid-filled nature of the cystic group of swel-

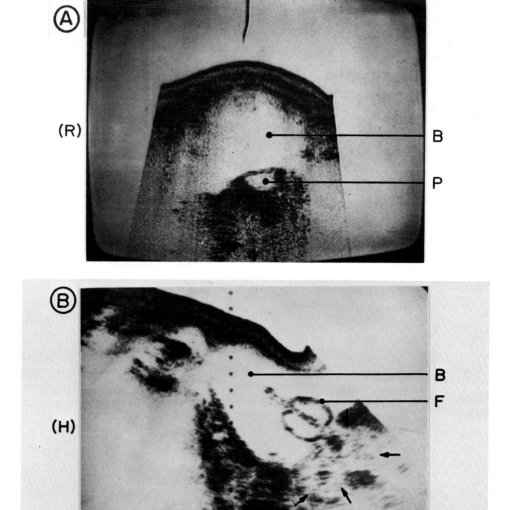

Figure 29. *A*. Transverse ultrasonogram taken in the supine position just above the symphysis pubis with the transducer angled sharply caudad demonstrates an enlarged prostate gland (P) visualized beneath the urine-filled bladder (B). *B*. Longitudinal ultrasonogram of another patient shows a markedly enlarged prostate (arrows). Note clearly defined image of a water-filled Foley catheter (F).

lings is readily distinguished from the solid pattern of testicular tumors and the attenuated ultrasonic pattern of bowel-containing hernial sacs (Figure 30).

When a hydrocele is found, an attempt should be made to demonstrate the underlying testis, since some testicular tumors will first be seen as a hydrocele. The testis is displayed ultrasonically as multiple uniform echoes (Figure 31). In tumors, an asymmetrical cluster of internal echoes arising from an area of localized or generalized testicular enlargement is found (Figure 32).

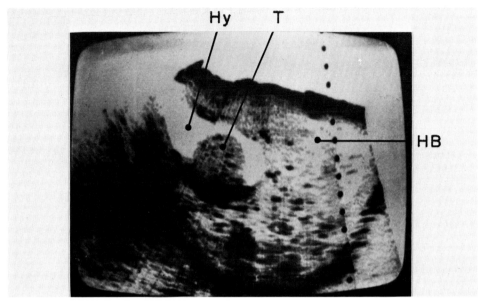

Figure 30. Hydrocele-hernia. Longitudinal scrotal image. The testes (T) is seen as a smoothly outlined echo-producing structure surrounded by a fluid-filled sac (Hy) representing a hydrocele. Surrounding both of these structures and filling the rest of the scrotum is a large echo-producing structure without recognizable anatomic outline, representing a large hernia (HB).

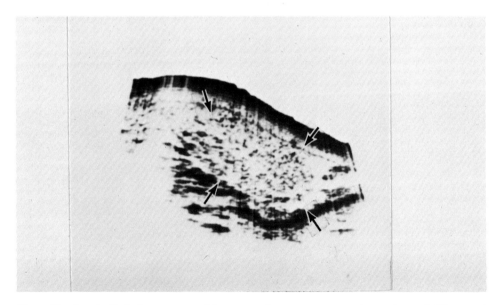

Figure 31. Longitudinal ultrasonogram of the scrotum demonstrates a normal testes (arrows). The normal testicle is an echo-producing smoothly outlined structure surrounded by a fibrous envelope, the tunica albuginea.

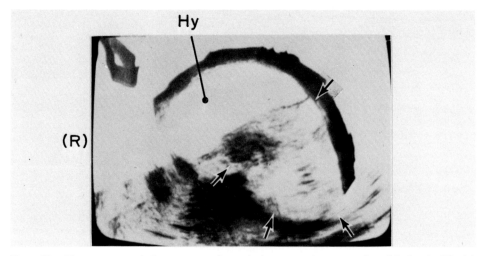

Figure 32. Transverse scrotal ultrasonogram of a testicular tumor plus a contralateral hydrocele. The left side of the scrotum contains a large irregular nonuniform echo-producing solid mass (arrows), representing a testicular tumor. The median raphe which separates the right and left halves of the scrotum is located eccentrically. In the right half of the scrotum is seen a large hydrocele (Hy). The right testes is not visualized in this section.

When the beam is attenuated before passing completely through the scrotal sac, it suggests that either air is present in herniated bowel or that calcification is present. The attenuation produced by calcified masses, however, tends to be spotty and, if fluid is present, a cystic structure will still be appreciated. Calcified walls most often are seen in hematoceles.

Doppler ultrasound is valuable in the diagnosis of testicular torsion (16). Since the Doppler principle can be used to detect the presence of a moving surface, such as the movement of blood within an artery or vein, it can readily indicate the absence of blood flow in the torsed testis. The procedure is simple, reliable, and free of known complications. The transducer is applied to the scrotal skin and the testis systematically examined, while changes in sound intensity are noted. This technique, although relatively new, gives every indication of assuming an important role in facilitating the often difficult differential diagnosis of testicular torsion versus epididymitis. Penile blood pressure also may be measured by means of the Doppler technique, and it has been found to be reduced in some cases of impotence.

REFERENCES

1. Sample WF: Personal communication.

2. Birnholz J: Ultrasound imaging of adrenal mass lesions. *Radiol* **109**:163, October 1973.

3. Pond GD, Haber K: Echography—a new approach to the diagnosis of adrenal hemorrhage in the newborn. *J Canad Ass Radiol* **27**:40, March 1976.

4. Ororashi B, Holmes JH: Grey scan sonography of an adrenal mass. *J Clin Ultrasound* **4**:121, April 1976.

5. McCullough DL, Leopold GR: Diagnosis of retroperitoneal fluid collections by ultrasonography: series of surgically proved cases. *J Urol* **115**:656, June 1976.

6. Ackerman LV: Tumors of the retroperitoneum, mesentery and peritoneum, in *Atlas of Tumor Pathology*, sect. 6. Washington, DC, Armed Forces Institute of Pathology, 1954.

7. Jacobson JB, Redman HC: Ultrasound findings in a case of retroperitoneal fibrosis. *Radiol* **113**:423, November 1974.

8. Bree RL, Green B, Keiller DL, Genet EF: Medial deviation of the ureters secondary to psoas muscle hypertrophy. *Radiol* **118**:691, March 1976.

9. McLaughlin IS, Morley P, Deane RF, Barnett E, Graham AG, Kyle KF: Ultrasound in the staging of bladder tumors. *Brit J Urol* **47**:51, February 1975.

10. Pedersen JF, Bartrum RJ, Grytter C: Residual urine determination by ultrasonic scanning. *Am J Roentgen* **125**:474, October 1975.

11. Harrison NW, Parks C, Sherwood T: Ultrasound assessment of residual urine in children. *Brit J Urol* **47**:805, 1975.

12. Watanabe H, Igari D, Tanahashi Y, Harada K, Sartoh M: Transrectal ultrasonotomography of the prostate. *J Urol* **114**:734, November 1975.

13. Miller SS, Garvie WH, Christie AD: The evaluation of prostate size by ultrasonic scanning: a preliminary report. *Brit J Urol* **45**:187, April 1973.

14. Walls WJ, Lin F: Ultrasonic diagnosis of seminal vesicle cyst. *Radiol* **114**:693, 1975.

15. Shawker T: B-mode ultrasonic evaluation of scrotal swellings. *Radiol* **118**:417, February 1976.

16. Levy BJ: Diagnosis of torsion of testicle using Doppler ultrasonic stethoscope. *J Urol* **113**:63, January 1975.

12

Aspiration-Biopsy Techniques

Barry B. Goldberg, M.D.
Professor of Radiology
Director, Division of Diagnostic Ultrasound
Thomas Jefferson University Hospital
Philadelphia, Pennsylvania

Howard M. Pollack, M.D.
Professor of Radiology
University of Pennsylvania
Hospital and School of Medicine
Philadelphia, Pennsylvania

While the preceding chapters have been devoted to the uses of ultrasound as a noninvasive diagnostic tool, this chapter will deal with its use as an aid in diagnostic procedures requiring the use of a needle for the removal of fluid or the biopsy of tissues. Diagnostic ultrasound has assumed an important role in aspiration and biopsy techniques since the first publication on the subject in the American literature in 1972 (1). Work in this field has been carried out by two major groups, one in Europe and the other in this country, resulting in numerous articles describing the multiple uses of ultrasound-assisted aspiration and biopsy techniques (2, 3, 4, 5, 6, 7, 8, 9, 10).

Using standard ultrasonic procedures, it is possible to localize an area of interest prior to its aspiration or biopsy, and then, using the information available on the ultrasonogram, determine the exact size of the area and its depth beneath the skin surface. The proper angle for needle placement also can be ascertained. Before the availability of ultrasound many needling procedures were performed totally blind, with the ever-attendant possibility of trauma to adjacent structures. With the use of ultrasound, however, these potential dangers usually can be avoided, thus reducing the complication rate. By using a specially developed aspiration-biopsy transducer (UABT) which contains a central lumen through which a needle can be passed, it is possible to record echoes arising from the region of the needle tip after it has been inserted into the body through the transducer lumen (Figure 1). This allows for continuous monitoring of the aspiration procedure. In this chapter the techniques used for various abdominal and retroperitoneal aspiration-biopsy procedures will be described.

TECHNIQUE

The technique for performing an aspiration or biopsy is the same whether or not ultrasound is used. The main advantage of ultrasound-aided needling is the additional information provided which, in general, makes the procedure easier and safer to carry out. Essentially, the area of interest is localized using two-dimensional B-scan ultrasound. The exact depth, position, and size of the mass or fluid collection is then determined from the ultrasonograms. The angle at which the needle should be inserted to orient it perpendicularly to the mass also is measured (Figure 2). The skin over the

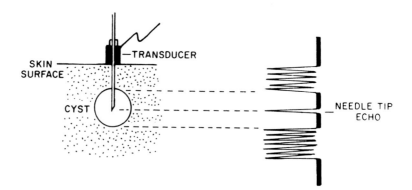

Figure 1. Diagrammatic representation showing needle having been inserted through central lumen of the aspiration-biopsy transducer into a cyst. A-mode representation shows needle tip echo.

342

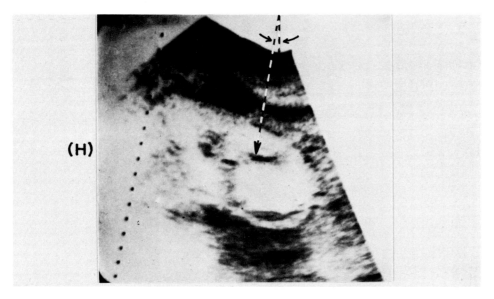

Figure 2. Longitudinal gray scale ultrasonogram of a lower pole renal cyst used to obtain the proper depth and angle for passage of the needle.

area of interest is marked either by using the transducer to exert pressure on the skin or by actually marking the skin. A small scratch can be made if it is desired that the mark be of a more permanent nature.

The area selected is prepared and draped using standard techniques. A gas-sterilized aspiration-biopsy transducer is then positioned over the site previously selected prior to sterilization of the field, for confirmation of the earlier measurements (Figure 3). The reconfirmed site is marked by applying pressure to the skin. When the transducer is removed, a "bull's-eye" impression, resulting from the hole in the transducer, will be seen. The local anesthetic then should be injected subcutaneously at this site, care being taken that no air is injected with the anesthetic agent, since the high reflectivity of air will prevent adequate penetration of the ultrasonic beam. If air is present it usually can be removed by applying pressure over the area and rubbing when the transducer is reapplied. For purposes of acoustic coupling between transducer and skin, sterile lubricating jelly may be employed. This is available commercially in multiple or single application sized tubes. Sterile saline or even the antiseptic solution used for skin prepping also may be used. The only difference between these is that reapplication of the water-type solution often is needed due to drying, which is not the case with the jelly.

Selection of the proper length of needle is accomplished by determining on the ultrasonogram the depth of the mass beneath the skin surface, taking into account the predetermined angle. To this distance is added the height of the aspiration-biopsy transducer. A needle stop, which is commercially available, may be positioned along the shaft of the needle at the designated distance, which is the sum of the height of the transducer and the calculated distance of the mass from the skin surface (Figure 4). The needle is now ready for insertion into the body. The shaft initially is passed through the lumen in the transducer, and the needle tip inserted through the skin for a short distance (Figure 5).

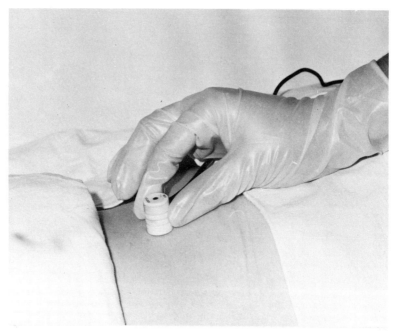

Figure 3. Aspiration-biopsy transducer positioned on the skin over the site previously selected from the information provided in Figure 2.

Once through the skin, the final repositioning of the transducer is made to insure proper angling. The needle is then advanced along the predetermined pathway quickly up to the needle stop. A fairly rapid advance increases the chances of puncturing rather than just invaginating the walls of a mass and also decreases the chances of pushing the mass aside.

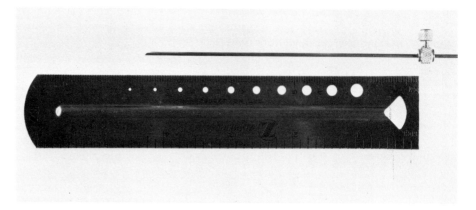

Figure 4. A needle stop has been placed along the shaft of the needle at the designated distance which is the sum of the height of the transducer and the distance from the skin surface to the area of interest. A sterilizable metal ruler is used for these measurements.

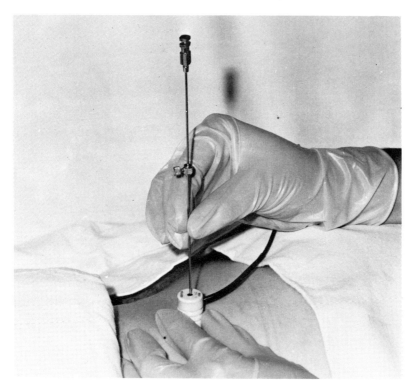

Figure 5. The needle with the needle stop in place has been inserted through the lumen of the aspiration-biopsy transducer into the skin.

Once the needle tip has entered a fluid-containing structure, an echo, representing the region of the needle tip, should be observed at the predetermined depth on the oscilloscopic screen (Figure 6). For best results, an A-mode type of display should be utilized because a vertical deflection is easier to visualize than a dot (B-scan). The strength of the echo produced at the needle tip is approximately that of a solid-solid interface and thus high sensitivity settings usually are needed to visualize the needle-tip echo adequately (11). When the inner core of the needle is removed and fluid travels up through the needle core, the strength of the needle-tip echo usually will increase, making it easier to monitor the aspiration procedure. With solid masses, the needle-tip echo often is lost within the reflections arising from the multiple echo-producing interfaces that are characteristic of a solid mass and only can be seen using M-mode (motion) display (Figure 7).

With fluid-containing masses or collections, the fluid can be aspirated completely or predetermined amounts can be removed, depending on clinical considerations. With solid-tissue biopsy, either core or aspiration techniques can be used, again depending on the clinical requirements. Since initial ultrasonograms are obtained prior to any needling procedure, ultrasound is valuable as a baseline study against which to evaluate for any possible complications. Thus, for biopsy procedures, a follow-up ultrasonic examination is performed after completion of the biopsy and within 24 hours to detect such potential complications as hemorrhage. For fluid collections, long-term follow-up studies

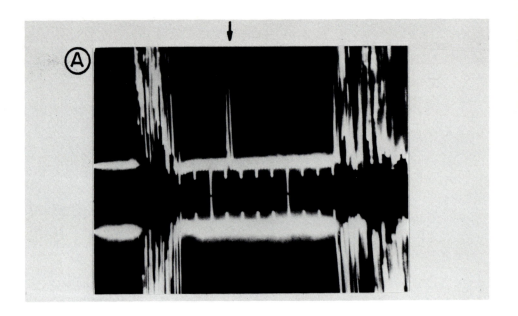

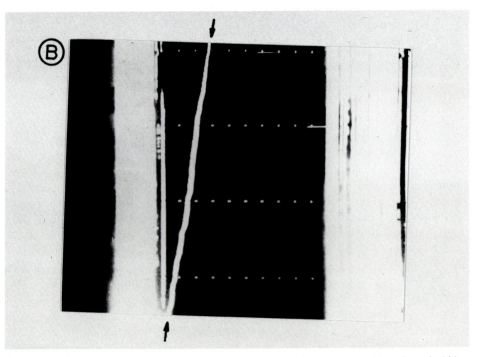

Figure 6. *A*. A-mode ultrasonogram shows echo arising from the needle tip (arrow) which is located within a fluid-containing structure. *B*. M-mode ultrasonogram shows the echo from the needle tip (arrows) as it is being advanced into the fluid-containing structure.

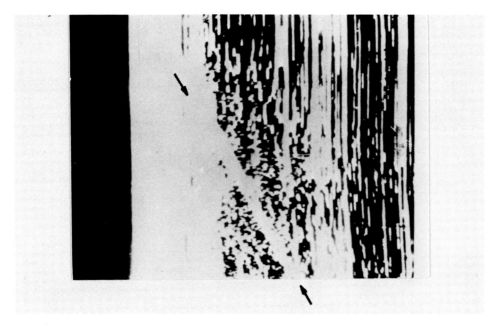

Figure 7. M-mode ultrasonogram shows needle tip echo (arrows) advancing through solid tissue that is producing multiple echoes, making it difficult to clearly define the needle tip.

often are performed to evaluate for any reaccumulation. It should be reemphasized that the aspiration or biopsy procedures followed are the same as they were prior to ultrasound and depend entirely on the techniques preferred by the physician-in-charge. Slight variations in technique will be described under the appropriate sections of this chapter.

ASPIRATION-BIOPSY TRANSDUCER DESIGNS

While it is true that a routine ultrasonic evaluation will supply the data needed (i.e., position, depth, and size) to perform an aspiration successfully, the use of a specially designed transducer containing a central lumen allows for more accurate needle placement. The central channel can be designed to accommodate any sized needle, although those commercially available usually will accept needles as large as 14 gauge. By using plastic inserts, the opening can be made smaller, thus helping to increase the stability of smaller gauge needles. The height of the transducer also can be increased by use of a special screw-on extension unit. This extension will provide more stability for very thin needles (i.e., 23 gauge) that need to be inserted very deeply within the body (Figure 8). The standard transducer has a frequency of 2.25 MHz; however, both lower and higher frequencies have been used experimentally. The higher frequency (i.e., 3–5 MHz) has proved successful for very superficial masses. Aspiration-biopsy transducers should be constructed specially to withstand high voltage and thus are tested under stresses in excess of 1000 volts for electrical leakage. This is important since the transducer is in contact with the patient and the presence of any electrical leak could be potentially dangerous.

The transducer, of course, must be sterilizable. While high-temperature sterilization is not feasible due to potential damage to the stability of the piezoelectric crystal, the transducer can be sterilized readily using established ethylene oxide or cold sterilization techniques (12). Ethylene oxide has been used for many years to sterilize plastic catheters and rubber anesthesia equipment. It has the advantage of instant availability and a dry format.

Aspiration-biopsy transducers are available in a variety of designs. The most commonly used one is a 2.25 MHz, either A-mode or B-scan. In fact, since the usual ultrasonic facility cannot obtain a large variety of transducers, the most versatile appears to be a B-scan aspiration-biopsy transducer with a separate cable so that it can be converted easily to an A-mode transducer when the need arises. Another variation is a transducer with a slot rather than a hole which allows the transducer to be removed without disturbing the needle (Figure 9). This type of arrangement is employed when, for example, long-term drainage of a fluid collection is desired.

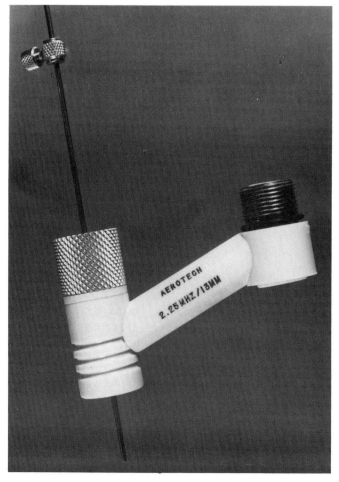

Figure 8.   B-mode aspiration-biopsy transducer with a metal extension (upper portion) used for providing more needle stability.

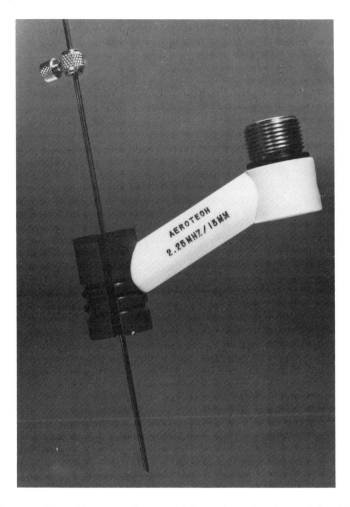

Figure 9. B-scan aspiration-biopsy transducer containing a slot rather than a hole which allows the transducer to be removed from around the needle.

RENAL CYST ASPIRATION

Ultrasound is used initially to determine if a renal mass is cystic in nature (Figure 10). From the ultrasonograms, as previously stated, the exact position and depth of the cyst beneath the surface can be learned (7, 13, 14). The proper angle for advancing the needle is determined easily. Standard aspiration techniques are followed as indicated above. The selected site is marked, usually with a wax pencil, and the area is cleansed. A sterilized aspiration-biopsy transducer is then repositioned over the area to confirm the initial site selection. The depth to the middle of the cyst (echo-free zone) is determined and a needle stop positioned along the shaft of the needle, taking into account the transducer height. A local anesthetic is applied, being careful not to introduce any subcutaneous air. The aspiration transducer is then reapplied and appropriately angled. The needle is first inserted through the transducer into the skin. The patient is asked to hold his breath in a neutral position while the needle is inserted to the needle stop. An echo arising from the needle tip should appear on the oscilloscopic screen if the needle is within the cyst (Figure 11). Removing the needle stylet will cause this echo to become stronger. On rare occasions, the cyst wall can be invaginated around the needle, resulting in visualization of the needle-tip echo without the return of fluid. It is important during passage of the needle that a fairly smooth, moderately rapid insertion be employed to break through the capsule and cyst wall. The absence of a needle-tip echo usually signifies that the needle has angled out of the field and is not within the cyst.

After entering the cyst, a portion of the fluid is removed and sent to the laboratory for cytology; culture (if infection is suspected); and chemical determinations, including LDH and lipids. The volume of fluid to be removed depends on the choice of the responsible physician, some preferring to remove only an aliquot of the fluid, while others remove as much of it as is possible. In any event the cyst volume may be estimated by using the formula $V \cong \dfrac{d^3}{2}$. This is a simplification of the formula for the volume of a sphere $V = \dfrac{4}{3} \pi r^3$. While not mathematically precise this modified formula is accurate enough for clinical purposes. After aspiration, contrast agents can be injected and roentgenograms taken to outline the internal cyst walls, (Figure 12).

Ultrasound has several advantages over other methods used for the aspiration of renal cysts. In particular, it is the only method that provides information about the depth of the lesion beneath the skin surface as well as the proper angle at which to insert the needle. With fluoroscopy, the depth of a mass is not readily appreciated, and it is generally not feasible to employ approaches requiring significant needle angulation. A direct posterior approach therefore must be used in almost all cases. This presents a problem in the case of upper pole renal masses, since the lower edge of the lung may not be appreciated with fluoroscopy and the possibility of pneumothorax exists. This is not

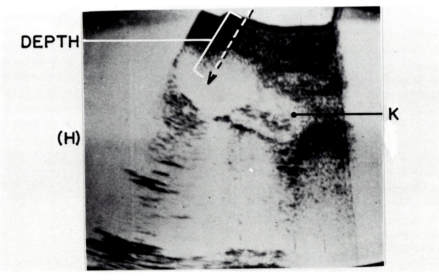

Figure 10.   Longitudinal B-scan of upper pole renal mass used to determine the exact position and depth beneath the skin surface (K = Kidney).

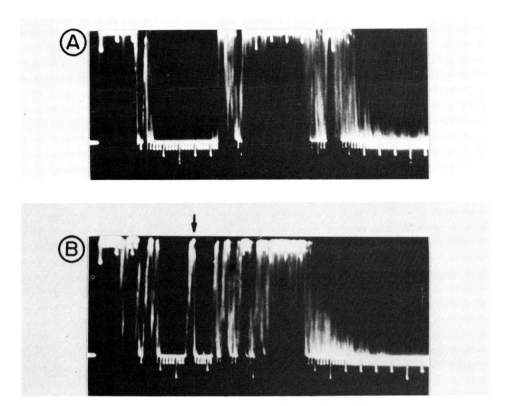

Figure 11. *A*. A-mode ultrasonogram showing cyst located between 3.5 and 7.5 cm beneath the skin surface (echo-free zone). *B*. A-mode ultrasonogram obtained during the aspiration of the renal cyst shows strong needle tip echo (arrow). The echo-free zone has decreased slightly as a result of removal of a portion of the fluid.

a consideration with ultrasound because the ultrasonic beam will be unable to penetrate if there is any air interposed between the transducer and the cyst. It is also difficult to aspirate an anteriorly located cyst without knowledge of its exact depth, since there is an ever-present danger that the needle will penetrate the intraabdominal cavity. Only with ultrasound is the exact depth known. The use of ultrasound makes for a much less cumbersome and more facile aspiration since it avoids the need for a fluoroscopy screen with its attendant dangers of both contamination and inadvertent bumping of the needle. Finally, by using ultrasound there is a significant reduction in irradiation both to the patient and the medical personnel in attendance.

The only major limitation of ultrasound is the inability of present equipment to clearly define cysts that are less than 2 cm in diameter. If a small cyst is seen and the patient cannot maintain quiet breathing, the movement of the kidney and thus the cyst will make it difficult to position the needle for aspiration. A combined ultrasound and fluoroscopic approach has been successful in such cases, with ultrasound determining the depth and angle and fluoroscopy the lateral movement (15). With this combined technique, the position of the needle can be altered continuously until the needle tip is within the cyst. The cyst, of course, must be large enough to be visible fluoroscopically, which also precludes this method in the aspiration of very small cysts.

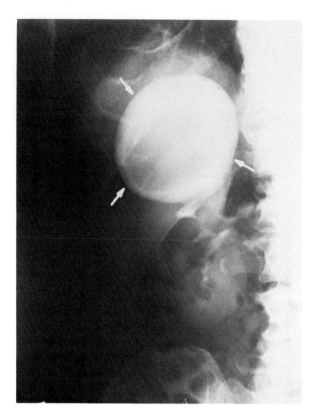

Figure 12.   Roentgenogram obtained after injection of water-soluble contrast material and air shows smooth walled upper pole renal cyst (arrows).

RETROPERITONEAL ASPIRATIONS

It is possible to guide a needle into any fluid-containing region in the body if an ultra-sonogram can define the area of interest. Thus, a cystic or predominantly cystic mass in the adrenal gland can be aspirated using the same techniques as previously described for aspirating renal cysts. Of course, the clinical indications for such an approach will vary considerably. In addition to an adrenal mass, the differential diagnosis of cystic or complex suprarenal masses includes pancreatic pseudocyst, abscess, splenic cyst, retro-peritoneal cyst, and even aortic aneurysm. Care must be taken not to diagnose the spleen as being a mass. Obviously, it is also possible to direct a needle into such fluid collections as hematomas or urinomas for the purpose of drainage.

In a similar fashion, antegrade pyelography can be performed in cases of hydro-nephrosis, when a retrograde study cannot be done. If it is desired to leave a catheter in place, a guide wire can be inserted through the needle, the needle pulled out, the transducer removed, and then a plastic catheter inserted over the guide wire into the hydronephrotic sac (16). Often this technique will obviate the need for surgical interven-tion.

Central renal cysts also can be aspirated under ultrasonic guidance (Figure 13). Although it is true that there is increased danger of encountering large blood vessels when needling central cysts as opposed to peripheral ones, there are times when the needle aspiration offers the best approach to these masses, and the only realistic alternative to surgery. The ultrasonic pattern for centrally located cysts is either cystic or complex with internal echoes produced by adjacent blood vessels. If a complex pattern is recorded, the recommended follow-up procedure to exclude a renal tumor is arteriography. If no abnormal vascularity is detected, the possibility that the mass might be a very poorly vascularized tumor still exists. Thus in these circumstances, since the only option left to the urologist is surgery, it is justifiable to attempt needle aspiration preoperatively. If clear fluid is found, which is negative on histochemical evaluation, and if the contrast cystogram reveals no irregularity, surgery can be avoided. If complications occur from entering a vessel, then surgery can be performed as originally planned.

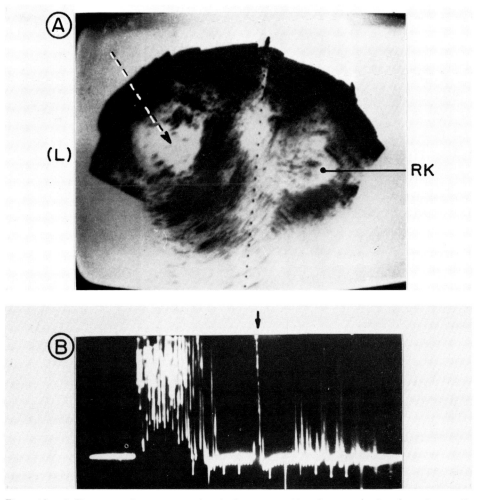

Figure 13.   *A*. Transverse ultrasonogram taken in the prone position shows predominantly cystic centrally located renal mass on the left (RK = Right kidney). *B*. A-mode ultrasonogram shows needle tip echo (arrow) within the central portion of the previously diagnosed central renal cyst. *C*. Roentgenogram shows water-soluble contrast material in a smooth-walled centrally located renal cyst (arrows). (*Continued on next page.*)

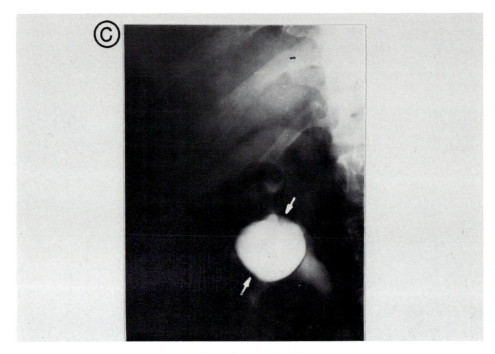

Figure 13.   (Continued)

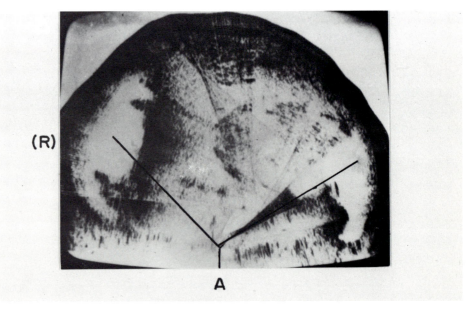

Figure 14.   Transverse supine ultrasonogram shows evidence of ascites (A) located in both flanks with gas-filled bowel centrally preventing penetration of the sound beam in this region.

Complications resulting from renal cyst aspiration are infrequent. In over 300 renal cyst aspirations we encountered only two patients with postaspiration bleeding severe enough to require hospitalization. In neither case was surgical intervention necessary. Another patient developed an intracystic infection which responded to antibiotics. Aside from those three patients there were no complications in our series.

SUPRAPUBIC BLADDER ASPIRATION

While suprapubic bladder aspiration is performed infrequently in adults, it is not uncommonly required in newborn and young children in order to obtain an uncontaminated urine sample. In the very young, catheterization usually is avoided because of the possibility of infection or urethral trauma. Since external collecting bag samples often prove unsatisfactory, the only remaining choice is a suprapubic approach. Ultrasound should be utilized prior to the attempt since it can easily determine the presence of urine within the bladder (8). Once urine is detected, the amount can be estimated using a formula similar to that for estimating the volume of any spherical mass, such as is used for a renal cyst [Volume $\cong$ ½ (diameter)^3].* A needle then can be directed into the bladder after appropriate cleansing of the suprapubic region. A bladder that is displaced or distorted, as a result of a fecal impaction or pelvic mass, for example, easily can be visualized ultrasonically. Thus, some complications such as trauma to bowel and other pelvic structure can be avoided.

INTRAABDOMINAL ASPIRATION TECHNIQUES

While the opportunity for aspirating intraabdominal masses does not arise often, it is not uncommon to use ultrasound as an aid in paracentesis. The presence of ascites easily can be detected ultrasonically using established techniques (Figure 14). Free fluid can be differentiated readily from loculated fluid by shifting the patient and rescanning. The optimal site for insertion of the trocar can be determined accurately. If there are air-filled loops of bowel interposed between the fluid and the transducer surface, the ultrasonic beam will not penetrate. Thus, a paracentesis can not be performed in an area of potential damage to the bowel.

* Formula for volume of a sphere.

$$v = \frac{4}{3}\pi r^3; \ r = \frac{1}{2}d$$

Therefore,

$$v = \frac{4}{3} \times \frac{22}{7} \times \left(\frac{1}{2}d\right)^3$$
$$v = \frac{4}{3} \times \frac{22}{7} \times \frac{1}{8}d^3$$
$$v \cong \frac{1}{2}d^3$$

where,

$$v = \text{volume}$$
$$r = \text{radius}$$
$$d = \text{diameter}$$
$$\pi = \frac{22}{7}$$

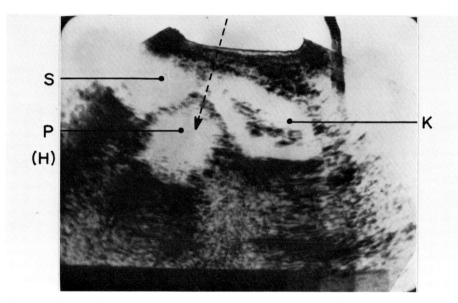

Figure 15.   Longitudinal prone ultrasonogram shows a cyst of the pancreas (P) situated between the spleen (S) and kidney (K). Arrow denotes pathway that would be followed for its aspiration.

It is possible to direct a needle under ultrasonic guidance into various fluid-containing structures within the abdomen, such as abscesses and pancreatic pseudocysts (17) (Figure 15). While there may be a small risk of injuring bowel by transperitoneal needling, there are circumstances, i.e., in severely debilatated individuals, when surgery is contraindicated and aspiration is the most realistic alternative. Under ultrasonic guidance, a needle can be directed easily into the cyst and the fluid removed. Ultrasound then can be used serially to detect any reaccumulation of fluid within a mass as well as to evaluate for any development of fluid within the peritoneal cavity. Ovarian cysts also can be aspirated using an abdominal approach or by positioning the aspiration transducer within the vaginal canal for deep-seated pelvic cysts. With this vaginal approach, pelvic abscesses also can be drained.

Since ultrasound can visualize the biliary system easily, including the gallbladder and dilated ducts, it can be used to guide a needle into place for transhepatic cholangiography (18). Because dilatation of the common bile duct, choledocholithiasis and dilatation of intrahepatic bile ducts all can be recognized ultrasonically with a high degree of accuracy, there has been a decrease in the need for transhepatic cholangiography. In carrying out splenoportagrams, ultrasound is used to locate the spleen initially and then to select the site for insertion of the needle.

Of course, ultrasound has been used successfully for aspiration of fluid-containing spaces and structures throughout the body, including thoracentesis, pericardiocentesis, and amniocentesis (5, 6, 19). It also has been used for the aspiration of cystic masses within the thyroid and the breast.

Ultrasonic aspiration techniques also have been used successfully in pediatric patients. Of particular interest is its use in renal transplants for aspiration of lymphoceles, which can develop after surgery. The lymphocele can be defined easily ultrasonically and its effect on the kidney, i.e. hydronephrosis, demonstrated easily. The exact depth, position,

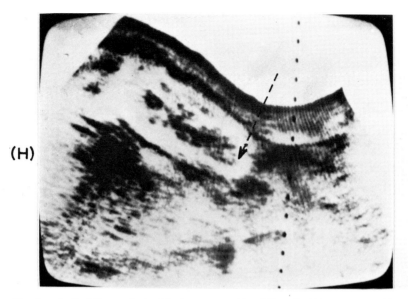

Figure 16.   Longitudinal B-scan obtained in the prone position defines the kidney prior to a biopsy with the arrow indicating the pathway for the biopsy of the lower pole.

and size of the lymphocele can be determined. With this information, a needle pathway can be selected away from vital structures. Ultrasound then can be used to evaluate for reaccumulation. The use of ultrasound in suprapubic bladder aspiration already has been described in a previous section.

BIOPSY PROCEDURES

Using B-scan ultrasound, two-dimensional images of the kidneys are obtained for localization prior to biopsy (Figure 16). The most common site for a routine biopsy is the lower pole of the kidney. Its depth can be measured easily as well as the angle that the longitudinal plane of the kidney makes with the skin (Figure 17). With this information, the biopsy needle can be angled in such a way that it will enter the lower pole perpendicular to its surface. This is a distinct advantage of ultrasonic localization over other methods which cannot easily determine the depth nor the angle that the kidney makes with the skin surface (10, 20). Isotope and x-ray techniques are able to provide adequate information only about the craniocaudal axis of the kidney. In fact, if the roentgenogram is not obtained with the beam centered directly over the area of interest, the effect of beam divergence reduces the effectiveness of this modality. Divergence and magnification factors increase the chances for incorrect placement of the needle.

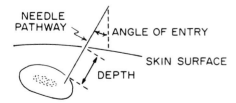

Figure 17.   Diagrammatic representation showing the needle pathway required for it to be perpendicular to the kidney. In order to do this, the angle of skin entry must be determined.

The biopsy procedure, whether it be for a core of tissue using a large-gauge needle or for a cellular aspirant using a very fine-gauge needle, is the same as that which the clinician would employ if ultrasound were not used. Two-dimensional ultrasound is utilized to obtain the initial measurement. A mark is then placed on the skin in the region determined to be optimal sonographically. The area is then prepped and

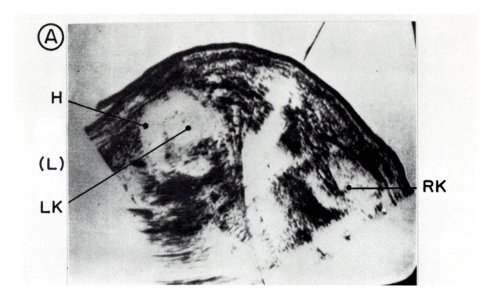

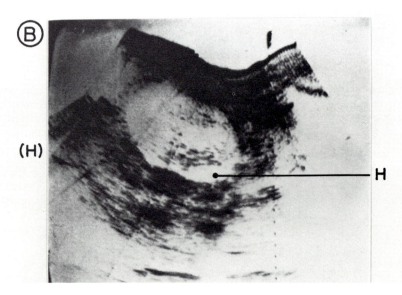

Figure 18.   *A.* Transverse ultrasonogram taken in the prone position shows a perirenal hematoma (H) surrounding the left kidney (LK). Note size of normal right kidney (RK). *B.* Longitudinal ultrasonogram of the same left kidney again shows the enlargement due to a perirenal hematoma (H).

anesthetized. Next, the biopsy needle is inserted through the aspiration-biopsy transducer and then through the skin with the proper angle being maintained. After puncture, the needle is inserted to the predetermined length. It is usually difficult to visualize the passage of the needle because of multiple echoes arising from the soft tissues through which it passes. An M-mode display usually is needed to record the echo produced by this type of needle tip during its transit through soft tissue. The larger the needle diameter the better the chance to visualize the moving needle echo within the solid tissue. If a slotted type of aspiration-biopsy transducer is available, it then can be removed while a core biopsy is obtained at the predetermined level. With an aspiration-type biopsy procedure, the needle is advanced to the desired depth following which a syringe is used to produce suction, aspirating the cells into the fine, usually 23-gauge, needle.

It is of importance after biopsy to obtain a follow-up ultrasonic examination of the area within 24 hours to evaluate for the development of hematoma (Figure 18). With respect to the kidney, postbiopsy hematomas should occur relatively infrequently, since the lower pole of the kidney can be localized accurately prior to insertion of the needle.

The same procedure is followed when it is desired to do a biopsy of any solid or complex renal tumor (9), except that the site selected for insertion of the needle is determined by the location of the tumor. If the tumor is necrotic, the needle-tip echo will be defined clearly on the A-mode display when the tip of the needle is within the mass. The core biopsy or aspirant is then obtained in a standard fashion. With masses having a liquid center, water-soluble contrast material can be injected to demonstrate the irregularity of the walls (Figure 19). Ultrasound also has been used successfully in the biopsy of renal transplants, following an approach similar to that used for routine renal

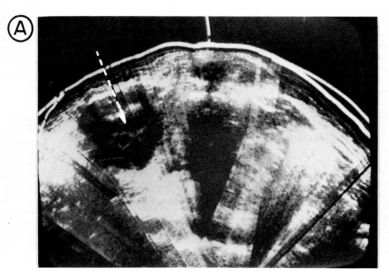

Figure 19. *A.* Transverse ultrasonogram obtained in the prone position demonstrates a complex renal mass having both cystic and solid components as a result of necrosis. Arrow denotes pathway for aspiration needle. *B.* A-mode ultrasonogram shows the needle tip echo (arrow) within the previously localized complex renal mass. *C.* Roentgenogram shows water-soluble contrast material injected into the complex renal mass, showing irregularity of the inner walls (arrows) as was suspected from the initial ultrasonograms. (*Continued on next page.*)

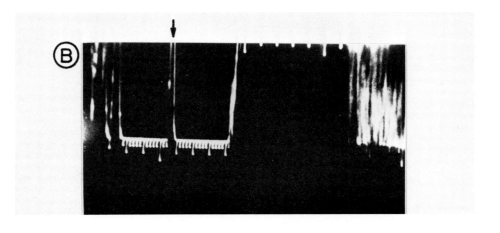

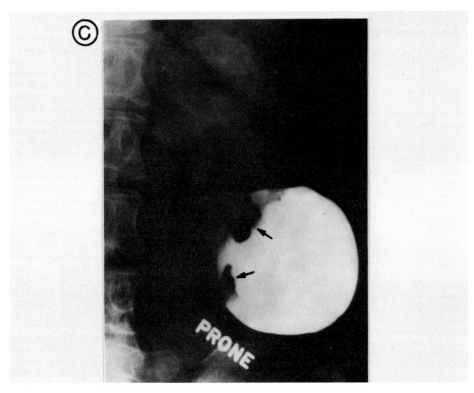

Figure 19.   (Continued)

biopsies. Biopsies of other retroperitoneal masses can be done if a definitive ultrasonic pattern can be recorded.

Various intraabdominal biopsy procedures have been accomplished under ultrasonic guidance. The most frequent is the biopsy of liver masses (4, 21). The procedure followed is quite similar to that employed to obtain a biopsy of other organs. First the mass is identified using two-dimensional B-scan ultrasound. Next the site for entrance of the needle through the skin is selected and marked. The depth and angle for passage of the needle is determined from the initial ultrasonograms (Figure 20). Entrance can be made from any angle determined by the site of the mass within the liver and the position of vital structures. The biopsy method can be either core or aspiration, although the latter is used more commonly. Using the initial ultrasonic information, the needle is passed through the aspiration-biopsy transducer into the body to the level of the needle stop previously positioned along the shaft of the needle. An echo usually will not be identified due to the multiple echoes produced by the solid tissue. However, the important information will already have been determined, that is, the depth, position, and angle. The biopsy is performed by applying suction on the syringe following which the needle is rapidly withdrawn. Biopsies of multiple lesions can be carried out with the sites selected from the initial ultrasonograms.

Biopsies of masses within the pancreas and environs also have been successfully performed under ultrasonic guidance (22, 23). Here again, as with the liver, B-scan ultrasound is used to localize the mass (Figure 21). As with any intraabdominal procedure the possibility of penetrating bowel and other vital structures is always present. Since many of these patients are quite sick, surgery is contraindicated. Treatment, however, often is delayed due to the lack of definitive proof of malignancy. The needle, usually 23-gauge, can be inserted into the mass using ultrasound and a cellular aspirant obtained. As with all biopsy procedures, follow-up ultrasonic examination is recommended within 24 hours to evaluate for complications, the most common of which is hemorrhage.

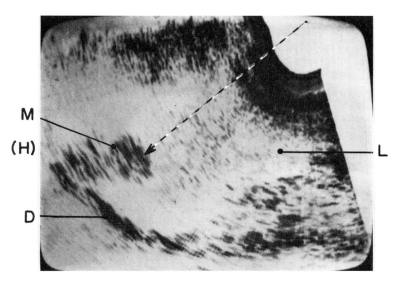

Figure 20. Longitudinal ultrasonogram taken in the supine position of the liver (L) shows a posteriorly located mass (M) Arrow denotes pathway and depth for passage of the biopsy needle (D = diaphragm).

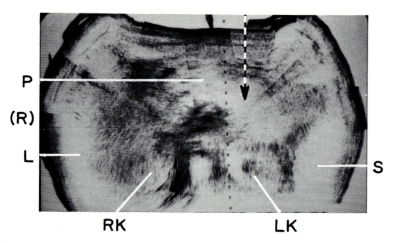

Figure 21. Transverse ultrasonogram taken in the supine position shows an enlarged tail of the pancreas consistent with tumor. Arrow denotes pathway for needle biopsy (P = Pancreas; S = Spleen; L = Liver; RK = Right kidney; LK = Left kidney).

In summary, ultrasound has been used successfully as an aid in the aspiration of fluid-containing structures and in the biopsy of solid masses and organs. It provides information not usually available with other localization procedures. Its ability to localize the mass prior to aspiration or biopsy and to then detect any complications such as bleeding makes it an important medical technique.

REFERENCES

1. Goldberg BB, Pollack HM: Ultrasonic aspiration transducer. *Radiology* **102**:187–189, January 1972.

2. Holm HH, Kristensen JK, Rasmussen SN, Northeved A, Barlebo H: Ultrasound as a guide in percutaneous puncture technique. *Ultrasonics,* March 1972, pp 83–86.

3. Goldberg BB, Pollack HM: Ultrasonic aspiration-biopsy transducer. *Radiology* **108**:67–671, September 1973.

4. Rasmussen SN, Holm HH, Kristensen JK, Barlebo H: Ultrasonically-guided liver biopsy. Preliminary Communications. *Brit Med J* **27**:500–502, May 1972.

5. Goldberg BB, Pollack HM: Ultrasonically guided pericardiocentesis. *Am J Card* **31**:490–493, April 1973.

6. Bang J, Northeved A: A new ultrasonic method for transabdominal amniocentesis. *Am J Obstet Gynecol* **114**:599–601, November 1972.

7. Goldberg BB, Pollack HM: Ultrasonically guided renal cyst aspiration. *J Urol* **109**:5–7, January 1973.

8. Goldberg BB, Meyer H: Ultrasonically guided suprapubic urinary bladder aspiration. *Pediatrics* **51**:70–74, January 1973.

9. Kristensen JK, Holm HH, Rasmussen SN, Barlebo H: Ultrasonically guided percutaneous puncture of renal masses. *Scand J Urol Nephrol* **6**:49–56, 1972.

10. Goldberg BB, Pollack HM, Kellerman E: Ultrasonic localization for renal biopsy. *Radiology* **115**:167–170, April 1975.

11. Goldberg BB, Ziskin MC: Echo patterns with an aspiration ultrasonic transducer. *Investigative Radiology* **8**:78–83, March–April 1973.

12. Engley FB, Metzgar MT: Ethylene oxide sterilization: a necessity for inhalation therapy departments. *Inhal Therap* **15**:9–13, 1970.

13. Leopold GR, Talner LB, Asher WM, Gosink BB, Ruben FG: Renal ultrasonography: an updated approach to the diagnosis of renal cyst. *Radiology* **109**:671–678, December 1973.

14. Doust BD, Maklad NF: Control of renal cyst puncture by transverse ultrasonic B scanning. *Radiology* **109**:679–681, December 1973.

15. Raskin MM, Roen SA, Serafini AN: Renal cyst puncture: combined fluoroscopic and ultrasonic technique. *Radiology* **113**:425–427, November 1974.

16. Pedersen JF: Percutaneous nephrostomy guided by ultrasound. *J Urol* **112**:157–159, August 1974.

17. Smith EH, Bartrum RJ: Ultrasonically guided percutaneous aspiration of abscesses. *Am J Roentgenology* **112**:308–312, October 1974.

18. Burcharth F, Rasmussen SN: Localization of the porta hepatis by ultrasonic scanning prior to percutaneous transhepatic portography. *Brit J Radiology* **47**:598–600, September 1974.

19. Sandweiss DA, Hanson JC, Gosink B, Moser KM: Ultrasound in diagnostic location and treatment of loculated pleural empyema. *Ann Int Med* **2**:1, January 1975.

20. Kristensen JK, Bartels E, Jorgensen HF: Percutaneous renal biopsy under the guidance of ultrasound. *J Urol Nephrol* **8**:223–226, 1974.

21. Lutz H, Weidenhiller S, Rettenmaier G: Targeted fine-needle aspiration biopsy of the liver employing ultrasonic control. *Schweiz med Wschr* **103, 29**:1030–1033, 1973.

22. Smith EH, Bartrum RJ, Chang YC: Ultrasonically guided percutaneous aspiration biopsy of the pancreas. *Radiology* **112**:737–738, September 1974.

23. Smith, EH, Bartrum RJ, Chang YC, D'Orsi CJ, Kokich J, Abbruzzese A, Dantono J: Percutaneous aspiration biopsy of the pancreas under ultrasonic guidance. *New Engl J Med* **292**:825–828, April 1975.

Index